D1531643

A Guide to Understanding and Living with Epilepsy

A Guide to Understanding and Living with Epilepsy

Orrin Devinsky, MD
Chairman, Department of Neurology
Hospital for Joint Diseases
Director, Comprehensive Epilepsy Center
New York University—Hospital for Joint Diseases
Associate Professor
New York University School of Medicine
New York, New York

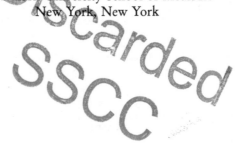

F. A. DAVIS COMPANY • Philadelphia

F. A. Davis Company
1915 Arch Street
Philadelphia, PA 19103

Printed in the United States of America

Last digit indicates print number: 10 9 8 7 6 5 4 3 2 1

Medical Editor: Robert W. Reinhardt
Medical Developmental Editor: Bernice M. Wissler
Production Editor: Crystal S. McNichol
Cover Design By: Donald B. Freggrens, Jr.

Cover art, *Poplars at Saint-Remy*, oil on canvas, 1889, 61.6 × 45.7 cm, Vincent van Gogh, Dutch, 1853–1890. © The Cleveland Museum of Art, bequest of Leonard c. Hanna, Jr., 58.32.

Library of Congress Cataloging in Publication Data

Devinsky, Orrin.
   A guide to understanding and living with epilepsy/Orrin Devinsky.
  Devinsky.
      p.   cm.
  Includes bibliographical references.
  ISBN 0-8036-2556-1 (soft: alk. paper)
  1. Epilepsy—Popular works. I. Title.
  [DNLM: 1. Epilepsy. WL 385 D495g 1994]
RC372.D48 1994
616.8'53 dc20
DNLM/DLC
for Library of Congress
                                              94-10823
                                                CIP

To all my patients, for all they've taught me about epilepsy.

Foreword

In 1977, the executive vice president of the Epilepsy Foundation of America wrote the Foreword to a 116-page book about epilepsy for the general public, entitled *The Epilepsy Fact Book*. At the time there were no similar books for lay people. In an effort to fill that gap, the *Fact Book* offered its readers the opportunity to learn, to explore, and to understand something of the complexity of this often misunderstood disorder.

The *Fact Book* was later joined by other books for lay people. Some concentrated on parenting issues and the problems of epilepsy in the early years. Others proposed alternative therapies or sought to immerse the reader in the personal experience of epilepsy. All helped to illuminate a condition that for far too long remained something that people didn't talk about.

Now, 17 years later, this new book about epilepsy is being offered to the public. Its scope and comprehensiveness mirror the enormous progress that has been made in epilepsy management. It also reflects the philosophy of its author, a philosophy long held by the Epilepsy Foundation of America and its professional advisors, that lay people will understand medical information when it is presented well and that they will act on it in their own best interests and those of their family members with epilepsy.

Dr. Devinsky's *A Guide to Understanding and Living with Epilepsy* is a most welcome addition to what is becoming a new literature of empowerment for individuals and families. This book takes the position that understanding epilepsy means being aware of a whole range of medical and social factors—everything from how the brain works and the kinds of issues that influence choice of treatment to family issues, sports participation, and school planning. It seeks to allay parental guilt while also encouraging a full life for children with seizures without overprotection. It takes the same comprehensive, detailed approach to the social issues associated with epilepsy as it does to the medical ones—a welcome development, because social issues are often more overwhelming for individuals and families than the medical condition itself.

Indeed, quality of life is a pervasive theme of the book, not surprisingly, perhaps, as the author is one of the primary investigators of how the experience of having epilepsy affects the ability of people to achieve their goals in life. Other Epilepsy Foundation of America staff and I have watched this book take shape over several months and were pleased to have the opportunity to comment and make a few suggestions along the way. We knew this was going to be a major book, covering in authoritative detail an enormous number of the kinds of questions we get every day from people with epilepsy and their families. Now that it has been completed, we welcome it as a valuable new reference and educational tool for everyone who works in this field—and especially for the families and the person with epilepsy who just want to *know*.

William M. McLin
Executive Vice President
Epilepsy Foundation of America

Preface

Vincent Van Gogh's "Poplars at Saint-Remy" appears on the cover of this book because that great artist is an example of a person who fulfilled his potential in spite of epilepsy. Because we often fear the unknown, the uncertainties created by a diagnosis of epilepsy may give individuals more difficulty than do the seizures themselves. The main goal of this book is to help people with epilepsy—whether they have a new diagnosis or are living with epilepsy—to understand the disorder and learn about the nature and diversity of seizures, the psychological and social implications of seizures and the diagnosis of epilepsy, the educational and vocational aspects of the disorder, and the medical and surgical therapies for seizures. The real motivation for writing this book, however, was to empower people with epilepsy by offering facts that would remove the fears caused by misinformation, by encouraging these individuals to assume a greater role in their medical care, by helping them to understand the importance of independence and self-esteem, and by giving them information that they can use to work toward achieving a better quality of life. Although most of my medical information about epilepsy comes from medical textbooks, medical articles, and professional lectures, the people I have cared for—my patients—have proved my greatest source of knowledge about living with epilepsy.

Knowledge is power: Education about epilepsy is key. People with epilepsy, or parents of children with epilepsy, should understand the types of seizures, the risks and benefits of the various antiepileptic drugs, the factors that can cause seizures or help prevent them, and which activities are safe and which are dangerous. Education about epilepsy can come from books, videotapes, and written materials from the Epilepsy Foundation of America, epilepsy support groups, libraries, and health care workers.

A little knowledge, however, can be confusing and frightening. For instance, anyone who reads the *Physician's Desk Reference*, which describes all the prescription drugs on the market, will be surprised to learn about the many adverse effects of antiepileptic drugs. The list seems almost endless. Some of these adverse effects are serious, even fatal. The risks, however, must be weighed against the benefits. For a child who is having so many absence seizures that the ability to learn, play, and socialize with other children is affected, the benefits of ethosuximide or valproate outweigh the risks. An antiepileptic drug may have a 1 in 100,000 chance of causing death, and although the fear of this chance is real, it should not deter someone from using the drug if the potential benefits are substantial.

Persons with epilepsy should become advocates for themselves or their children who have epilepsy. They should speak out if the medical care seems wrong or violates common sense. If they are dissatisfied with the seizure control or the adverse effects of therapy, they should discuss it with the doctor. The current regimen may truly be the best possible one, but sometimes a second opinion is helpful. Parents of a child with epilepsy must make sure the child's educational needs are met. Public Law 94-142 secures the education of special children. Adults with epilepsy must make sure that the privilege to drive and their rights to employment are fairly considered. The new Americans with Disabilities Act provides legal safeguards against discrimination.

This book is organized so that either it can be read from cover to cover or selected chapters or sections can be chosen. Because epilepsy presents different problems and challenges at different stages of life, information pertaining to infants, children, adolescents, adults, women of childbearing age considering parenthood, and the elderly are treated separately. The four appendices provide additional information that will help the reader to understand the terminology used in talking or writing about epilepsy, to become familiar with the different antiepileptic drugs and their indications for use, to find resources that may be helpful to persons with epilepsy, and to learn more about the disorder from suggested readings.

I hope people with epilepsy everywhere will find this book informative and useful. If it answers their questions about epilepsy, removes their doubts and dispels their fears of the disorder, and builds their confidence through knowledge, then it will have served its purpose.

Orrin Devinsky, MD

Acknowledgments

I have never been ashamed to ask for help. In writing this book, I asked for and received more help than I ever have on any other project. I thank those people with epilepsy, their family members, and professional colleagues who have so generously shared their thoughts and time: Helene Abramson, Robert Clancy, Barbara Clayton, Esther Cohen, Joyce Cramer, Joan Dauhajre, Lawrence Davis, Pat Dean, Michael and June Furlan, Patricia Gibson, Peter and Katherine Gogolak, Jayne Goldberg, Bruce Hermann, Gregory Holmes, Steve Kepniss, Steve Lasher, Catherine Ledwith, Richard Mattson, Roseanne Mercandetti, Martha Morrell, Nancy and Paul Novograd, Kenneth Perrine, Judy Rogers, Steven Schachter, and George Smith.

I also thank Linda Weinerman, who provided editorial suggestions and help, and Margarita Hernandez, who coordinated the typing and provided consistently superb secretarial oversight to the project. For their dedicated and professional attention to the production of this work, I thank Sandy Reinhardt, Bernice Wissler, Herb Powell, and Crystal McNichol of F. A. Davis.

Very special thanks go to Ann Scherer, William McLin, and others at the Epilepsy Foundation of America for sharing materials and providing valuable advice.

And, finally, my deepest appreciation goes to my wife Deborah and my daughters Janna and Julie, who waited patiently while I disappeared into the study to write.

Contents

CELONTIN® KAPSEALS®

PARKE-DAVIS

537* 150 MG

525* 300 MG

(methsuximide)

DEPAKENE®

ABBOTT

250 MG

(valproic acid capsules)

DEPAKOTE®

ABBOTT

NT* 125 MG

NR* 250 MG

NS* 500 MG

(divalproex sodium)
delayed-release tablets

DEPAKOTE® SPRINKLE

ABBOTT

125 MG

(divalproex sodium)
coated particles
in capsules

DILANTIN® KAPSEALS®

PARKE-DAVIS

365* 30 MG

362* 100 MG

(phenytoin sodium)

DILANTIN® KAPSEALS® with 1/4 gr. PHENOBARBITAL

PARKE-DAVIS

375* 100 MG / 16 MG (1/4 GR)

(phenytoin sodium,
phenobarbitol)

DILANTIN® KAPSEALS® with 1/2 gr. PHENOBARBITAL

PARKE-DAVIS

531* 100 MG / 32 MG (1/2 GR)

(phenytoin sodium,
phenobarbital)

DILANTIN® INFATABS®

PARKE-DAVIS

007* 50 MG

(phenytoin)

FELBATOL®

WALLACE LABORATORIES

0430* 400 MG

0431* 600 MG

(felbamate)

KLONOPIN®

ROCHE

0.5 MG

1 MG

2 MG

(clonazepam)

LAMICTAL®

BURROUGHS WELLCOME

100 MG

150 MG

200 MG

(lamotrigine)

MESANTOIN® TABLETS

SANDOZ

78/52* 100 MG

(mophenytoin)

MILONTIN®

PARKE-DAVIS

393* 500 MG

(phensuximide)

MYSOLINE®

WYETH-AYERST

431* 50 MG

430* 250 MG

(primidone)

*Manufacturer's product identification code

NEURONTIN®

PARKE-DAVIS

100 MG

300 MG

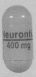

400 MG

(gabapentin)

PARADIONE®

ABBOTT

150 MG

300 MG

(paramethadione)

PEGANONE®

ABBOTT

AD* 250 MG

AE* 500 MG

(ethotoin tablets)

PHENOBARBITAL®

WARNER CHILCOTT

699* 15 MG

700* 30 MG

607* 60 MG

698* 100 MG

(generic)

TEGRETOL®

BASEL

27* 200 MG

(carbamazepine)

TEGRETOL® CHEWABLE

BASEL

52* 100 MG

(carbamazepine)

TRANXENE®-SD™ HALF STRENGTH

ABBOTT

TX* 11.25 MG

(clorazepate dipotassium)

TRANXENE® SD™

ABBOTT

TL* 22.5 MG

(clorazepate dipotassium)

TRANXENE® T-TAB™

ABBOTT

TL* 3.75 MG

TM* 7.5 MG

TN* 15 MG

(clorazepate dipotassium)

TRIDIONE®

ABBOTT

AM* 300 MG

**LE*150 MG
DULCET® TABLET**

(trimethadione)

VALIUM®

ROCHE

2 MG

5 MG

10 MG

(diazepam)

VALRELEASE®

ROCHE

15 MG

(sustained release diazepam)

ZARONTIN®

PARKE-DAVIS

237* 250 MG

(ethosuximide)

*Manufacturer's product identification code

Medical Aspects of Epilepsy

CHAPTER 1

Modern Facts about Epilepsy

about epilepsy

Epilepsy has afflicted human beings since the dawn of our species and has been recognized since the earliest medical writings. We now understand that epilepsy is a common disorder resulting from seizures that cause temporary impairment of brain function. Few medical conditions have attracted so much attention and generated so much controversy. Throughout history, people with epilepsy, as well as their families, have suffered unfairly because of the ignorance of others. Fortunately, the stigma and fear generated by the words "seizures" and "epilepsy" have progressively diminished during the past century, and the majority of people with epilepsy now lead normal lives.

The Greek physician Hippocrates wrote the first book on epilepsy, titled *On the Sacred Disease*, around 400 BC. Hippocrates recognized that epilepsy was a brain disorder, and he refuted the ideas that seizures were a curse from the gods and that people with epilepsy held prophetic powers. False ideas die slowly, though, and for centuries epilepsy was considered a curse of the gods, or worse. For example, in a handbook on witch-hunting, *Malleus Maleficarum*, written by two Dominican friars under papal authority in 1494, witches were identified by the presence of certain characteristics, including seizures. The *Malleus* brought about a wave of persecution and torture and led to more than 200,000 women being put to death. In the early 19th century, people who had severe epilepsy and people with psychiatric disorders were cared for in asylums, but the two groups were separated because seizures were thought to be "contagious."

The modern medical era of epilepsy began in the mid-19th century, under the leadership of three English neurologists: Russell Reynolds, John Hughlings Jackson, and Sir William Richard Gowers. Still standing today is Hughlings Jackson's definition of a seizure as "an occasional, an excessive, and a disorderly discharge of nerve tissue on muscles." Hughlings Jackson also recognized that seizures could alter consciousness, sensation, and behavior.

The past century has brought an explosion of knowledge about the functions of the brain and about epilepsy. Research in epilepsy continues at a vigorous pace, with investigations ranging from how microscopic particles in the cell trigger seizures, to the development of new antiepileptic drugs, and to a better understanding of how epilepsy affects social and intellectual development.

PEOPLE WITH EPILEPSY ARE NOT "EPILEPTICS"

The word "epileptic" should not be used to describe someone who has epilepsy, as it defines a person by one trait. A label is powerful and can create a limiting and negative stereotype. It is better to refer to someone as "a person with epilepsy" or to a group of people as "people with epilepsy."

PEOPLE WITH EPILEPSY ARE NOT NECESSARILY BRAIN-DAMAGED

Epilepsy is a *disorder of brain function* that may or may not be associated with damage to brain structures. Temporarily disturbed brain function can also occur with extreme fatigue; with the use of sleeping pills, sedatives, or general anesthesia; or with high fever or serious illness. "Brain damage" implies that something is permanently wrong with the brain's structure. It may occur with head trauma, cerebral palsy, or stroke. Injuries to the brain are the cause of seizures in some, but by no means all, persons with epilepsy. Brain injuries range from undetectable to disabling. Although brain cells cannot regenerate, most people make substantial recoveries after brain injuries. Brain damage, like epilepsy, carries a stigma, and some people may unjustly consider brain-injured patients "incompetent."

PEOPLE WITH EPILEPSY USUALLY ARE NOT RETARDED

Many people mistakenly believe that people with epilepsy are also mentally retarded. In the large majority of cases, this is not true. Like any other group of people, people with epilepsy have different intellectual abilities. Some are brilliant and some score below average on intelligence tests, but most are somewhere in the middle.

The majority of people with epilepsy have normal intelligence and lead productive lives. In some people, however, epilepsy is associated with brain

injuries that cause neurological impairments, including mental retardation. With only very rare exceptions, seizures do not cause mental retardation.

PEOPLE WITH EPILEPSY ARE NOT VIOLENT OR CRAZY

The belief that people with epilepsy are violent is an unfortunate image that is both wrong and destructive. The vast majority of people with epilepsy have no greater tendency toward irritability and aggressive behaviors than do other people in the general population. Many features of seizures and their immediate aftereffects can be easily misunderstood as "crazy" or "violent" behavior. Unfortunately, police officers and even medical personnel may confuse seizure-related behaviors with other problems. However, these behaviors merely represent semiconscious or confused actions resulting from the seizure. During seizures, some persons may not respond to questions, may speak gibberish, repeat a word or phrase, crumple important papers, or may appear frightened and scream. Some persons are confused immediately after a seizure, and if they are restrained or prevented from moving about, they can become agitated. Some persons may be able to respond to questions and carry on a conversation fairly well, but several hours later they will have no recollection of the conversation.

Anxiety and depression may be slightly more common among people with epilepsy than in the general population. In some people, problems associated with epilepsy, such as injury to specific brain areas or sensitivity to certain medications, can contribute to aggressive or confused behavior. The issue of aggression and epilepsy is discussed in Chapter 27.

SEIZURES DO NOT CAUSE BRAIN DAMAGE

Single seizures do not cause permanent brain damage. Although tonic-clonic (grand mal) seizures lasting longer than 30 to 60 minutes may injure the brain, there is no evidence that shorter seizures, lasting less than 30 minutes, cause permanent injury to the brain. Prolonged episodes of other types of seizures also are unlikely to injure the brain.

Some persons have difficulty with memory and other intellectual functions after a seizure. These problems may be caused by the aftereffects of the seizure on the brain, by the effects of antiepileptic drugs, or both. Usually, however, these problems do not mean that the brain has been damaged by the seizure.

EPILEPSY IS NOT NECESSARILY INHERITED

Most cases of epilepsy are not inherited. However, some types of epilepsy, most of them easily controlled with medications, are genetically transmitted, that is, passed on through the family.

EPILEPSY IS NOT A LIFE-LONG DISORDER

Most persons with epilepsy do not have seizures or require medication all their lives. The majority of childhood forms of epilepsy are outgrown by adulthood. For most forms of epilepsy in children and adults, when the person has been free of seizures for 2 to 4 years, medications can often be slowly withdrawn and discontinued under a doctor's supervision.

EPILEPSY IS NOT A CURSE

Epilepsy has nothing to do with curses, possession, or other supernatural processes. Like asthma, diabetes, and high blood pressure, epilepsy is a medical problem.

EPILEPSY SHOULD NOT BE A BARRIER TO SUCCESS

Epilepsy is perfectly compatible with a normal, happy, and full life. The person's quality of life, however, may be affected by the frequency and severity of the seizures, the effects of medications, and associated neurological disorders. Some types of epilepsy are harder to control than others. Successfully living with epilepsy requires a positive outlook, a supportive environment, and good medical care.

Acquiring a positive outlook may be easier said than done, especially for those who have grown up with insecurity and fear. This difficulty highlights the importance of instilling in children with epilepsy a sense of self-esteem. Many children with epilepsy have low self-esteem, perhaps caused in part by the reactions of others and in part by parental concern that fosters dependence and insecurity. Children develop strong self-esteem and independence through praise for their accomplishments and emphasis on their potential abilities.

CHAPTER 2

The Brain and Epilepsy

The human brain is an intricate and extraordinarily complex organ that controls life-support functions such as breathing and temperature regulation, primitive survival behaviors such as eating and drinking, and sleep-wake cycles, emotions, sensations, movements, and intellect. From an evolutionary perspective, the newest part of our brain—the part that differs most from the brain of other animals—is the *cerebral cortex*, which forms the large outer surface of the upper brain. The outer surface contains numerous folds *(sulci)* that increase the surface area and allow more cerebral cortex to be packed into the skull (Fig. 1).

ANATOMY OF THE BRAIN

The Cerebrum

The upper brain, or *cerebrum*, is composed of white matter and gray matter (Fig. 2). The gray matter forms the cerebral cortex and consists largely of nerve cells *(neurons)* and supportive cells *(glial cells)*. The white matter lies beneath the cerebral cortex and is composed of nerve fibers. The nerve fibers act like telephone wires, connecting different areas of the brain, spinal cord, muscles, and glands.

The cerebrum is divided into the left and right hemispheres, which are connected by a large white fiber bundle called the *corpus callosum* (see Fig. 1B). Each cerebral hemisphere contains four lobes: frontal, parietal, temporal, and occipital. Each lobe contains many different areas that have different functions. For example, in almost all right-handed persons, the area that controls speech lies in the left frontal lobe, and the area that controls comprehension of spoken and written language lies in the left temporal lobe. Some brain functions are fairly well confined to specific areas, but most others rely on a network of related areas. For functions requiring an integrated network, damage to one area of the network can often be compensated for by other areas. For example, the ability to pay attention involves

7

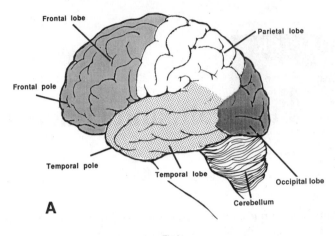

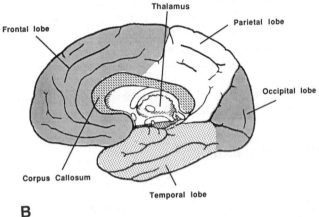

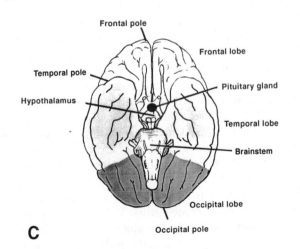

FIGURE 1. Three views of the brain. (*A*) Outer surface (*side view*). (*B*) Inner surface (*cross-sectional view*). (*C*) Lower surface (*bottom view*).

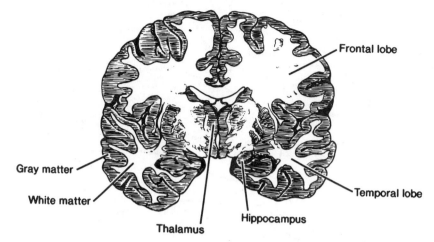

FIGURE 2. Cross-section of the brain showing the gray matter and the white matter.

both cerebral hemispheres, as well as other brain areas located in the brainstem (see below). Damage to or disrupted function in certain critical areas of the "attention network" (interconnected brain areas that help us focus our attention and concentrate) can severely disrupt our ability to stay focused and not get distracted. Disruption of function or damage to other, less critical areas in this network will cause only a mild and temporary disorder of attention.

The right half of the brain controls the left side of the body, and the left half of the brain controls the right side of the body. Therefore, an injury to the left cerebral cortex from a head injury or a stroke can cause weakness and loss of sensation on the right side of the body if the motor (movement) or sensory areas of the left cerebral cortex or the fiber bundles that connect these areas with other parts of the brain are damaged.

The cerebral cortex contains some areas that are evolutionarily new, such as the language areas of the left cerebral hemisphere. Other areas developed much earlier in our evolution. For example, the deep, central portions of the frontal and temporal lobes contain the limbic cortex, which controls emotions and memory (see Fig. 3C). The limbic cortex is particularly important in epilepsy, as it is commonly the area from which partial seizures arise. The functions of the different parts of the brain are summarized in Figure 3.

Injury or disordered function of either newer or older areas of the cerebral cortex can cause seizures. If seizures arise from a specific area of the brain, then the initial symptoms of the seizure often reflect the functions

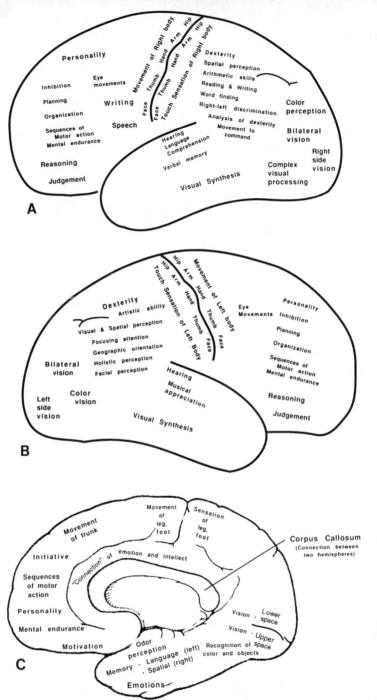

FIGURE 3. Areas of the human brain responsible for specific functions. (*A*) Left hemisphere (*side view*). (*B*) Right hemisphere (*side view*). (*C*) Inner surface (*cross-sectional view*). The areas in the frontal lobe and the lateral parietal lobe are not so precisely distributed as the drawings indicate, and the areas overlap in their control of some functions.

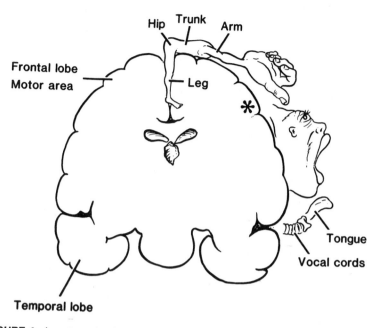

FIGURE 4. A cartoon showing the parts of the body whose movements are controlled by various areas of the motor cortex in the right hemisphere; the asterisk indicates the hand area.

of that area. For example, if a seizure starts from the motor area of the right hemisphere that controls movements in the left thumb, then the seizure may begin with jerking movements of the left thumb or hand. The motor cortex of each hemisphere is organized so that groups of muscles are controlled by specific areas. The lowest part of this brain area controls the vocal cords and mouth, the middle part controls the hand and arm, and the upper part controls the leg on the opposite side of the body (Fig. 4).

The Brainstem and Spinal Cord

The lower part of the brain contains the *brainstem* (Fig. 5), which controls sleep-wake cycles, breathing, and heartbeat. The upper part of the brainstem contains the thalamus and hypothalamus (see Figs. 1B and 1C). The lower part of the brainstem contains the cerebellum. The spinal cord begins as a continuation of the lower part of the brainstem.

The Thalamus

The *thalamus* serves as a relay station to send messages about bodily sensations (for example, a touch on the left hand or the sounds and visual

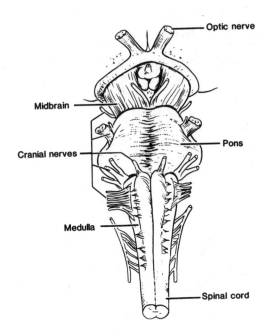

Optic nerve

Midbrain

Cranial nerves

Pons

Medulla

Spinal cord

FIGURE 5. The brainstem.

impressions of a car) to the cerebral cortex for conscious awareness. The thalamus is also important in pain perception and in regulating the level of consciousness; patients with damage to the thalamus may enter a nearly continuous sleeplike state from which they are difficult to arouse. Some of the generalized epilepsies may arise in the thalamus.

The Hypothalamus

The *hypothalamus* regulates endocrine functions through its control over the pituitary gland, the "master" endocrine, or hormone, gland. Hormones are proteins made and released by an endocrine gland into the bloodstream to influence the activity of other parts of the body. The hormones released by the pituitary gland control the activity of other endocrine glands, such as the ovaries, testicles, thyroid, parathyroid, and adrenal glands. The limbic areas of the temporal lobes influence the hypothalamus, which in turn alters pituitary gland functions. This may explain alterations in certain hormone functions in people with epilepsy, causing, for example, irregular menstrual cycles. Hormones also influence the limbic areas. For example, the stress hormone cortisol and the sex hormones estrogen, progesterone, and testosterone all attach to cells in the limbic areas and affect the functions of these cells. This may explain why some women with epilepsy are more prone to seizures at certain times during their menstrual cycle.

The Brainstem and Cerebellum

The Lower Brainstem

The lower part of the brainstem (see Fig. 5) controls movement and sensation of the face, eye movements, taste, heartbeat, breathing, and other bodily functions, such as how much acid is produced by the stomach.

The Cerebellum

The cerebellum, located behind the brainstem, helps coordinate movement.

The Spinal Cord

The *spinal cord* receives and sends information to the body about sensation and movement. For example, cells in the motor area of the left cerebral cortex send fibers, or "brain wires," down through the brainstem. In the lower brainstem, these fibers cross over to the opposite (right) side and then continue downward into the right side of the spinal cord. This explains why the right cerebral cortex controls movements of the left side of the body—the fibers cross in the lower part of the brainstem. In the spinal cord, these fibers activate other cells, which in turn send fibers into the nerves that pass into the arm and which directly activate the muscles to make the hand move.

Similarly, there are touch receptors in the hand. When these receptors are activated by touch, they excite nerve impulses to flow up the same nerves in the arm. However, in contrast to the muscle impulses that pass from the spinal cord to the muscles of the hand, the sensory impulses pass from the hand to the spinal cord. This sensory information then passes up the spinal cord to the lower brainstem, where there is a "relay station." The relay station is a group of nerve cells that receive the information and then pass it on to a new fiber called an axon, which crosses over to the opposite half of the brainstem and goes up to another relay station in the thalamus. This crossing-over explains why touch information from the right hand ends up in the left cerebral cortex.

From the thalamus, the information finally makes its way to the parietal lobe of the brain, the area that brings touch sensation to conscious awareness. The motor and touch sensation areas of each hemisphere communicate with each other. This communication allows us to make precise complex movements and to know instinctively where our hand or other body part is in space. Without it there would be no basketball stars or concert pianists.

The Central and Peripheral Nervous Systems

The brain and spinal cord comprise the central nervous system. The nerves in the face, arms, and legs make up the peripheral nervous system. Epilepsy is a disorder of the central nervous system, specifically the brain. Although some chiropractors maintain that problems in the spinal cord or in the blood vessels associated with the spinal bones of the neck may contribute to epilepsy, there is absolutely no evidence to support these claims, except in extremely rare cases of strokes from blockages of these blood vessels that are followed by epilepsy. In such cases, however, chiropractic manipulation of the neck can be dangerous.

NERVE CELLS OF THE BRAIN

Neurons (nerve cells) are the building blocks of the brain. Nerve cells are so small that a microscope is needed to see them. There are approximately 14 billion nerve cells in the brain and spinal cord. Nerve cells are usually composed of three parts: the cell body, axon, and dendrites (Fig. 6). The *soma* (cell body) contains the enzymes and chemicals that regulate the metabolism of the cell and genetic information to power and direct the cell's activities. The *axon* is the long portion of a nerve cell that resembles a wire. Axons are the critical, "transmitting" parts of the nerve fibers in both the central and peripheral nervous systems. The axons that go from the motor area in the cerebral cortex to the leg area in the spinal cord can be longer than 4 feet. The message to wiggle your toes quite literally goes down the axon. Axons carry chemicals known as *neurotransmitters* (chemical messengers) from the cell body to the end of the axon, where they are passed on to other nerve cells. Therefore, axons serve as the "copper wires" of the brain's telephone system. The space between the end of the axon and either the adjacent muscle fiber or the dendrite of another nerve cell is called the *synapse*. The neurotransmitters released from the axon travel across the synapse to interact with receptors on the muscle or dendrite.

Myelin, the fatty covering that surrounds most axons, serves the same function that plastic does around telephone wires—to insulate the wires from each other and prevent "cross-talk" between the different wires. The heavier the coating of myelin, the faster an axon transmits its messages. The fastest axons in the nervous system transmit messages at a rate of approximately 350 feet per second.

Dendrites serve as the cell's receiving antennas. Neurotransmitters released by the axon attach to or, more precisely, fit into receptors on the dendrite's membrane. This is analogous to a key (the neurotransmitter) fitting into a lock (the receptor). A specific key is needed for a specific lock—

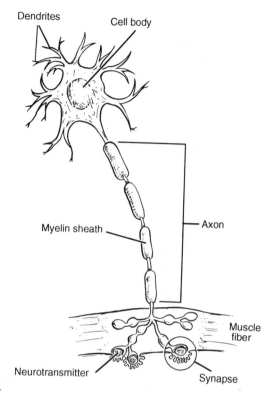

FIGURE 6. A neuron (nerve cell).

there are no "master keys" in the brain. These chemical neurotransmitters may increase or decrease the cell's activity and thereby cause changes in the electrical activity and chemical composition of the cell. Thus, both electrical and chemical systems are critical for nerve cell functions and for the transmission of information in the nervous system. Many of the drugs used to treat epilepsy and other brain disorders such as Parkinson's disease and insomnia bind to, or with, the receptors on the dendrites, thus increasing or decreasing the activity in this nerve cell.

NEUROTRANSMITTERS

Neurotransmitters are the chemical messengers of the brain. These substances are produced in the nerve cell body, carried down the inside of the axon, and released at the end of the axon. The neurotransmitters then cross the synapse, a tiny junction between the walls of the axon and dendrite, to bind to receptors located on the dendrite.

There are a variety of neurotransmitters, but individual nerve cells produce only one major neurotransmitter, for example, gamma-aminobutyric acid (GABA). Some of the neurotransmitters are carried a long distance within the nervous system, whereas others have local effects; that is, they are produced by and released onto cells that are close to each other. Neurotransmitters are important in diseases of the nervous system. In Parkinson's disease, for example, there is degeneration of the cells in the brainstem that manufacture dopamine, an important neurotransmitter in the regulation of movement. Loss of nerve cells may contribute to the *development* of epilepsy in some cases. For example, prolonged lack of oxygen may cause a selective loss of cells in the hippocampus (see Fig. 2), which may lead to epilepsy.

Some of the major brain neurotransmitters can be classified as excitatory (they stimulate or increase brain electrical activity; that is, they cause nerve cells to fire) or inhibitory (they shut off or decrease brain electrical activity; that is, they cause nerve cells to stop firing). According to one theory, epilepsy is caused by an imbalance between neurotransmitters that cause nerve cells to fire and those that cause them to stop firing; either a deficiency of inhibitory neurotransmitters such as GABA or an excess of excitatory neurotransmitters such as glutamate increases the likelihood that a seizure will occur. This is an area in which much research is being conducted. Many of the new drugs being developed to treat epilepsy act by increasing activity in the inhibitory systems that turn cells off or by decreasing activity in the excitatory systems that turn cells on.

SEIZURES—A STORM OF BRAIN ELECTRICAL ACTIVITY

The nerve cells of the brain communicate through electrical and chemical messages. The communication processes are interwoven: changes in chemical activity cause changes in electrical activity and vice versa. The brain is organized so that there is a fine balance between excitation and inhibition of electrical activity. Further, there are systems in the brain that limit the spread of electrical activity.

During an epileptic seizure, the regulatory systems that maintain the normal balance between excitation and inhibition of the brain's electrical activity break down. For example, there may be a loss of inhibitory nerve cells (cells that turn off other cells when they become too active) or an overproduction of a neurotransmitter (a chemical that stimulates cells to discharge electrical signals).

For an electrical discharge in the brain to alter a person's behavior, the brain cells must be functionally or structurally abnormal. In most seizures, a small group of abnormal cells cause changes in neighboring cells or in cells with which they have strong connections. Ultimately, groups of cells are activated synchronously. That is, the electrical discharges of many cells become linked, creating a storm of activity.

The question often arises, if an injury to the brain (for example, oxygen deprivation at birth or head trauma) caused the epilepsy, why was there an interval of many years between the actual injury and the first seizure? We now have some insights into this period of epileptogenesis, or the process leading to the development of seizures. An animal model of epilepsy known as kindling may shed some light on this question. In this model, an area of an animal's brain is stimulated once a day with a small current of electricity. At first, the stimulations may cause no measurable change in the brain's electrical activity or the animal's behavior. After a week, there may be a small, local storm of electrical activity after the stimulation. There may or may not be any change in the animal's behavior. After several weeks, the storm may be followed within seconds by storms in the same area of the opposite hemisphere or in areas adjacent to the original storm of activity. When these electrical storms occur, the animal may show clinical signs of a seizure such as facial grimacing or staring with unresponsiveness. After additional stimuli, the electrical and clinical signs of the seizure become more intense and ultimately culminate in a tonic-clonic (grand mal) seizure. Finally, in some animals, tonic-clonic or other seizures may occur spontaneously, that is, without the electrical stimulation. Thus, a "fire" has been "kindled" in the brain. In more advanced species, such as baboons and rhesus monkeys, the kindling process proceeds slowly. In humans, kindling caused by a brain injury may progress over a period of years, thereby explaining the delay in the development of epilepsy.

CHAPTER 3

Classification of Seizures

A seizure is not a disease. Rather, a seizure is a symptom of many different disorders that can affect the brain. A person with diabetes in whom the blood sugar becomes extremely low or high can have a seizure. A person who drinks too much alcohol can have seizures, especially during the first several days after drinking is stopped. High fevers, especially in infants and young children, can cause seizures. Head injury, stroke, brain tumors, and brain infections can also cause seizures.

DEFINITION OF SEIZURES AND EPILEPSY

A *seizure* is a brief, excessive surge of electrical activity in the brain that causes a change in how a person feels, senses things, or behaves. Seizures can cause an incredible range of effects, including, for example, a sensation of "pins and needles" in the thumb for a few seconds, a smell of burnt rubber and a strange feeling in the belly, a ringing sound that keeps increasing in volume, staring with loss of awareness for several minutes, or convulsive movements.

Epilepsy is a disorder in which a person has two or more seizures without a clear cause, such as alcohol withdrawal. The seizure may be the result of a hereditary tendency or of a brain injury, such as severe head trauma or stroke, or the cause may be unknown. The condition of *recurrent and unprovoked seizures* is referred to as *epilepsy*. It is a common misconception that all seizures, regardless of their cause, can be referred to as epilepsy.

For many persons, the diagnosis of "epilepsy" seems more serious and frightening than "seizure disorder." However, epilepsy is a seizure disorder. Accepting the condition for what it is, name and all, is often the first step toward leading a normal life.

IMPAIRMENT OF CONSCIOUSNESS DURING SEIZURES

A simple definition of "consciousness" is the ability to respond and to remember. In some cases, persons with absence seizures, complex partial seizures, or, occasionally, tonic-clonic seizures have no recollection of the seizure. In other cases, they are aware that they had a seizure, but are absolutely convinced that they had no loss or impairment of consciousness, when, in fact, they did. Therefore, it is helpful to have a family member or friend test the person during a seizure by asking him or her to follow commands such as "show me your left hand" and "remember the color yellow." If the person can follow the command and remember the word, consciousness is preserved, at least during the time tested.

Although neurologists describe consciousness during seizures as "impaired" or "preserved," the two categories are not as clearly separate as one might imagine. The degree of impairment and preservation of consciousness varies from seizure to seizure. Consciousness is affected if either responsiveness or memory is impaired during an attack, but these two criteria do not have the same functional importance. For example, someone may have a seizure in which he or she can respond to most commands but later is unable to recall some details of the seizure. It is possible that, in certain cases, that person could safely operate dangerous equipment. Some seizures, however, may impair someone's ability to move voluntarily. The person is unable to speak or raise his or her hand to someone else's request but may be able to recall the entire event and, therefore, did not have impaired consciousness, but only impaired motor control.

CLASSIFICATION OF SEIZURES

Seizures can be broadly separated into two groups: (1) primary generalized seizures and (2) partial seizures (Table 1). Primary generalized seizures begin with a widespread, excessive electrical discharge simultaneously involving both sides of the brain. In contrast, partial seizures begin with an abnormal electrical discharge restricted to one region of the brain. Distinguishing primary generalized seizures from partial seizures is important because the types of tests needed and the medications used to treat these disorders differ. A description of what happened before, during, and after the seizure, as well as recordings of the brain waves, helps the doctor to determine the type of seizure. Brain waves, electrical activity generated by the brain, are recorded with an electroencephalograph machine; this test, called an electroencephalogram (EEG), can detect abnormal electrical im-

TABLE 1. CLASSIFICATION OF EPILEPTIC SEIZURES

Primary Generalized Seizures
  Absence seizures
    Typical
    Atypical
  Myoclonic seizures
  Atonic seizures
  Clonic seizures
  Tonic seizures
  Tonic-clonic seizures

Partial Seizures (Seizures Originating in Specific Parts of the Brain)
  Simple partial seizures (consciousness not impaired)
    With motor symptoms (jerking, stiffening)
    With somatosensory (touch) or specialized sensory (smell, hearing, taste, sight)
      symptoms
    With autonomic symptoms (heart rate change, internal sensations)
    With psychic symptoms (*déjà vu*, dreamy state)
  Complex partial seizures (consciousness impaired, automatisms usually present)
    Beginning as simple partial seizures
    Beginning with impairment of consciousness
  Partial seizures secondarily generalized to tonic-clonic seizures

---

pulses in people with epilepsy (see Chapter 8). In primary generalized epilepsy, the EEG shows a widespread increase in electrical activity. In partial seizures, the brain waves show a more restricted, or local, increase of electrical activity. However, the EEG may be normal in people with epilepsy, and occasionally shows "epilepsy waves" in people who have never had a seizure. Hereditary factors are more important in primary generalized seizures than in partial seizures. In some cases, it can be difficult to distinguish primary generalized seizures from partial seizures, as many of their features overlap. For example, a tonic-clonic seizure may begin as a primary generalized seizure or as a partial seizure, and a staring spell can be an absence seizure (a type of primary generalized seizure) or a complex partial seizure.

Primary Generalized Seizures

Primary generalized seizures begin simultaneously from both sides of the brain. The principal types of primary generalized seizures are absence seizures, atypical absence seizures, myoclonic seizures, atonic seizures, clonic seizures, tonic seizures, and tonic-clonic seizures.

Absence Seizures

Frank, a 7-year-old boy, often "blanks out" for a few seconds, and sometimes for 10 to 20 seconds. His teacher calls his name, but he doesn't seem to hear her. He usually blinks a few times, and his eyes may roll up a bit, but with the short seizures he just stares. Then he is right back where he left off. Some days he has more than 50 of these spells.

Absence (petit mal) seizures are brief episodes of staring with impairment of awareness and responsiveness. The episode usually lasts less than 10 seconds, but may last as long as 20 seconds. The seizure begins and ends suddenly. There is no warning before the seizure, and immediately afterward the person is alert and attentive and usually unaware that a seizure has occurred. In the majority of cases, these spells begin in children between 4 and 14 years of age. In approximately 75% of children, absence seizures resolve and do not continue after 18 years of age. Absence seizures are often provoked by rapid breathing (hyperventilation), and they can usually be reproduced in the doctor's office with this technique if the patient is not taking medication. For some reason, however, absence seizures are uncommon during exercise with rapid breathing. Children with absence seizures have normal development and intelligence.

Simple absence seizures are just "stares." However, most spells are complex absence seizures, in which staring is accompanied by some change in muscle activity, especially if the seizure lasts more than 10 seconds. The most common movements are eye blinks, but others include slight tasting movements of the mouth, automatic hand movements such as rubbing the fingers together, and contraction or relaxation of the muscles.

The EEG is extremely helpful in diagnosing absence seizures. In the majority of cases, a characteristic finding is three-per-second spike-and-wave discharges, especially during hyperventilation (see Fig. 13). Tests that show images of the brain, called computed tomography (CT) and magnetic resonance imaging (MRI) (see Chapter 8), are normal in children with absence seizures, and in most typical cases it is not necessary to obtain these tests.

Atypical Absence Seizures

It is hard for me to tell when Kathy is having one of her staring spells. During the spells, she doesn't respond as quickly as at other times. The problem is that she often doesn't respond so quickly, and she often just stares when she is not having an absence seizure.

The staring spells of *atypical absence seizures* also occur predominantly in children, and usually begin before 6 years of age. In contrast with absence seizures, atypical absence seizures often begin and end gradually (over seconds), often last more than 10 seconds (the usual duration is 5–30 seconds), and are not provoked by rapid breathing. The child stares but often has only a partial reduction in responsiveness. Eye blinking or slight jerking movements of the lips may occur. Children who have these seizures are more likely to have lower-than-average intelligence. In some children, especially those with intellectual deficits, atypical absence seizures may be difficult to distinguish from the child's usual behavior.

Most children with these seizures have an abnormal EEG, which reveals slow spike-and-wave discharges, even when they are not having a seizure. The EEG abnormality is not provoked by hyperventilation.

Myoclonic Seizures

> In the morning I get these "jumps." My arms just go flying up for a second. Occasionally my mouth shuts for a split second. Sometimes I get a few of these jumps in a row. Once I have been up for a few hours I never get any more of these jumps.

Myoclonic seizures occur as brief, shocklike jerks of a muscle or group of muscles. Myoclonus may occur in people who do not have epilepsy. For example, as many people fall asleep, their body suddenly jerks, which is referred to as sleep jerks, sleep starts, or benign nocturnal myoclonus. Among the abnormal forms of myoclonus are both epileptic and nonepileptic types.

Epileptic myoclonus usually causes abnormal movements on both sides of the body at the same time. The neck, shoulders, upper arms, body, and upper legs are usually involved. Myoclonic seizures occur in a variety of epilepsy syndromes, and the prognosis for control of these seizures varies among the different syndromes (see Chapter 4).

Myoclonic seizures in the Lennox-Gastaut syndrome often occur along with atonic and other seizure types. During these attacks, the person may fall. In addition to the areas of the body mentioned above, these seizures may involve the muscles of the face. As with other seizures in patients with the Lennox-Gastaut syndrome, myoclonic seizures are often difficult to control with medication.

Myoclonic seizures in the juvenile myoclonic epilepsy syndrome most often involve the neck, shoulders, and upper arms. The seizures most commonly occur in the early morning hours, shortly after awakening. The attacks are usually well controlled with medication, which almost always needs to be continued throughout the person's life.

Progressive myoclonic epilepsy refers to a group of disorders associated with neurological deterioration. These disorders are rare in comparison with the other types of myoclonic seizures.

Atonic Seizures

Bob's "drop" seizures are his biggest problem. He falls to the ground and often hits his head and bruises his body. Even if I'm right next to him and prepared, I may not catch him. The helmet is great, but he often forgets to put it on before he gets out of bed. Even with carpet in the bedroom and mats in the bathroom, he gets hurt.

The brief spells of *atonic seizures*, lasting less than 15 seconds, are associated with a sudden loss of muscle strength, causing the eyelids to droop, the head to nod, or an object to be dropped, or causing a fall to the ground. Atonic seizures usually begin in childhood. Because of possible sudden falling, injury is common.

Clonic Seizures

Generalized convulsive seizures may involve jerking (clonic) movements on both sides of the body without a stiffening (tonic) component. *Clonic seizures*, in contrast with the more common tonic-clonic seizures, are not followed by a prolonged period of confusion or tiredness after the seizure has ended.

Some tonic-clonic seizures are preceded by a series of jerking movements. These seizures are referred to as clonic-tonic-clonic seizures and are common among people with juvenile myoclonic epilepsy (see Chapter 4).

Tonic Seizures

Jeff just stiffens up. Both arms are raised over his head, and his face has this grimace, like someone is pulling on his cheeks. The episodes last less than a minute, but if he is standing he may lose his balance and fall. These seizures don't knock him out like the grand mals, but if he has a few close together, he is often tired.

Tonic seizures, usually lasting less than 20 seconds, are associated with sudden stiffening movements of the body, arms, or legs, and involve both sides of the body. They are more common during sleep. Tonic seizures are most common in children who have lower-than-average scores on intelligence tests, but can occur in any child or adult.

Tonic-Clonic Seizures

These are the seizures that frighten me. They last only a minute or two, but it feels like an eternity. I can often tell they are coming because she is more cranky and out of sorts. When it starts, Heather suddenly shrieks with this unnatural cry, then she falls, and every muscle in her body seems to be activated. Her teeth clench. I know she can't, but I still worry about her swallowing her tongue. At the very beginning, she is pale, and later, a slight bluish color. Shortly after she falls, her arms and upper body start to jerk while her legs are more or less still stiff. This is the longest part of the seizure. Then it finally stops and she passes into a deep sleep.

Tonic-clonic (grand mal) seizures are convulsive seizures. The person briefly stiffens and loses consciousness, falls, and often utters a cry. It is not a cry from pain, but is caused by air being forced through the contracting vocal cords. The stiffening is followed by jerking of the arms and legs. The seizures usually last 1 to 3 minutes. There may be excessive saliva production, sometimes incorrectly described as "foaming" at the mouth. Biting of the tongue or cheek may cause bleeding. Loss of urine or, rarely, a bowel movement may occur. After the convulsion the person may be tired and confused for a period of minutes to hours and often goes to sleep, but he or she may be agitated or depressed. The time immediately after the seizure is called the postictal period. First aid for tonic-clonic seizures is discussed in Chapter 9.

When tonic-clonic seizures last more than 30 minutes or recur in a series of three or more seizures without the person returning to a normal state in between, a dangerous condition called *convulsive status epilepticus* has developed. *When tonic-clonic seizures last longer than 5 minutes, medical help should be obtained* (see Chapter 9).

Partial Seizures

Partial seizures begin with an abnormal burst of electrical activity in a restricted area of brain tissue. Most partial seizures arise from the temporal or frontal lobes. Less commonly, partial seizures begin in the visual (occipital lobe) or sensory (parietal lobe) areas of the brain. Head injury, brain infections, stroke, and brain tumors are common causes of partial seizures. In some cases, hereditary factors are also important. In the majority of cases, no cause can be identified.

Partial seizures are divided into two main types, depending on whether consciousness is fully preserved. During *simple partial seizures* the person is alert, able to respond to questions or commands, and can remember what occurred during the seizure. During *complex partial seizures*, the ability to pay attention or to respond to questions or commands is impaired. Often, there is no memory of what happened during all or part of the seizure. The distinction between simple and complex partial seizures is critical, because the ability to drive, operate dangerous equipment, swim alone, and perform other activities usually has to be restricted in people with uncontrolled complex partial seizures.

Simple Partial Seizures

> I almost enjoy them. The feeling of *déjà vu*, like I have lived through this moment, and I even know what is going to be said next. Everything seems brighter and more alive.

> It is a pressure that begins in my stomach and then rises up to my chest and throat. When it reaches my chest, I smell the same odor, something burnt, definitely unpleasant. At the same time I feel nervous, not because of the aura, I just get anxious.

Simple partial seizures can cause a remarkably diverse group of symptoms. In some cases, the symptoms are not recognized as a seizure, because many symptoms of partial seizures can also be caused by other factors. For example, abdominal discomfort is likely to be the result of a gastrointestinal disorder, but it also can be a symptom of a partial seizure arising in the temporal lobe. Tingling in the little finger that spreads to the forearm may come from a seizure, migraine, or nerve disorder.

Motor seizures involve a change in muscle activity. Most often, the body stiffens, or the muscles begin to jerk in one area of the body such as a finger or the wrist. The abnormal movements may remain restricted to one body part or spread to involve other muscles on the same side or both sides of the body. Some partial motor seizures cause weakness of one or more body parts, including the vocal apparatus, which affects the ability to speak.

Sensory seizures cause changes in sensation. Most often, a person has a hallucination, or the sensation of something there that is not there, such as a feeling of "pins and needles" in a finger or seeing a red ball. The abnormal sensations may remain restricted to one area of the body or spread to other areas. There also may be an illusion or the distortion of a true sensation. For example, a car that is standing still may appear to be moving farther away, or a person's voice may be muffled and difficult to understand. Hallucinations and illusions can involve all types of sensations, including touch (numbness, pins and needles), smell (often an unpleasant odor), taste, vision (a spot of light, a scene with people), and hearing (a click or ringing, a person's voice).

Autonomic seizures cause changes in the part of the nervous system that automatically controls bodily functions. The autonomic nervous system is formed by groups of cells and fibers in the hypothalamus, lower brainstem, spinal cord, and peripheral nervous system. However, parts of the cerebral cortex, especially the limbic regions, can strongly influence activity in the autonomic nervous system. This is the reason why strong emotions such as fear are associated with increases in the heart rate and breathing rate, sweating, and a sinking feeling in the chest. The connection between the limbic system and the autonomic nervous system may also be the physiological basis of why we say such things as "In my heart, I feel it's right," or "I just have this feeling in my gut." These visceral sensations are probably linked with the emotions in limbic structures. Partial seizures commonly arise from the limbic system. Therefore, autonomic changes are common during partial seizures. Autonomic partial seizures can cause a strange or unpleasant sensation in the abdomen, chest, or head. There may be heart rate or breathing rate changes, sweating, or goose bumps that come on for no reason. Autonomic partial seizures are common.

Psychic seizures cause changes in the brain that affect how we think, feel, and experience things. These seizures can cause problems with language function, such as garbled speech, inability to find the right word, and difficulty understanding spoken or written language, as well as with time perception and memory. One type of psychic seizure causes sudden emotions such as fear, anxiety, depression, or happiness. These emotions are spontaneous; they do not result from the person seeing, hearing, or thinking about something that might trigger the emotion. Other psychic seizures can cause feeling as if one has experienced or lived through this moment before (*déjà vu*), feeling as if familiar things are strange and foreign (*jamais vu*), feeling as if one is not one's self (depersonalization), and feeling as if the world is not real, or as if one is in a dream (derealization). Psychic seizures arise from the limbic areas or more highly advanced areas of the cerebral cortex.

Complex Partial Seizures

Harold's spells begin with a warning; he says he is going to have a seizure and usually sits down. I ask him what he feels, but he either doesn't answer or just says, "I feel it." Then he makes a funny face, like he is both surprised and a bit distressed. He just stares. I call his name, and he may look at me when I call, but he never answers. During this part, he may make these mouth movements, like he is tasting something. He often grabs the arm of the chair and squeezes it. Other times, he touches his shirt, as if he is picking lint off, even though it's clean. The whole thing lasts a couple of minutes, and then as he comes back he keeps asking questions. He never remembers that he has a warning, and never remembers what he asks or says right after the seizure. He looks tired afterward; if he has two of these spells in the same day he often goes to sleep after the second one.

Susan's seizures usually occur during sleep. She makes this grunting sound, like she is clearing her throat. She sits up in bed, opens her eyes, and stares. She sometimes clasps her hands together. I ask her what she is doing, but she doesn't say a word. After a minute or so, she lies back down and goes back to sleep.

With *complex partial (psychomotor or temporal lobe) seizures*, consciousness is impaired but not lost. The person typically stares and is unable to respond to questions or commands, or responds incompletely and inaccurately. Automatic movements (automatisms) occur in most complex partial seizures. Automatisms can involve the mouth and face (lip smacking, chewing, tasting, and swallowing movements), the hands and arms (fumbling, picking, tapping, or clasping movements), vocalizations (grunts, repetition of words or phrases), or more complex acts (walking or mixing foods in a bowl). Other, less common automatisms include screaming, running, shouting, bizarre and sometimes "sexual"-appearing movements, and disrobing. Complex partial seizures usually last from 30 seconds to 3 minutes. Auras, or warnings, which are actually simple partial seizures, are common and typically precede the alteration of consciousness by seconds. After the seizure, lethargy and confusion are common, but usually last less than 15 minutes. Complex partial seizures occur in persons of all ages, from infants to the elderly.

Some people are unaware that they have had a complex partial seizure. Many of the symptoms are so subtle that others may just think their friend or relative is "thinking about something," "daydreaming," or "spacing out." These episodes can cause memory lapses, and someone who has a complex partial seizure may perform fairly complex activities and later have no recall of them. One of the earliest reported medical cases was that of a doctor. One day he found himself walking away from a ward and realized that he was supposed to examine a patient. He found the patient's bed and examined the woman. To his amazement, when he went to write his note, he found that he had been there just before and had written down the correct diagnosis—pneumonia in the bottom of the left lung—but had no recollection of ever having seen the woman. In this case, it is likely he examined the woman and made his notes either just before or after the complex partial seizure, but the seizure "wiped out" his memory for a short period.

The unusual automatic behaviors of complex partial seizures can be a source of great embarrassment and concern. For some persons, these "automatisms" are typical for their seizures. Others may have more usual automatisms, but occasionally have embarrassing behavior such as disrobing at work. This was a problem, for example, in a person I cared for who worked in an elementary school. As with most other aspects of epilepsy, special precautions can be taken to help minimize the negative effects of such behaviors.

Secondarily Generalized Seizures

They start with a tingling in the right thumb. Then the thumb starts jerking. In a few seconds, the whole right hand is jerking, and I learned to start rubbing and scratching my forearm. Sometimes I can stop the seizure this way. Other times the jerking spreads up the arm. When it reaches the shoulder, I pass out and people tell me that my whole body starts to jerk.

I see this colored ball on my right side. The ball seems to grow and fill up my whole view. As the ball grows, everything becomes like a dream, and I don't feel real. It is the strangest feeling. The seizure can just stop, and my vision is just a little blurry, or it can go all the way, so that I fall to the floor and have a grand mal.

When a restricted burst of excessive electrical activity spreads to involve both sides of the brain, the partial seizure may become a *secondarily generalized tonic-clonic seizure*. Patients may or may not recall an aura, and witnesses may first observe a complex partial seizure that progresses to a tonic-clonic seizure. A secondarily generalized tonic-clonic seizure may be difficult to distinguish from a primary generalized tonic-clonic seizure, especially if it is not witnessed or occurs during sleep. The EEG and MRI are often helpful in distinguishing the seizures.

THE POSTICTAL PERIOD

The period immediately after a seizure, called the postictal period, varies depending on the type, duration, and intensity of the seizure, as well as other factors. Absence seizures are not followed by any symptoms—when the seizure ends, the person resumes activity as if nothing happened. After most complex partial seizures, the person is slightly confused and tired, usually for less than 5 to 15 minutes. After tonic-clonic seizures, the person often complains of muscle soreness and headache, and of pain in the tongue or cheek if those areas were bitten. The person may be confused and tired, often awakening briefly after the seizure and then going to sleep.

Other symptoms follow some seizures. Todd's paralysis, first described in the mid-1800s as muscle weakness affecting one side of the body, may occur as weakness of an arm after a partial motor or tonic-clonic seizure. Seizures may also be followed by impairments in vision, touch sensation, language, and other functions. Often, the nature of the postictal problem can help identify the area from which the seizure began. For example, weakness in the right arm and leg may follow a seizure that began in the motor area of the left hemisphere.

CHANGE IN SEIZURE PATTERNS

Many people have more than one type of seizure. For example, someone may have simple and complex partial seizures, simple and complex partial and secondarily generalized tonic-clonic seizures, absence and my-clonic seizures, or myoclonic and tonic-clonic seizures. In addition, the fea-tures of a given type of seizure may change from seizure to seizure, or more commonly, over a period of months or years. For example, a person's simple partial seizures that precede tonic-clonic seizures may change from an un-pleasant smell and a strange stomach sensation to simply a sensation of chest discomfort, or there may be no warning at all.

Changes in a person's seizures may result from changes in the patterns of spread of the abnormal electrical discharge. In the case of the person whose aura (simple partial seizure) no longer precedes the tonic-clonic sei-zure, the area from which the seizure begins and the intensity of the dis-charge have probably not changed. Rather, the electrical activity may have taken other pathways, allowing it to spread more rapidly. In this case, the seizure is no more severe, although the absence of a warning may prevent the person from avoiding injury.

Milder forms of seizures, such as simple partial or absence seizures, may be followed by tonic-clonic seizures. In some instances, the change in seizure type may be caused by provocative factors such as missed medica-tion or lack of sleep. In other cases, it is the natural history of the person's disorder; he or she has always had a small chance of having a tonic-clonic seizure.

The exact reasons why seizure patterns change over time are not known. There may be some changes in the brain such as reorganization of connections or an increase or decrease in the concentrations of certain chem-icals related to epilepsy or to the cause of epilepsy. If seizures become more frequent or more severe, a medical checkup is advisable.

CHAPTER 4

Classification of Epileptic Syndromes

When a disorder is defined by a characteristic group of features, it is called a syndrome. These features may be symptoms or signs of the disorder. Symptoms are problems the patient notices or complains about to the doctor. Signs are what the doctor observes during the examination or with laboratory studies.

Epileptic syndromes are defined by a cluster of features such as the seizure types, age when seizures begin, electroencephalogram (EEG) findings, and prognosis, or future outlook, for the disorder. Classifying an epileptic syndrome often provides information on how long the seizures will persist and what medications are most helpful. Some of the most common or well-defined epileptic syndromes are febrile seizures, infantile spasms, Lennox-Gastaut syndrome, benign rolandic epilepsy, juvenile myoclonic epilepsy, progressive myoclonic epilepsy, reflex epilepsies, temporal lobe epilepsy, and frontal lobe epilepsy.

FEBRILE SEIZURES

Tommy was just 14 months old. He caught a bad cold from one of the children in the playgroup. He had a fever and runny nose. He was taking a nap when I heard this strange banging sound. I ran into his room, and his whole body was stiff and shaking. The whole thing probably lasted less than 10 minutes. They were the longest 10 minutes of my life. He had never had another one, and didn't need any seizure medication. Now when he has a fever I give him Tylenol, and if it doesn't break quickly, I also use cold compresses.

Children aged 3 months to 5 years may have tonic-clonic seizures when they have a high fever. These are called febrile seizures and occur in 2% to

5% of children. There is a slight familial (hereditary) tendency toward febrile seizures. Therefore, if parents, brothers or sisters, or other close relatives have had febrile seizures, the chances are slightly increased that a child will have febrile seizures. The usual situation is a healthy child with normal development, aged 6 months to 2 years, who has a viral illness with high fever. As the child's temperature rapidly rises, he or she has a tonic-clonic seizure. The seizure usually involves muscles on both sides of the body. In contrast with tonic-clonic seizures in later childhood and adulthood, febrile seizures often last longer than 5 minutes. In most instances, hospitalization is not necessary, although a prompt medical consultation is essential.

The prognosis for febrile seizures is usually excellent. There is no reason for a child who has had a single febrile seizure to receive antiepileptic drugs, unless the seizure was unusually long or other medical conditions warrant it. Recurrence rates for febrile seizures vary from 50% if the seizure occurred before age 1 year to 25% if the seizure occurred after age 1 year. The vast majority of children with febrile seizures do not have seizures without fever after age 5 years. Risk factors for later epilepsy include (1) abnormal development before the febrile seizure; (2) complex febrile seizures (seizures lasting longer than 15 minutes, more than one seizure in 24 hours, or movements restricted to one side); and (3) a history of seizures without fever in a parent or brother or sister. If no risk factors are present, the chances of later epilepsy are the same or nearly the same as in the general population; if one risk factor is present, the chances of later epilepsy are 2.5%; if two or more risk factors are present, the chances of later epilepsy range from 5% to 10%.

Prevention of febrile seizures is important. If a child who has had a febrile seizure subsequently has a fever, he or she should have a cool bath or cool cloths applied to the body and head and should be given acetaminophen (Tylenol). Aspirin should not be used in young children because of the potential risk of precipitating a serious disorder called Reye's syndrome.

The decision to treat a child that has recurrent febrile seizures with antiepileptic drugs is difficult, as there is no consensus among experts. Children who have had more than three febrile seizures or prolonged seizures, or who have seizures when they have no fever, are often treated, usually with phenobarbital. More recently, rectal diazepam (Valium) has been used effectively in children with recurrent febrile seizures. This medication is only administered at the time of fever.

INFANTILE SPASMS

At first I thought Chris was just having the little body jerks when he was moved or startled, like my other children had when they were infants. But then I knew something was wrong. The jerks became more violent, and his tiny body was thrust forward and his arms flew apart. They only lasted a few seconds but started to occur in groups lasting a few minutes. It was so hard to see such a young baby having these things.

Infantile spasms (West's syndrome), a very uncommon form of epilepsy, begin between 3 and 12 months of age and usually stop by the age of 2 to 4 years. The seizures, or spasms, consist of a sudden jerk followed by stiffening. With some spells, the arms are flung out as the body bends forward ("jackknife seizures"), whereas other spells have more subtle movements limited to the neck or other body parts. In 60% of the cases, some brain disorder or brain injury, such as birth trauma with oxygen deprivation, precedes the seizures, but in the remaining cases, there is no injury and the child's development is normal. The future course of the disorder and the child's subsequent development are related to the cause of the seizures, the state of the child's intellectual and neurological development before the seizures (the better the condition at that time, the better the prognosis), and whether the seizures are controlled quickly or persist.

Infantile spasms are often treated with adrenocorticotropic hormone (ACTH) or prednisone, a steroid hormone. Some authorities recommend a trial of antiepileptic drugs before hormonal therapy. The sooner therapy is begun, the better the results. ACTH is a hormone made by the pituitary gland that stimulates the adrenal glands to make and release additional cortisol, which acts much like prednisone. Interestingly, many experts believe that ACTH is more often and more rapidly effective than prednisone. However, ACTH must be given as an injection, initially once a day, and after several weeks, every other day, whereas steroid hormones like prednisone can be given by mouth. ACTH stops seizures in more than half of the children with infantile spasms. When the spasms stop, many children will later develop other seizures. Even without any form of treatment, infantile spasms will stop in more than 90% of children by the age of 5 years. However, many of the untreated children will have frequent spasms for many years and later have partial or generalized seizures or other epileptic syndromes. Approximately one fifth of the cases of infantile spasms will evolve into the Lennox-Gastaut syndrome.

LENNOX-GASTAUT SYNDROME

The first time I heard Tommy's diagnosis, Lennox-Gastaut syndrome, the words had no meaning. I asked the doctor for information, and he said there wasn't much written for parents. So I went to a medical library and spent the afternoon with a few textbooks and a medical dictionary. Sometimes, I had to ask one of the students to explain the definitions. I was in tears when I left. It sounded totally hopeless; Tommy had no future. Ten years later, Tommy's seizures are under much better control. He loves school (special education classes), has lots of friends, is an incredibly important part of our family, and gives us all great pleasure. He can almost beat me at tennis!

The parent of a child with Lennox-Gastaut syndrome needs lots of patience. Kathy has been on every medication, many of them three or four times. Nothing has ever controlled the seizures well. As the doctors kept going up on the doses, she would either undergo terrible personality changes, turn into a zombie, or look like a drunk. We have finally come to accept the seizures and her mental handicaps. We also have part-time help at home so that we and our other kids could have a more normal life. The more we let go of some our unrealistic hopes and accepted Kathy for who she is, the more our time with Kathy changed from disappointment to joy.

The Lennox-Gastaut syndrome, defined by the triad of difficult-to-control seizures, mental retardation, and a slow spike-and-wave pattern on the EEG, is a serious, but uncommon, epileptic syndrome. The seizures usually begin between 1 and 6 years of age, but can begin later. The syndrome involves some combination of tonic, atypical absence, myoclonic, and tonic-clonic seizures that are usually resistant to medications. The majority of children with the Lennox-Gastaut syndrome have intellectual impairment ranging from mild to severe. Behavioral problems are also common and probably relate to a combination of the neurological injury, seizures, and antiepileptic drugs. The EEG pattern of slow spike-and-wave discharges is typically the predominant activity.

Although children with the Lennox-Gastaut syndrome often have delayed intellectual and behavioral development, the prognosis is variable. Development in children whose seizures come under fair to good control may be nearly normal, but in those who have frequent seizures and take high doses of multiple antiepileptic drugs, it may be severely delayed.

The course of the seizures varies markedly, because some children will later have fairly good seizure control, and others will grow up to have drop attacks and partial and tonic-clonic seizures. In children or adults with frequent, poorly controlled seizures, it is often wise to avoid high doses of antiepileptic drugs, because they often compound the behavioral, social, and intellectual problems, especially when two or more drugs are used together. It may be better to tolerate slightly more frequent seizures in order to have a more alert and attentive child whose quality of life is much improved.

A new antiepileptic drug, felbamate, appears to better control the seizures of the Lennox-Gastaut syndrome and improve behavior, especially when it is substituted for multiple-drug therapy. Other medications that are commonly used for the Lennox-Gastaut syndrome include valproate (valproic acid), carbamazepine, phenobarbital, phenytoin, and clonazepam.

BENIGN ROLANDIC EPILEPSY

We heard a thud from Timmy's room one night. We rushed in and saw him on the floor, having a whole body seizure. The next day, the pediatrician asked if Timmy had ever had any tingling or jerking movements in his face or body. We were shocked when Timmy said yes, sometimes his tongue would tingle or his cheek would jerk for a little while. The doctor did an EEG and said it was "rolandic epilepsy," and said that Timmy didn't have to be treated. That's what we wanted to hear. It's been 5 years now, and except for a few tingles and twitches, Timmy has been doing great.

Benign rolandic (sylvian) epilepsy is a common childhood seizure disorder, with seizures beginning between 2 and 13 years of age. A hereditary factor is often present. The most characteristic attack is a partial motor seizure (twitching) or a sensory seizure (numbness or tingling sensation) involving the face, but tonic-clonic seizures may occur, especially during sleep. The seizures are infrequent, however, and many patients need no medication. In others, the seizures are easily controlled with low to moderate doses of carbamazepine, phenytoin, or valproate, which are usually continued until age 15, when the seizures spontaneously stop in almost all patients.

The EEG shows a characteristic pattern over the central and temporal regions of the brain (Fig. 7) and often shows abundant abnormal activity,

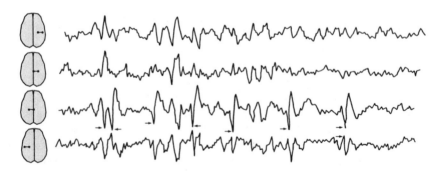

FIGURE 7. EEG revealing centrotemporal spikes (abnormal epilepsy waves recorded over the central and temporal regions) (*arrows*) from a boy with benign rolandic epilepsy. The brain figures on the left of the diagram indicate the area from which each recording was obtained.

especially during sleep. This is unusual because the child may have had no seizures, or only a single seizure. Thus, the abundance of epileptiform activity (brain waves that are markers for increased brain electrical activity and are usually found only in people with epilepsy) on the EEG has no correlation with the severity of the disorder.

JUVENILE MYOCLONIC EPILEPSY

I have always had these little jerks, ever since I was 12 or 13 years old, but I assumed everybody had them. They never really bothered me until one day I had a big one and fell down. I had a couple of grand mal seizures and was put on medication for a few years, and then the drugs were stopped. During college, whenever I stayed up all night or drank too much, the next day I would get lots of those jerks, and sometimes a big seizure right after the jerks. I never thought much of those jerks; in fact, my wife, who doesn't have epilepsy, gets them sometimes as she is falling asleep.

Juvenile myoclonic epilepsy (JME) was first described in the late 1950s and is now recognized to account for about 4% of the cases of epilepsy. The syndrome is defined by myoclonic seizures with or without tonic-clonic or absence seizures. Seizures usually begin shortly before or after puberty, although some may begin in early adulthood. Seizures usually occur in the early morning, shortly after awakening. The intellectual functions of persons with JME are the same as those in the general population, and range from superior to normal or slightly below average.

In most cases, the seizures are well controlled with medication, but the disorder is usually lifelong. Valproate is the treatment of choice. Myoclonic seizures may be controlled with valproate, acetazolamide, clonazepam, or phenobarbital. Carbamazepine may actually worsen the myoclonic jerks. Absence and tonic-clonic seizures can be treated with the standard medications (see Table 2).

In most cases, a characteristic EEG pattern of spike-and-wave discharges is present. The CT and MRI scans of the brain are normal and are not needed in typical cases.

REFLEX EPILEPSIES

It was only later that I realized he was sitting under a fluorescent light that was flickering when he had his first seizure. All three of his seizures have happened when there have been flashing or flickering lights. The last seizure was when they did the EEG with the flashing lights. Now we keep Dan away from any light flickers. Even driving through shaded areas where the light filters down through the leaves and flickers—we just give him a pair of dark sunglasses and he keeps his head down.

Reflex epilepsies are triggered by certain things in the environment. The most common form of reflex epilepsy is photosensitive epilepsy, which usually begins in childhood and is often outgrown before adulthood. In this disorder, flashing lights trigger absence seizures (staring), myoclonic seizures (jerking of the eyes, head, or arms), or tonic-clonic seizures. Avoiding flashing lights is desirable. Even driving through a series of trees in which the sun passes through can produce the same effect as a strobe light. For some people, certain rates of blinking or colors are most likely to provoke seizures. Recently, there has been great interest in the safety of video games for children or adults with epilepsy. Certain video games can provoke seizures, but this has been reported in only a small number of persons with epilepsy (see Chapter 14).

Other environmental triggers in reflex epilepsy include sounds such as church bells, a certain type of music or song, or a person's voice; reading; doing arithmetic; certain movements such as writing; and even thinking about specific topics. Because of unavoidable environmental triggers, or in some cases, the occurrence of seizures without detectable causes, many persons with reflex epilepsy require treatment. Valproate is effective for photosensitive and other reflex epilepsies. Other successful medications are carbamazepine, phenytoin, and phenobarbital.

The reflex epilepsies are usually categorized as primary generalized epilepsy, which accurately describes photosensitive epilepsy. Other forms of reflex epilepsy are classified as partial epilepsy.

TEMPORAL LOBE EPILEPSY

I get the strangest feeling; most of it can't be put into words. The whole world suddenly seems more real at first; it's as though everything becomes crystal clear. Then I feel as if I'm here but not here, kind of like being in a dream. It's as if I've lived through this exact moment many times before. I hear what people say, but they don't make sense. I know not to talk during the episode, since I just say foolish things. Sometimes I think I'm talking but later people tell me that I didn't say anything. The whole thing lasts a minute or two.

This description of a partial seizure depicts some of the unusual features of seizures beginning in the temporal lobe. The features of temporal lobe seizures are extremely varied, although certain patterns are common (see the discussion of simple and complex partial seizures in Chapter 3).

The experiences and sensations that accompany these seizures are often impossible to describe, even for the most eloquent adult. In children, it is even more difficult to obtain an accurate picture of what they are feeling. Temporal lobe seizures are often composed of a mixture of different feelings, emotions, thoughts, and experiences that may be familiar or completely foreign. In some cases, a series of old memories resurfaces; in others, the person may feel as if everything—including his or her room and family—appears strange. Hallucinations of voices, music, people, smells, or tastes may occur.

Experiences during temporal lobe seizures vary in intensity and quality. Sometimes, the seizures are so mild that the person may barely notice. In other cases, the person may be consumed with fright, intellectual fascination, or even pleasure.

Dostoyevsky, the 19th-century Russian novelist, who himself had epilepsy, gave vivid accounts of apparent temporal lobe seizures in his novel *The Idiot* (see Appendix 4):

> *He remembered that during his epileptic fits, or rather immediately preceding them, he had always experienced a moment or two when his whole heart, and mind, and body seemed to wake up with vigour and light; when he became filled with joy and hope, and all his anxieties seemed to be swept away for ever; these moments were but presentiments, as it were, of the one final second ... in which the fit came upon him. That second, of course, was inexpressible.*

> *Next moment something appeared to burst open before him: a wonderful inner light illuminated his soul. This lasted perhaps half a second, yet he distinctly remembered hearing the beginning of a wail, the strange, dreadful wail, which burst from his lips of its own accord, and which no effort of will on his part could suppress. Next moment he was absolutely unconscious; black darkness blotted out everything. He had fallen in an epileptic fit.*

Complex partial seizures, most often with automatisms, or automatic behavior, such as lip smacking and rubbing the hands together, are the most common seizure type in temporal lobe epilepsy. Some 75% of people with this disorder also have simple partial seizures, and approximately 50% have tonic-clonic seizures at some time. In some individuals, however, temporal lobe epilepsy may be associated only with simple partial seizures.

In most instances, the temporal lobe seizures begin in the deeper portions of the temporal lobe, part of the limbic system, which controls emotions and memory (see Fig. 3C). In some individuals with temporal lobe epilepsy, especially when seizures have occurred for more than 5 years, there may be problems with memory. In the overwhelming majority of cases, these memory problems are not severe.

In most cases, the seizures can be fully or well controlled with the medications for partial seizures. When not controlled with antiepileptic drugs, temporal lobe seizures can often be controlled with surgery. Temporal lobectomy is the most common and successful form of epilepsy surgery (see Chapter 11).

FRONTAL LOBE EPILEPSY

My head starts jerking toward the right side. I try, but can't stop it. Then my right hand goes up and my head turns toward the hand. I may just stay in that position for half a minute and it's over, or it can become a grand mal seizure.

Usually I don't get any warning, I just have tonic-clonic seizures. Occasionally I get a momentary warning before the seizure—a strange feeling in my head.

I spend the night watching Molly sleep sometimes. She will have 5 or 10 seizures in a single night. They are short, usually less than 20 seconds. Her body starts to rock, like she is adjusting her position in the bed, and then she may start to make these kicking movements with her legs, like she is riding a bicycle.

After temporal lobe epilepsy, frontal lobe epilepsy is the next most common type of epilepsy featuring partial seizures. The frontal lobes are large (see Fig. 1A, B) and include many areas that do not have a precisely known function. Therefore, when a seizure begins in these areas, there may be no symptoms until it spreads to other areas or to most of the brain, causing a tonic-clonic seizure. When motor areas of the frontal lobe are affected, abnormal movements occur on the opposite side of the body. Seizures beginning in frontal lobe motor areas can result in weakness or the inability to use certain muscles, such as the muscles that allow someone to speak.

Complex partial seizures may also begin in the frontal lobes. In comparison with temporal lobe complex partial seizures, those beginning in the frontal lobe tend to be shorter (usually lasting less than 1 minute, whereas temporal lobe complex partial seizures usually last more than 1 minute), are less likely to be followed by confusion or tiredness, more often occur in a cluster or series, and are more likely to include strange automatisms such as bicycling movements, screaming, or even sexual activity. Although the features may suggest that the seizures begin in the frontal (or temporal) lobes, definitely determining where the seizures begin requires an EEG recording during the seizure.

In most cases, the seizures can be fully or well controlled with medications for partial seizures. When they are not controlled with antiepileptic drugs, frontal lobe seizures may be surgically treated (see Chapter 11).

RARE EPILEPSY SYNDROMES

Progressive Myoclonic Epilepsies

At first the doctors just thought Avi had a seizure because he was growing so fast. He had more grand mal seizures, and they started him on medication. Each drug seemed to work for a while and then it was as if his body became immune to it. They tried more and more drugs, two or three at a time, and the seizures just became more frequent. The worst part was that Avi was slipping—he was changing. He was not as sharp and quick as he had been. We blamed it on the drugs, but it just got worse and worse. Over a 3-year period, after the seizures began, Avi's mind seemed to get slower and slower. Then came the little seizures that would cause his speech to sputter and hesitate and his mind to turn on and off, like someone was taking a light switch and flicking it up and down.

The rare, often hereditary, progressive myoclonic epilepsies are characterized by a combination of myoclonic and tonic-clonic seizures. In addition, unsteadiness, muscle rigidity, and mental deterioration are often present. Inherited errors of metabolism may lead to the disorder, but in many cases test results are normal, and the cause remains unknown.

The medical treatment of progressive myoclonic epilepsy is often successful only for a few months or years. As the disorder progresses, drugs become less effective, and adverse effects may be more severe as more drugs are used at higher doses. The adverse effects are then superimposed on the neurological deterioration of the condition. In such cases, it is often worthwhile trying to reduce the doses of the medications. The patients may require more than one drug. Valproate is most commonly used, but phenytoin, clonazepam, phenobarbital, and carbamazepine are also used. Zonisamide, a new drug tested mainly in Japan, has been reported to be helpful in controlling seizures in progressive myoclonic epilepsies (see Chapter 10). The Epilepsy Foundation of America (EFA) (see Appendix 3) can provide information on trials of this medication.

Landau-Kleffner Syndrome

The Landau-Kleffner syndrome (acquired aphasia with seizure disorder in children) is a rare disorder. It is characterized by a loss of speech milestones and the presence of epilepsy waves on the EEG. In the typical case, a child between 3 and 7 years of age develops language problems, with or without a history of seizures. The language disorder may start suddenly or slowly; it usually affects auditory comprehension (understanding spoken language) the most, but may also affect spoken language together with comprehension, or spoken language alone. Seizures are usually infrequent and often occur during sleep. Simple partial motor seizures are most common, but tonic-clonic seizures can also occur. Seizure control is rarely a problem.

The EEG is often the key to the diagnosis. A normal EEG, especially one done when the child is awake, does not exclude the diagnosis. Sleep activates the epilepsy waves, and therefore sleep recordings are extremely important.

The boundaries of the Landau-Kleffner syndrome are imprecise. Some children may have a delay in language development followed by a loss of speech milestones. This syndrome—or a variant—may also occur in selected children who never develop language function. The exact relationship between the epilepsy waves on the EEG and the language disorder is imprecise, although in some cases the epilepsy activity may contribute to the language problems.

Standard antiepileptic drugs are ineffective in treating the language disorder. Steroids are effective in some children, improving both the EEG abnormalities and language disorder. A new form of epilepsy surgery, multiple subpial transections (see Chapter 11), has been reported to improve both the EEG abnormalities and language disorder in a small number of children. Confirmation of this finding from other epilepsy centers is pending. Further study is needed to help to define fully this syndrome and its treatment.

Rasmussen's Syndrome

Rasmussen's syndrome almost always begins between 14 months and 14 years of age and is associated with slowly progressive neurological deterioration and seizures. Seizures are often the first neurological problem. In one fifth of cases, the first seizure is an episode of partial or tonic-clonic status epilepticus. Simple partial motor seizures are the most common seizure type.

Although the disease is rarely fatal, its effects are devastating. Progressive weakness on one side (hemiparesis) and mental retardation are common, and language disorder (aphasia) often occurs if the disorder affects the side of the brain dominant for language functions, which is usually the left side. Mild weakness of an arm or leg is the most common initial symptom besides seizures. These and other neurological problems often begin 1 to 3 years after the onset of seizures. On CT and MRI scans of the brain, there is evidence of atrophy (slowly progressive loss of brain substance). When sections of the brain are examined under a microscope, there are features that suggest a viral infection, although definitive proof of a viral cause is lacking.

Treatment of the disease with antiepileptic drugs is disappointing. Steroids may be effective, although additional studies are needed. Surgical therapy has also been used with occasional success. Removing portions of the frontal or temporal lobe has controlled seizures in a few patients. In children with severe weakness and loss of touch and vision on the opposite side of the involved hemisphere, a functional hemispherectomy (see Chapter 11) may be successful.

CHAPTER 5

An Overview of Epilepsy

Studies on large groups of people, known as epidemiological studies, have provided important information on epilepsy. These studies have helped us better define the frequency, causes, and future course of epilepsy.

EPILEPSY—MORE COMMON THAN YOU THINK

There are currently more than 1.5 million Americans who have active epilepsy. Active epilepsy is defined as epilepsy that has been treated with antiepileptic drugs during the past 5 years. The total number of active cases of a disorder existing at a certain time is called the prevalence. The prevalence of epilepsy is 0.65%; that is, 6.5 out of 1000 people have epilepsy. More men than women have epilepsy.

New cases of epilepsy are most common among children, with another peak occurring in the elderly. The highest rate of occurrence of new cases, or the incidence, of epilepsy is during the first year of life. The incidence of epilepsy declines over the first 20 years of life and then remains stable until age 55 to 60 years, when there may be an increase, largely related to stroke, brain tumors, and Alzheimer's disease. By age 80 years, the cumulative incidence of epilepsy is between 1.3% and 3.1%. In other words, there is a 1.3% to 3.1% chance that if you live to 80 years of age, you will have active epilepsy at some time during your life. By 40 years of age, there is a 1% to 2% chance of having had epilepsy.

CAUSES OF EPILEPSY

Epidemiological studies have identified numerous factors that cause epilepsy. Other factors, not the subject of epidemiological studies, also are clearly associated with an increased risk of seizures and epilepsy; some of these are brain tumors, abnormal collections of blood vessels in the brain, bleeding into the brain, and lack of oxygen or blood flow to the brain. Further, the causes of epilepsy vary with the age at which seizures develop (Fig. 8).

Babies who are small for gestational age (in other words, who have a low birth weight compared with other infants born after the same number of weeks of pregnancy) and infants with seizures in the first month of life have an increased risk of epilepsy.

Factors associated with a greater than 10-fold increase in the risk of developing epilepsy include head trauma involving a concussion with loss of consciousness for more than 30 minutes, some memory impairment after the injury (posttraumatic amnesia), abnormalities such as weakness or impaired coordination on the neurological examination, or skull fracture; central nervous system infections such as meningitis, encephalitis, or cerebral abscess; cerebral palsy and mental retardation; Alzheimer's disease; complicated (complex) febrile seizures; stroke resulting from blockage of arteries or veins; and alcohol abuse. Factors associated with a less than 10-fold increase in the risk of developing epilepsy include use of illegal drugs; a family history of epilepsy or febrile seizures; multiple sclerosis; and seizures occurring within days after head trauma ("early seizures").

Epidemiological studies have failed to establish a clear relationship between vaccination and epilepsy. In some cases, however, vaccination may cause a fever associated with a febrile convulsion.

HEREDITARY INFLUENCES AND EPILEPSY

Hereditary (genetic) factors are important in some cases of epilepsy. When epilepsy develops at a young age, there is an increased risk of epilepsy among the brothers and sisters and the affected person's children. Genetic factors are more commonly present in primary generalized epilepsy than in partial epilepsy.

Among patients with primary generalized epilepsy and the spike-and-wave abnormality on the electroencephalogram (EEG), the risk of epilepsy in a brother or sister is approximately 4%. When a child with absence or tonic-clonic seizures has an EEG showing a paroxysmal response to photic stimulation or multifocal spikes (that is, more restricted epilepsy waves coming from several separate areas) and one of that child's brothers or sisters has the spike-and-wave abnormality on the EEG, another child in the family has an 8% risk of developing epilepsy. When a parent and a child have primary generalized epilepsy, there is a 10% risk that the parent's other children will have isolated seizures or epilepsy.

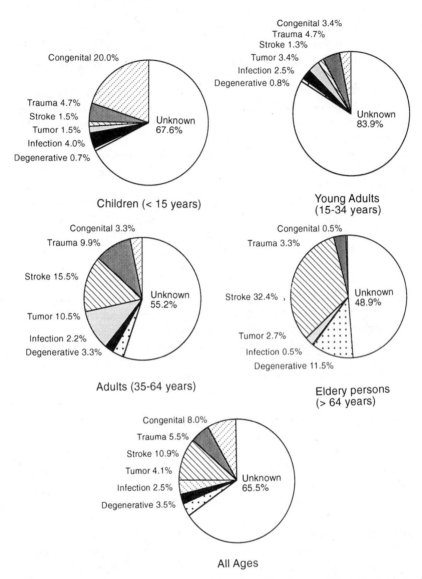

FIGURE 8. The percentage of cases of epilepsy resulting from various causes, shown for persons of all ages and different age groups. (From Hauser, WA: Seizure disorders: The changes with age. Epilepsia 33 (Suppl 4): S6-S14, 1992, with permission.)

Among individuals with partial epilepsy in whom a clear cause of seizures can be identified, such as serious head injury with loss of consciousness for longer than a day, there is evidence that the chance of developing epilepsy may be influenced by heredity. The rate of seizures is higher among the family members of people who develop epilepsy after head trauma than among the relatives of people who do not. The one form of partial epilepsy with a strong genetic component is the syndrome of benign rolandic epilepsy, in which there is as much as a 35% chance that one of the child's brothers and sisters will show the characteristic EEG abnormality, but only 5% of all brothers and sisters will develop seizures. Among those brothers and sisters with the characteristic EEG abnormality, however, 15% will develop seizures.

There is an increased risk of epilepsy in children of parents with epilepsy. Overall, the chance that a child of a parent with epilepsy will have unprovoked seizures by age 25 is 6%, compared with 1% to 2% in the general population. Epilepsy is roughly twice as common among the children of women with epilepsy than among the children of men with epilepsy.

In most cases where heredity is important, a single gene is not considered to be the sole determining factor. However, recent studies have linked the syndrome of juvenile myoclonic epilepsy to chromosome 6.

PROGNOSIS OF EPILEPSY

Risk of Recurrent Seizures after a First Seizure

After a single, unprovoked seizure, the risk of recurrent seizures varies from 16% to 61%. The risk of recurrence is higher among individuals who have a history of brain injury or other type of brain abnormality, partial seizures, or an abnormal EEG. When seizures do recur, they are most likely to occur within the first year. If someone experiences two seizures, chances are approximately 85% that he or she will have a third seizure.

After a single seizure, people with a known brain injury or abnormality (symptomatic epilepsy) have roughly twice the risk of having another seizure compared with people without a known brain injury (idiopathic epilepsy). People with a history of a much earlier injury to the brain (such as head trauma or brain infection) who had a seizure at the time of the injury have a higher risk of developing epilepsy than if they had no seizure at the time of the injury. People with abnormalities on the neurological examination appear to be at slightly greater risk of a second seizure than those with normal results.

The EEG is another important predictor of recurrence after a single seizure. People with abnormalities characteristic of epilepsy ("epileptiform" abnormalities), such as spike-and-wave discharges, spikes, or sharp waves, have approximately twice the chance of having another seizure compared with people with normal EEGs or with nonspecific abnormalities such as mild slowing on their EEGs (see Chapter 8). The presence of epileptiform activity on the EEG may be most predictive in cases in which there is no history of brain injury or abnormality.

The importance of a family history of epilepsy in predicting recurrence after a first seizure remains uncertain. Most studies have found either no increase or only a slightly increased recurrence rate among people with a family history of epilepsy.

Remission of Epilepsy and Risk of Relapse

After the diagnosis of epilepsy is made and effective therapy is prescribed, approximately two thirds of people will be seizure-free for 5 years. The longer the time between seizures, the greater the chances of permanent remission (freedom from seizures). Twenty years after the diagnosis of epilepsy, approximately three quarters of people will have been seizure-free for 5 years. However, the longer that people continue to have seizures after the diagnosis of epilepsy is made, the lower the chances of a remission.

Factors that predict a higher chance of remission include primary generalized seizures, especially tonic-clonic seizures, and younger age when the diagnosis of epilepsy is made. Therefore, children with epilepsy are more likely to stop having seizures than are adults. The remission rate may be higher in the absence of a known brain injury or abnormality and when the neurological examination results are normal.

The role of the EEG in predicting whether epilepsy will go into remission remains uncertain. The characteristic EEG pattern of centrotemporal spikes (see Fig. 7) in benign rolandic epilepsy virtually guarantees remission by age 16 years. People with the widespread spike-and-wave EEG pattern that is characteristic of some types of primary generalized epilepsy are less likely to become seizure-free than are those without these abnormal patterns. However, the value of other patterns of epilepsy waves on the EEG in predicting remission is uncertain.

People with epilepsy who become seizure-free for 5 years may subsequently relapse and have seizures. Overall, about 1.5% of people who have been seizure-free for 5 years have another seizure. The chances of relapse are more likely in people with complex partial seizures and in those who are more than 20 years old.

There is some risk of relapse after antiepileptic drugs are discontinued, but they may also play a role in the remission of epilepsy. More than 100 years ago, the English neurologist Sir William Richard Gowers suggested that "seizures beget seizures." That is, once you have one seizure, you are more likely to have another simply because your brain "learns" how to have a seizure. Although his concept remains unproved, there is anecdotal, or informal, evidence that he may have been right. The longer someone remains seizure-free while taking antiepileptic drugs, the better chance he or she has of remaining seizure-free when the medication is stopped. Just as the brain learns to have seizures, it may also "forget" to have seizures. Antiepileptic drugs may enhance the forgetting process by controlling seizures. This effect of antiepileptic drugs, however, is unproven.

A majority of people who are seizure-free for 2 to 4 years can safely discontinue their medications without having further seizures. The rate of seizure recurrence after medication withdrawal varies from approximately 20% to 35% in children and approximately 30% to 65% in adults. Currently, most neurologists consider withdrawing antiepileptic drugs after someone has been seizure-free for approximately 2 years. However, various factors may influence the doctor's decision of when it is appropriate to consider withdrawing the antiepileptic drugs (see Chapter 10).

EPILEPSY AND LIFE SPAN

The average person with epilepsy lives a normal life span. People with infrequent seizures have death rates comparable to the general population. Overall, however, epilepsy is associated with a slight reduction in life span. In part, this reduction reflects seizure-provoking conditions such as stroke and brain tumors, which can shorten survival. The increased risk of death associated with epilepsy is almost entirely limited to the first 10 years after the diagnosis is made.

Fatal Seizures

Convulsive (tonic-clonic) status epilepticus is a medical emergency and may cause permanent injury or death if treatment is delayed or ineffective. Single seizures that impair consciousness are almost never fatal. However, fatalities from epilepsy can occur in a variety of scenarios; for example, a tonic-clonic seizure may cause someone to fall in front of a train, or a complex partial seizure may cause a person to cross a busy street without caution. The most dangerous setting for someone with episodes of impaired consciousness is driving a motor vehicle, where a brief lapse can prove deadly. Fatal accidents and traumas are increased for people with epilepsy. Death from drowning is also more common among people with epilepsy.

Seizures causing a fatal injury are *extremely rare*. Unfortunately, they can occur. Prevention is the best medicine. For people with seizures that impair consciousness or motor control, avoiding situations that place them at risk is important. However, the reality is that activities of daily living—crossing streets, taking trains, and taking subways—can be dangerous. There must be balance between safety and leading an active, productive, and enjoyable life. For the vast majority of people with epilepsy, this balance can be achieved.

Unexplained Death in Epilepsy

There is a mysterious, rare condition in which young or middle-aged persons with epilepsy die without a clearly defined cause. They are often found dead in bed without signs of having had a convulsive seizure. In many cases, their blood levels of antiepileptic drugs are low. The cause of death, by definition, is unknown, but some researchers suggest that a seizure causes an irregularity in the heart rhythm. It is important to understand that such cases are *extremely rare*.

ACKNOWLEDGMENT

Much of this chapter was derived from the authoritative book, *Epilepsy: Frequency, Causes, and Consequences* (see Appendix 4).

CHAPTER 6

Seizure-Provoking Factors

Many persons with epilepsy can identify certain factors that increase their chances of having a seizure. The medical world has not thoroughly examined this subject, which remains ripe for study. Proving or refuting an association between seizures and a certain factor such as menses or a full moon is more complicated than it seems, and therefore few formal studies have addressed the issue.

MISSED MEDICATION

Most people do not think of missed medication as a problem that can lead to seizures. However, it is almost certainly the most common cause of both "breakthrough" seizures and life-threatening convulsive status epilepticus, prolonged seizures that require emergency medical treatment. When status epilepticus occurs in this setting, it is usually after antiepileptic medications are abruptly stopped. Medications are missed for many different reasons. Perhaps the most common and benign instance of missed medication is occasionally missing a single dose, which is more likely to cause seizures if the medication is taken only once daily than if it is taken two to four times a day. Missing several doses in a row increases the likelihood of a breakthrough seizure. Some patients go away for a weekend, forget to pack their medication, and hope they can "get away without medication for a few days."

Different strategies can be used to prevent missed medication. The patient should never have less than a 1- to 2-week supply of medication. For those who order large quantities of antiepileptic drugs by mail, it is wise to have a spare 2- to 4-week supply of medication. It is a good idea to keep extra medication at work and in the car. When going on a trip, it is smart to pack two separate supplies of medication: one for a carry-on bag and one for luggage that is checked. The hand-carried medications are "insurance" just in case the checked bag is misplaced or stolen.

Patients can help themselves to remember to take all their medication as prescribed by establishing some cues. Their daily pattern can be helpful in determining what time of day or activity would be a good point to stop and take the pills. Is there a specific time of day, such as 8 AM or 8 PM? Can the pills be taken with meals, two or three times daily? Can dosing be linked with taking a shower, shaving, or some other bathroom activity? On days when the routine is interrupted, such as by sleeping late or skipping lunch, the person should make a special effort to remember to take the pills. There are many pill boxes available for organizing medication by day of the week and time of day. There are even wrist watches and pill boxes that can be easily programmed as a reminder to take the medication.

Some persons with epilepsy decide to discontinue their medication without a doctor's advice. This is a dangerous decision. Abruptly stopping some antiepileptic drugs can cause withdrawal symptoms, including prolonged tonic-clonic seizures, even if they have never occurred before. Further, changes in one drug can dramatically alter the blood levels and effectiveness of other drugs, and in some cases cause serious adverse effects. Medications should never be stopped suddenly unless the doctor recommends it. In the case of a rash, for example, the doctor may feel that it is unsafe to continue taking the medication, but if suddenly stopping the drug poses a risk of status epilepticus, he or she may prescribe another medication, or the person may be hospitalized during the time the drug is withdrawn.

The patient should always be comfortable enough with the doctor to discuss his or her wants and needs. No matter why the patient wants to discontinue the medication—because the adverse effects are intolerable, or because of plans to get pregnant—he or she should discuss it with the doctor. If the doctor feels it is too dangerous or unwise to stop the drugs, and the patient still feels strongly, it may be necessary to obtain a second opinion, but the medication should not be stopped without a doctor's advice.

Refilling the Prescription

When the supply of pills is dwindling, and there are refills on the last prescription, another supply should be obtained from the pharmacy. If there are no refills left, the doctor will telephone the pharmacy if asked. Patients must never, *ever*, wait until the last minute to call the doctor or pharmacy.

If the patient finds himself or herself with no medication, or only a few pills, he or she can always get more medication in almost any location.

Most doctors and clinics are available to speak with patients 24 hours a day. A patient will rarely need to call a doctor at 3 AM for a refill, but it can be done if it is an emergency. If not, the patient should wait until morning and call the doctor. If it is a weekend, it is best not to wait until Monday to call if it means running out of pills. If the doctor is unavailable, and no other doctor is taking calls and seeing patients until the doctor returns, the patient might consider calling or visiting a 24-hour doctor service, outpatient clinic, or even an emergency room. If the patient needs antiepileptic drugs in a foreign country, the patient's doctor can telephone a pharmacy or hospital there. If that is impossible, the patient can go to a doctor or hospital in the foreign country. Where there is a will, there is always a way—patients with epilepsy must not run out of medications.

Traveling Across Time Zones

When traveling across time zones, it is important that the amount of medication taken over a 24- or 48-hour period remain the same as if the patient were at home, and the interval between doses should be approximately the same.

Each drug has a half-life, the time required for the concentration of the drug in the blood to decline to half of its original value. Medications with a short half-life, such as carbamazepine and valproate, pose a slightly greater problem than those with a longer half-life, such as phenytoin or phenobarbital. For drugs with a short half-life, it is important to keep the interval between doses as close to the usual routine as possible. Otherwise, the person risks adverse effects from high blood drug levels or seizures from low blood drug levels. However, an alarm clock does not have to be used to take the medications at exactly the same interval. For example, a man takes carbamazepine, 200-mg tablets, four times a day (one after each meal and one at bedtime). He is planning a trip from New York City to London; the flight departs from New York at 8 PM and arrives in London at 8 AM. He should take the after-dinner dose as usual, and then take the bedtime dose on the plane at approximately the usual bedtime. He might be tempted to take a pill after eating breakfast on the plane, but because there is a 5-hour time difference, he should delay taking this dose for several hours. Otherwise, he would be taking it only 4 hours after the bedtime dose, which would push his blood drug level too high. Next, he should delay the rest of the doses for that day by 1 to 2 hours, and on the following day resume the usual schedule.

That was an easy example, but here is a slightly more difficult scenario (Fig. 9). The man's business next takes him from London to Milan, Italy; then, to return home, he takes an 11 AM flight from Milan, which arrives

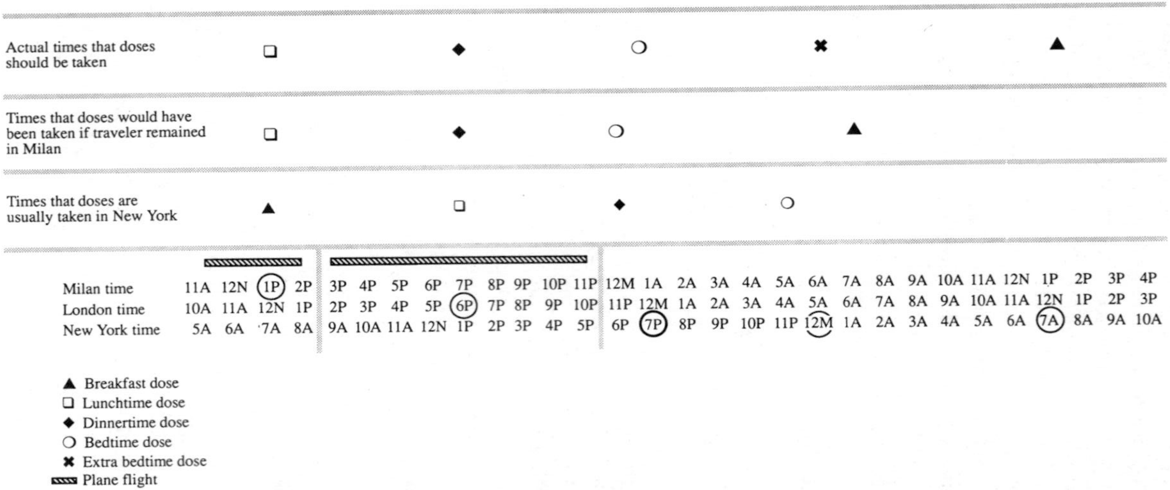

FIGURE 9. Example of alterations in the schedule for taking antiepileptic drugs required by time changes during international travel. Scheme shows the schedule for taking medications during a flight from Milan, via London, to New York. The circled times at the bottom show the local time when each dose is taken.

in London at 1 PM, and then another flight from London, which leaves at 2 PM and arrives in New York City at 5 PM. Now there is a 6-hour time difference going west. He should take his usual lunchtime dose at about 1 PM Milan time (noon London time, 7 AM New York time); take the next (dinnertime) dose in the middle of the flight to New York City (about 6 hours after the lunchtime dose, which would be about 6 PM London time and 1 PM New York time); and take the bedtime dose at 7 PM New York time (6 hours after the dinnertime dose). Next, he should try to take an extra bedtime dose around midnight New York time, and then resume his usual schedule the next day. If he is not awake to take an extra bedtime dose at midnight New York time, he should try to wake up at 2 or 3 AM to take an extra dose, then take his breakfast dose around 8 or 9 AM, with the remaining doses taken preferably 5 to 6 hours apart.

With medications that have a long half-life, the timing is less critical, because the blood drug levels do not fluctuate as much in the intervals between doses.

If the seizures have been difficult to control, if there are problems with dose-related adverse effects, or if the time differences are confusing, the patient should ask the doctor about taking medications during travel.

SLEEP DEPRIVATION

Sleep deprivation, or lack of sleep, can trigger a seizure. Indeed, some people suffer a single seizure for the only time in their entire life after doing an "all-nighter" at college or after a prolonged period of poor sleep associated with a major life stress. For persons with epilepsy, lack of proper sleep can increase their chances of having a seizure, or even increase the intensity and duration of a seizure. Doctors take advantage of this phenomenon by asking persons with suspected epilepsy to stay up all night before having an EEG to "activate the brain" and make it more likely that abnormal brain electrical activity will be revealed. Similarly, when doctors in an epilepsy center are using video-EEG to study seizures, they will often ask the patient to stay up all night to provoke a seizure.

The reason sleep deprivation provokes seizures is not known. The sleep-wake cycle is associated with prominent changes in brain electrical activity. There is often a clear relationship between seizures and the sleep-wake cycle. Some persons have all of their seizures while sleeping, some have most of their seizures just before or shortly after they wake up, others have seizures as they are falling asleep or waking up, and still others have seizures randomly spread throughout the day or night.

Most doctors recommend that persons with epilepsy get adequate sleep. Defining "adequate sleep" is difficult, but a simple definition is a night's sleep that leaves a person feeling refreshed the next day. Although it is hard to specify a minimum number of hours, in general, persons with epilepsy should try to sleep at least 7 hours a night.

For persons who have problems with falling asleep and staying asleep, some simple measures may be helpful: Make sure the sleeping environment is quiet and dark, go to bed at least half an hour before trying to fall asleep, avoid caffeinated beverages within 6 hours of going to sleep, have no more than one alcoholic beverage a day, exercise daily but do not exercise shortly before going to sleep, and read in bed as opposed to watching television. Some people find that reading a good novel keeps them up and TV puts them to sleep, however, and they should turn on the TV.

Sleeping pills should only be used under a doctor's supervision and almost never for more than 2 or 3 weeks. Even with short-term use, they must be handled carefully, because stopping certain types of sleeping pills, especially the benzodiazepines such as flurazepam (Dalmane), triazolam (Halcion), and temazepam (Restoril), can trigger seizures in susceptible persons. However, for those who are exposed to tremendous stress, such as loss of a job or a relationship, the judicious use of sleeping pills for several nights can help to prevent a seizure from sleep deprivation.

Persons who have come to depend on sleeping pills should consult their doctors about getting off of them. Gradual reduction of the sleeping pill dosage, possible substitution of non–habit-forming medications that promote sleep, and the simple measures just described can be helpful.

Younger children require more sleep than adults. The pediatrician can offer guidance on how much sleep the average child requires at different ages and tips on helping to maintain a regular sleep routine. A good book on this subject is *Solve Your Child's Sleep Problems* (see Appendix 4). If a child consistently has more seizures when he or she does not sleep enough, the parents should try to recognize and avoid the things that cause sleep deprivation.

ALCOHOL USE

A relationship between alcohol use and increased seizure frequency has been recognized for centuries. During the past century, however, the role of alcohol in epilepsy has been more clearly defined. Alcohol actually has properties to counteract seizures (that is, alcohol has antiepileptic effects), but it should never be consumed in the hope of controlling seizures. Alcohol does not often provoke seizures while the person is drinking but may cause "withdrawal" seizures 6 to 72 hours later, after drinking has stopped. Withdrawal seizures are most common among persons who have abused alcohol for years. When alcohol consumption is suddenly stopped or markedly reduced over a short period of time, a seizure may occur. In a similar way, the abrupt withdrawal of barbiturates, such as phenobarbital and primidone, or benzodiazepines, such as diazepam and clonazepam, may cause a seizure after prolonged use.

The use of alcohol by persons with epilepsy is controversial. In general, they are less likely than others to use or abuse alcohol. This largely reflects the doctor's restrictions and the warnings on their medication bottles not to take drugs and consume alcohol. Several studies, however, have demonstrated that adults with epilepsy may have one or two alcoholic beverages a day without any worsening of their seizures or changes in the blood levels of their antiepileptic medications.

There is also good evidence that consumption of three or more alcoholic beverages over a short period of time by persons with epilepsy can cause a worsening of their seizures 6 to 72 hours after the alcohol consumption has stopped. Moderate to heavy alcohol consumption is never recommended for persons with epilepsy. Finally, those who consume large amounts of alcohol tend to forget to take their antiepileptic drugs and to sleep poorly.

Persons with epilepsy and a history of alcoholism or drug abuse should not drink alcohol. Long-standing alcohol abuse can cause seizures. In such cases, the relative roles of alcohol withdrawal, alcohol intoxication, head injury, and malnutrition remain uncertain. It is likely that all of these factors contribute to some degree to the development of seizures in people who chronically abuse alcohol.

DRUG ABUSE

Cocaine can cause seizures. All forms of cocaine consumption, including snorting, injecting it into the skin or veins, and smoking crack with a pipe, can cause seizures. Seizures can occur within seconds, minutes, or hours after the cocaine has been consumed. Seizures caused by cocaine are uniquely dangerous and may be associated with heart attacks, interruption of the heart's normal rhythm (cardiac arrhythmia), and death. Seizures caused by cocaine can occur in someone who has never had a seizure, as well as in persons with epilepsy. Those who have epilepsy definitely should avoid cocaine.

Amphetamines, like cocaine, are brain stimulants. They are often prescribed to treat attention deficit disorder, hyperactivity, and narcolepsy.

When used under a doctor's supervision, amphetamines or other stimulants do not appear to increase the likelihood of seizures in persons with epilepsy. When amphetamines and related drugs are abused, they can lead to sleep deprivation, confusion, and major psychiatric disorders, which can cause persons with epilepsy to forget to take their antiepileptic drugs, thereby increasing the risk of seizures. Very high doses of amphetamines can cause severe tonic-clonic seizures, heart attacks, and death.

Marijuana (cannabis, pot) is obtained from the flowering tops of hemp plants. The active ingredient in marijuana is tetrahydrocannabinol (THC). Studies in animals have suggested that THC has some antiepileptic properties. However, THC, which is used in some cancer patients to treat the nausea caused by chemotherapy, causes a variety of adverse effects and is not recommended for the treatment of epilepsy. First, there is no evidence that it is effective in treating seizures in people. Second, even if THC were found to have some antiepileptic effects in humans, as is the case with alcohol, abrupt withdrawal of the substance after recreational use may increase the likelihood of seizures.

Heroin and related *narcotics* (drugs derived from opium and manufactured drugs that are chemically similar to opium) are dangerous when abused. Narcotics are also used medically to treat severe pain. These drugs do not directly affect the chances that someone with epilepsy will have a seizure. However, narcotic use often leads to failure to take prescribed antiepileptic medications. Further, when taken in large amounts, narcotics can cause serious oxygen deprivation to the brain. These problems can lead to seizures.

Nicotine (in tobacco) and *caffeine* (in coffee, tea, chocolate, and other foods) are drugs that are often used and abused in our society. There is no evidence that nicotine or caffeine affects seizure control. However, cigarette smoking can be dangerous in persons who have seizures that impair consciousness or motor control, because a dropped cigarette can cause a fire.

MENSES

Approximately half of the women of childbearing age who have epilepsy report an increase in seizures around the time of their menses, or monthly period. Seizures occurring predominantly around the time of menstruation are referred to as *catamenial epilepsy*. Seizures may occur shortly before menstruation, during and immediately after menstruation, or at the time of ovulation (midcycle).

The hormonal changes associated with the menstrual cycle are well defined and are the most likely cause of changes in the seizure frequency.

The steroid sex hormones can easily cross the barrier that separates the blood and the brain (the blood-brain barrier). The brain contains numerous nerve cells that are directly affected by estrogen and progesterone, the main sex hormones in women. Studies in animals have shown that estrogen can cause or worsen seizures, whereas progesterone tends to act like an anti-epileptic drug.

Control of seizures that occur mainly around the time of menstruation remains a difficult problem. For women who have regular menstrual cycles, a slight increase in the dosage of the antiepileptic drugs before the time of increased seizure frequency may be helpful. Some doctors recommend also taking acetazolamide (Diamox), a mild diuretic and antiepileptic drug, but there is no proof of its effectiveness for catamenial epilepsy, particularly when taken on a daily basis. It may help to reduce the water retention that occurs in the premenstrual period. A few doctors have advocated the use of hormonal agents such as progesterone or birth control pills for women with catamenial epilepsy, but the efficacy and safety of hormonal therapy for this type of epilepsy remain to be established.

STRESS

Stress can affect brain function in many ways. Stress is associated with a variety of unpleasant emotions such as worry, fear, depression, frustration, and anger. Stress can cause sleep disorders and commonly occurs with sleep deprivation or disrupted, fragmented sleep. Stress and anxiety can trigger an increase in the breathing rate, known as hyperventilation. Hyperventilation is a well-recognized means of precipitating seizures in certain patients, especially those with absence seizures. Stress and preoccupation with problems may also cause some people to miss their medication. Stress can cause hormonal changes such as an increase in the steroid hormone cortisol, which may also influence seizure activity.

The final effect of stress, and the most difficult to prove, is a direct effect of negative emotions on the brain, such as worry or fright, causing seizures. There is a plausible mechanism for this effect. Because the limbic system (deep parts of the temporal and frontal lobes) regulates emotional functions and is one of the most common places for a seizure to arise, it makes sense that dramatic changes in the activity of the limbic system, as may occur with intense or prolonged emotional states, could increase the susceptibility to seizures.

If stress appears to provoke seizures, it may be helpful to avoid stressful situations and learn relaxation techniques. However, stress is part of everyone's life, and none of us can completely avoid it. Unfortunately, the worst stresses—the death of a loved one, serious injury, loss of a job, or financial hardship—are often unpredictable. At these times, it is important for persons with epilepsy to obtain adequate sleep and not to miss medications.

Parents should try to recognize what is stressful to their child who has epilepsy, particularly if the seizures are difficult to control for unexplained reasons. They should realize that the parental perspective and the child's perspective are different. What seems trivial to a parent may be stressful to a child. The child can be asked if there are things that worry him or her, or situations that feel uncomfortable. Simply stopping those activities is a bad idea, however, as that may signal to the child that he never has to do anything that he does not like to do. It is best to work out some compromise that reduces the stress but also encourages the child to be active. If the stress is serious, a psychological consultation may be necessary.

OVER-THE-COUNTER DRUGS

Some over-the-counter drugs (drugs that can be bought without a doctor's prescription) can occasionally cause first-time seizures or increase the frequency of seizures in people with epilepsy (see Table 9). Some cold and sleep preparations contain phenylpropanolamine and diphenhydramine (e.g., Benadryl). Phenylpropanolamine is also present in some diet pills, and diphenhydramine is also used for coughs and itching, as well as for nasal congestion; these drugs should be avoided by people with epilepsy. Medications for runny and stuffed noses containing pseudoephedrine or phenylephrine appear to be safe; there are no well-documented reports of seizures caused by these drugs. Diphenhydramine ointment applied to the skin for itching also appears to be safe for people with epilepsy.

For aches and pains, acetaminophen (e.g., Tylenol, Panadol, Excedrin Aspirin Free) is probably the safest medication. Aspirin also appears safe, but it should not be used in children, and prolonged high doses of aspirin should be avoided by persons taking phenytoin. Persons with high blood levels of valproate or phenytoin may experience adverse effects when taking aspirin, as the result of drug interactions. Ibuprofen (e.g., Motrin, Advil) can also interact with phenytoin, leading to increased blood phenytoin levels and possible adverse effects. Propoxyphene, another pain reliever found in over-the-counter preparations, when taken with carbamazepine, can lead to increased blood carbamazepine levels and possible adverse effects.

NUTRITIONAL DEFICIENCIES

Many people are extremely interested in pursuing dietary changes or taking nutritional supplements to improve seizure control. Foods can alter brain function, but information on which to make recommendations is scarce. Very low levels of sugar in the blood can cause seizures in some people, especially people with diabetes who take too much insulin, so it is reasonable to recommend that persons with epilepsy try to eat regularly and eat a balanced diet. There is no proof, however, that "hypoglycemia" diagnosed by a low blood sugar level (before eating or on a glucose tolerance test) has any relationship to seizures or epilepsy.

Various amino acids, vitamins, or herbs are often used to treat seizures, but there is no evidence that any of these nutritional supplements clearly improve seizure control. Research studies have been unable to confirm the thousands of reports of persons who have appeared to respond to these nutritional substances. That is not to say that promising therapies should be ignored, even if they are not in the Western tradition of drug therapy, but persons with epilepsy would be wise not to embrace a treatment until there is some solid proof that it works. Most nutritional supplements are, in effect, drugs. Steroids, for example, whether taken for cancer, arthritis, or to build muscles, can be claimed as a natural therapy, because steroid hormones are naturally found in the body. There is nothing natural, however, about extremely high doses of steroids, or of vitamins, amino acids, or other organic compounds. They may even be dangerous, and probably most often have no real effect on seizure control.

Vitamins

Vitamins are chemicals that are manufactured either by our bodies or by plants or animals that we eat. In modern Western societies, vitamin deficiencies are rare. Human beings evolved in environments with limited sources and varieties of nutrition. Although our current diet may be unhealthy because of too much fat, sugars, and processed foods, vitamin deficiencies are uncommon unless the diet is seriously restricted. In rare cases the body is unable to manufacture or absorb vitamins, and the result is a vitamin deficiency, but even then, seizures are rare.

The only vitamin deficiency known to cause or worsen seizures is a vitamin B_6 (pyridoxine) deficiency. This deficiency occurs mainly in newborns and infants and causes difficult-to-control seizures. To test whether a baby with seizures has a vitamin B_6 deficiency, doctors will often prescribe a small dose of the vitamin to see if the seizures stop or decrease in frequency. In some cases, the doctor may administer the vitamin intravenously to a young baby while recording the EEG, which will improve dramatically if there is a vitamin B_6 deficiency. Some doctors may also try vitamin B_6 in older children with difficult-to-control seizures, although there is no solid evidence that the vitamin is helpful in them.

Some unconfirmed reports claim that Vitamin E improves seizure control in children, but the response is variable and rarely dramatic. Citing the effectiveness of a therapy on the basis of case reports can be misleading. Vitamin therapies deserve further study in controlled clinical trials.

Phenytoin and phenobarbital can cause a deficiency of the vitamin folic acid (folate). Folate is important in the production of blood cells and may be important for peripheral nerves. Folate deficiency can cause a predisposition to certain birth defects. Women of childbearing age and persons with anemia or other blood-cell disorders who are taking antiepileptic drugs should supplement their diet with folate. Although there are reports that folate may reduce the effectiveness of some antiepileptic drugs, there is no solid evidence to support this claim.

Valproate can deplete the liver's stores of carnitine, a substance that functions like a vitamin to help in the metabolism of fats. Although there is no clear evidence of this effect, some believe that carnitine supplementation can help prevent the rare cases of liver damage caused by valproate. Because serious liver damage from valproate is extremely rare, supplementation should only be considered in individuals at great risk, such as children under 2 years old who are being treated with valproate as well as other antiepileptic drugs. (This is the group with the highest rate of valproate-associated liver damage.) There are isolated reports of carnitine supplementation helping older children and adults with other adverse reactions to valproate, such as tremor and tiredness. However, studies confirming or refuting these preliminary reports have yet to be done.

Minerals

Minerals are essential nutrients obtained in the diet. Some minerals are essential for manufacturing vitamins, and others, such as iron, are essential for the manufacture of red blood cells.

Low levels of sodium, calcium, and magnesium can alter the electrical activity of brain cells and cause seizures. Dietary deficiency of these minerals is rare unless there is severe general malnutrition. Low sodium levels may be caused by medications such as diuretics (water pills) or carbamazepine, by excessive water intake, or by hormonal disorders. Low calcium levels most often result from kidney disease or hormonal disorders. Because magnesium levels alter the body's regulation of calcium, low magnesium levels often contribute to or cause low calcium levels.

It is rare for persons with epilepsy to require supplementation of sodium, calcium, or magnesium. However, for those who have low levels of these minerals, dietary alterations or mineral supplements are reasonable after a medical examination has excluded an underlying disorder.

Certain adverse effects of valproate may be alleviated by mineral supplementation. Inflammation of the pancreas (pancreatitis), which is a rare but serious adverse effect of valproate, may be prevented by selenium supplementation. Selenium at a dose of 100 micrograms per day has been used to prevent valproate-induced pancreatitis in a child who previously had this problem when taking valproate. Selenium (10–20 micrograms per day) and zinc (30–50 milligrams per day) may help to counteract the hair loss that some people experience when taking valproate or other drugs. These dosages are available in many over-the-counter high-potency multivitamins.

Glycine and Herbs

Glycine, a naturally occurring amino acid, is thought to be a neurotransmitter, with a role in seizure control. Correcting a deficiency of glycine by the administration of dimethylglycine has been reported to control some seizures, although controlled studies have not been done.

Herbs have been used for centuries by numerous cultures to treat seizures. Again, as in the case of other nonmedical treatments, there is little evidence to support or refute the use of specific herbs.

CYCLES OF THE MOON

The moon's effect on certain behaviors has been alleged since the dawn of civilization. The words "lunatic" and "lunacy" are derived from the word "lunar," meaning "related to the moon." The moon affects the magnetic and gravitational activities of the Earth. Tidal changes are the most dramatic example of its gravitational effects. The role of magnetic energy in animal behavior has only recently been recognized.

The moon has been implicated in seizure occurrence for centuries. The moon's role in epilepsy was "proved" and "disproved" on numerous occasions before the modern age of scientific study. Modern neurology rarely even considers the moon's cycles as a possibility. Nevertheless, some persons and parents of children with epilepsy are absolutely convinced that seizures are more likely to occur during certain phases of the moon.

The role of the moon in epilepsy is the subject of considerable study in the former Soviet Union, but has received little attention in modern Western medical studies. The notion of a relationship between the moon's phases and human behavior is worthy of closer study.

PART TWO

Diagnosis and Treatment of Epilepsy

CHAPTER 7

The Health Care Team

Health care is a partnership. The notion that doctors and other health care professionals give orders and patients blindly follow them is out of date. The person with epilepsy must become part of the health care team. All the members of the team depend on what the patient tells them. The diagnosis depends largely on the information given in the patient's medical history. Decisions about therapy are influenced by the patient's communication of concerns or fears. The choice of antiepileptic drugs, for example, may depend on the patient's feelings about the drugs' adverse effects and their expense, or on the patient's willingness to make lifestyle changes, such as not driving.

THE DOCTOR AND PATIENT

A good relationship between the doctor and the patient is one of the cornerstones of good medical care. The doctor and patient are partners in the health care process; they share a common goal but have different responsibilities in achieving that goal. For some patients, the doctor's visit is a passive event; the doctor checks them over and makes recommendations. It should be an interactive one, however, because the doctor needs to know the patient's concerns and desires. Some patients will do anything to avoid taking medications, including giving up driving. Others want to avoid seizures at almost any cost. These are personal decisions that work best for a specific person in a specific situation. When a person's situation in life changes, such as a new job that requires a lot of driving, marriage, or loss of health insurance, the treatment may need to change.

Communication is central to the doctor-patient relationship. The patient and family members must provide the doctor with the information he or she needs to make a correct diagnosis and to prescribe the most effective and best-tolerated treatment. The doctor should discuss with the patient, in understandable language, why tests are being obtained, what the tests in-

65

volve, and perhaps most important, the risks and benefits of therapy. Ideally, the relationship should be comfortable and based on trust. The past several decades have seen a major shift toward greater communication between doctor and patient. Doctors are now much more willing to share information about choices, medical facts, and potential risks. Doctors in earlier generations, however, were more available (house calls are now ancient history in most areas) and more able to spend time listening to their patients.

Time is often a limiting factor in communication between doctor and patient. Patients often feel rushed, and their questions go unasked or unanswered. The doctor may appear to be more concerned about moving patients in and out of the office, ordering tests, and prescribing drugs than about taking time to listen to the issues bothering the patient. Doctors, however, often complain that patients provide too much irrelevant information, which is time consuming. Further, some patients enjoy discussing social, political, and other unrelated topics with their doctors; patients should limit their comments to issues concerning their health, especially if the doctor's office is busy. There are several ways to help foster a more productive interaction with the doctor.

The First Visit

The patient's first consultation with a doctor often determines the nature of their relationship. The doctor may begin by asking about the main problem that brought the patient to the office and may then ask the patient to give a fairly detailed account of his or her symptoms. The doctor may question the patient carefully about events surrounding the seizure: Could it have been provoked by sleep deprivation, excessive use of alcohol, or some other factor? Did the episode occur shortly after standing? Was there a warning? Exactly what happened during the episode? What was the setting? How long did the episode last? Was the patient tired or confused after the episode? When did the patient first seek medical attention? What tests were done? What medication was prescribed? What was the response to the medication? Have there been subsequent episodes? What were they like?

It is helpful if the patient can briefly summarize his or her medical history in writing, or ask the referring doctor to write a letter summarizing it. Patients should bring with them all important medical records, such as notes from other doctors, seizure calendars (records of seizures), results of laboratory studies such as blood drug levels and electroencephalogram (EEG) and magnetic resonance imaging (MRI) reports, and the actual MRI films and EEG tracings, which can be borrowed. This information will help the doctor focus his or her questions and will provide important details that might otherwise be forgotten during the visit.

It is often helpful for patients to bring with them a written list of questions, particularly if the purpose of the visit is to define issues or provide specific answers. Questions are best asked at the end of the visit, after the doctor has had a chance to record the medical history, review previous laboratory studies, and perform a physical examination. It is best to limit the list to five questions; additional questions can be saved for a future visit. In some doctor's offices and clinics, a nurse reviews the doctor's information and recommendations. The nurse can answer many of the patient's questions and may provide reading materials on epilepsy. This is often helpful, especially if the patient did not understand the doctor's answers to some questions.

When the patient leaves the doctor's office, he or she should have a good understanding of the treatment plan. The patient should ask for written instructions, particularly on how to take the medications. The patient should know what to do if another seizure occurs or if medications are missed. The plan should make sense to the patient. If things do not make sense or important issues remain unresolved, the patient should ask the questions again. If important questions come up after the patient leaves the doctor's office, he or she can call up and ask them. In many cases, they can be answered by the nurse. Less important questions or bits of information, such as the fact that an uncle has epilepsy, can usually wait until the next visit.

Follow-up Visits

Follow-up doctor's appointments usually last 10 to 30 minutes. If the patient is seizure-free and having no adverse effects from the medications, the visit may be brief. If the seizures are worse, or the medications have caused new adverse effects, the visit often needs to be longer. Before the patient sees the doctor, a nurse may check blood pressure, review seizure control and dosage of medications, ask about adverse effects of the medications, and discuss any new social or medical problems that have arisen since the last visit. Many questions can be answered by the nurse at this time.

There is often a gap between the doctor's perception of how the patient is doing and how the patient feels he or she is doing. The doctor and patient share the same goal of having the person with epilepsy enjoy a good quality of life. If one tonic-clonic seizure a year or one complex partial seizure a month bothers the patient, or if the adverse effects of the medication are a problem, the patient should make sure the doctor knows of it. Often, there must be a balance between seizure control and adverse effects of the medication. Epilepsy can affect people in other ways. Some may fear a seizure because of embarrassment or possible injury. Discussing the patient's concerns helps the doctor understand the disorder and how it affects this patient, so that treatment strategies and recommendations can be tailored for his or her specific problems.

If there is a need to discuss special subjects, such as pregnancy, discontinuing antiepileptic drugs, or epilepsy surgery, a longer appointment may be required. If special needs are anticipated on a visit, the patient may want to schedule additional time with the doctor.

It is important that patients communicate their needs to the doctor. For example, some patients may have difficulty affording certain drugs and may prefer to take less expensive ones. (For information on ways to save on the costs of antiepileptic drugs, see Chapter 10). For others, prescription plans make the cost issue irrelevant. Some patients take less than the prescribed amounts of medication to stretch their supply or to avoid bothersome adverse effects. Patients should not adjust their medications without consulting the doctor. If a drug is unaffordable, or the medication is causing troublesome adverse effects, the patient should tell the doctor. If the doctor is not responsive, the patient should make sure the doctor understands how seriously this problem affects him or her, and should speak to the nurse if possible. If repeated efforts to make the doctor aware of the problems are unsuccessful, the patient should consider changing doctors.

Financial Issues and Insurance Coverage

Most doctors have office or business managers who can answer questions about financial concerns or insurance coverage. In cases of financial hardship, many doctors are willing to accept payment plans or reduced fees. As managed care and health maintenance organizations multiply in our country, the access to doctors both expands and contracts. It expands because people with these health care plans will have access to pediatricians, neurologists, and other physicians. It contracts because the number of doctors available in such plans is usually limited. For example, a specific plan may have only one neurologist and no epileptologist (a neurologist with special training in epilepsy). Fortunately, only a minority of persons with epilepsy need to see an epileptologist. Local Epilepsy Foundation of America (EFA) affiliates may be able to provide the names of doctors who accept insurance, those who accept Medicaid, Medicare, or worker's compensation, or doctors who are willing to see patients at reduced rates. They may also have the names, addresses, and telephone numbers of clinics where care is given free of charge.

The types of insurance that cover epilepsy vary tremendously. Many doctors do not accept patients with Medicaid, Medicare, or worker's compensation unless they are willing to pay personally, separate from those forms of coverage. Patients with Medicaid can often obtain good care at public clinics in teaching hospitals, where the coverage is accepted in full payment. At many teaching hospitals, a patient may be able to attend an epilepsy clinic supervised by an epileptologist. However, the doctors who directly provide the care at teaching-hospital clinics are often residents in training. The residents' fund of knowledge and experience varies tremendously. Most have a limited knowledge of how to diagnose and treat epilepsy. Residents should be supervised by an attending doctor. Therefore, a patient should try to speak with both the resident doctor and the attending doctor. In addition, residents' assignments usually rotate from month to month. Therefore, the patient can literally have a new doctor every month. The attending doctor usually has a more permanent position, so consulting with him or her briefly at each visit helps to maintain continuity of care.

Medicare reimburses doctors more fairly than Medicaid, and many doctors accept Medicare (see Chapter 30). All physicians who participate in Medicare are allowed maximum rates they can charge for services. These rates are often lower than the standard rates charged for a service to a person who does not have Medicare.

Worker's compensation programs (see Chapter 26) are regulated by the state and have fixed fees for medical services. Doctors who care for people with worker's compensation must accept the allowed fee as full payment. However, some doctors will not accept patients with this coverage.

Second Opinions and Changing Doctors

If the doctor is not meeting the patient's needs, it is worth considering obtaining a second opinion or even changing doctors. Before doing this, however, the patient should consider again the areas in which he or she feels uncertain. In many cases, by asking the doctor additional questions or raising certain issues, the patient may feel much more comfortable. When a second opinion about the case is obtained, the patient may find that the doctor has not left any stone unturned and the second doctor agrees with all aspects of the care. On the other hand, the second doctor may have helpful suggestions regarding tests or changes in the treatment regimen.

For a second opinion, it is probably best for the patient to ask the doctor for the name of an epileptologist. The patient may also get a list of names from the local affiliate of the EFA or from a friend or relative. It is important that care be coordinated. The referring, or primary, doctor and the second doctor should communicate, and the primary doctor should send copies of the patient's records to the second doctor. The patient may wish to continue care with the second doctor, but usually the primary doctor remains in charge of the case.

Changing doctors is often awkward and uncomfortable. In some cases, communication and trust between the patient and the doctor may break down. Problems can arise, for example, over time spent during the visit, finances, adverse effects of medication, failure to take medication as prescribed, or language difficulties. Relationships have a "chemistry," and sometimes the chemistry is not right. It is best for the patient to call the doctor's office and tell the secretary, office manager, nurse, or doctor that he or she is changing doctors and ask that the records be forwarded to the new doctor. If asked to give a reason for this desire to change doctors, the patient can simply say, "It is just something I want to do," or can nicely explain why. Patients should not burn bridges behind them, however. There may be only two neurologists in a community, and the patient may turn out to like the original one better than the second one. The patient will need to write a brief note asking that the records be forwarded to the new doctor or directly to the patient. Patients have a legal right to have a copy of their medical records. The note can be very simple: "Please forward all of my medical records to Dr. ——," and give the doctor's address. It is helpful to call the new doctor's office before the appointment to make sure that the records have arrived. If they have not, the patient should call the first doctor's office and find out if the records have been sent. Although it is uncommon, there may be a charge for copying the records, but there are limits on the charges.

Seizure Calendar

Patients with epilepsy should strongly consider keeping a seizure calendar. It is simple and can often help answer questions about changes in the type or frequency of seizures over time, the effect of different medications on seizure control, adverse effects of medications, and seizure-provoking factors. The most basic seizure calendar includes the date and time of the seizure, as well as the type of seizure. If a precipitating factor is suspected (e.g., lack of sleep, missed medication, stress, menstrual period), the patient should write it down. For women, it may be helpful to keep track of the relationship between seizures and the menstrual cycles. This can be done by recording the woman's basal body temperature (taking the temperature shortly after awakening), although this rarely provides essential information. It is also helpful to record the medication, dosage, and blood drug levels.

THE NURSE

Nurses are on the front line of medicine. In the emergency room, they are often the first ones to obtain information about a problem. In the office and clinic, they often greet the patient and review his or her current medical status. After the doctor orders tests or changes the medication regimen, the nurse more fully explains the test or describes exactly how to take the drugs. The nurse often serves, quite literally, as the translator between the doctor and the patient. In many offices, clinics, and hospitals, the nurse provides written instructions, and may distribute literature or even show video tapes, further explaining epilepsy and the doctor's recommendations.

In many doctor's offices, the nurse also answers questions over the telephone and in person. The nurse may spend more time with the patient than the doctor. The patient should feel comfortable talking with the nurse about a problem and should have confidence in the nurse's response. However, if the patient wishes to speak with the doctor, or wants the nurse to check with the doctor, he or she should feel free to ask the nurse to do this.

THE NURSE-CLINICIAN

In some doctor's offices and in many epilepsy centers, nurse-clinicians play a vital role in patient care. These specially trained nurses help to assess, coordinate, and implement patient education and care. They can answer routine questions over the telephone, such as those about laboratory results, upcoming tests, adverse effects of medications, dosage schedules, interactions between antiepileptic drugs and other medications, and the safety of activities. The nurse-clinician can also be helpful in making referrals to other members of the health care team, such as the social worker or the physical therapist. Because the doctor and nurse-clinician work closely together, their recommendations on specific issues and questions are usually quite similar.

THE NURSE PRACTITIONER

Nurse practitioners are nurses with advanced medical education. They are licensed by the state to take a medical history, examine patients, order tests, and prescribe medications, including narcotics and other restricted substances. Nurse practitioners can therefore serve as relatively independent practitioners who diagnose diseases and treat patients.

Nurse practitioners undergo extensive training and licensure examinations. They are supervised by doctors, who review the case histories and treatment plans at intervals specified by the state licensing board. The position of nurse practitioner is relatively new. Over the next decade, it is anticipated that the number and importance of these nurses will grow.

THE PHYSICIAN'S ASSISTANT

Physician's assistants are playing an increasing role in American health care. Their name describes their role: they assist doctors in obtaining the medical history, examining the patient, recommending therapy, drawing blood, ordering tests, speaking with consulting doctors, and many other functions.

THE SOCIAL WORKER–COUNSELOR

Social workers are valuable members of the treatment team for epilepsy. Unfortunately, social workers with expertise in epilepsy may only be available in comprehensive epilepsy programs. Social workers play many roles. In some centers, the social worker is one of the key providers of patient and family education about epilepsy. In addition, the social worker often provides the community outreach education programs. Often the social worker assists in identifying and obtaining precious resources. These resources include special education programs, respite centers (where a child or adult with special needs can spend some time to give the caregivers a rest), home health aides, medical insurance benefits, vocational rehabilitation centers, and referrals to psychologists and other mental health workers. Social workers may also be helpful in referring a person with epilepsy who has experienced discrimination to advocacy groups such as the local Protection and Advocacy Service, Legal Aid Society, or an attorney specializing in this subject. (The EFA may also be helpful in this regard.)

Social workers sometimes function as counselors, and their fees can be substantially below those of psychologists and psychiatrists. The counseling sessions provide an important place for persons with epilepsy to discuss social and personal issues that the physician may not have time to address. Counseling sessions may be especially beneficial for children, helping them to understand issues of independence, maturity, and personal growth. In some cases, the social worker can help to identify parents whose overprotectiveness is adversely affecting a child with epilepsy. Other problems of home life, such as a parent or spouse with substance abuse problems or a psychiatric disorder, living in a divorced family, or the death of a loved one, can be discussed, put in perspective, better understood, and coped with after counseling sessions.

Further, the social worker can inform the doctor about issues that may have a bearing on medical issues, thereby bringing about important changes in medical therapy or referral to a psychologist or psychiatrist. Social workers can also be helpful in crisis situations. They can help to refer patients to doctors or epilepsy centers that are best able to handle the problem.

THE EEG TECHNOLOGIST

The EEG is a recording of the electrical activity of the brain (see Chapter 8). The EEG technologist is the person who performs the EEG test. He or she explains the testing procedure to the patient, obtains some background information (age, diagnosis, medications, time of last meal, time of last seizure), and then applies the electrodes to the patient's scalp, records the EEG, and prepares the EEG record for the doctor's review. The EEG technologist is supervised by the director of the EEG laboratory.

Because the EEG session often takes more than an hour, the technologist spends a good bit of time with the patient and therefore may gather information about the patient's epilepsy that may be helpful to the doctor or other members of the health care team.

THE PHARMACIST

Pharmacists, who fill prescriptions and dispense drugs, play an important role in health care. They may have known individuals and families over many years, and they are often aware of both health and personal issues. Pharmacists can be helpful in discussing the potential adverse effects of medications, costs of drugs, and relative risks and benefits of generic versus brand-name drugs (see Chapter 10 for discussion of this issue; do not switch drugs without first checking with the doctor). For people who are taking several drugs, pharmacists can often provide information on potential drug interactions.

Many people feel more comfortable talking to their pharmacist than to their doctor. Pharmacists are knowledgeable and can provide expert information about medications. However, they cannot substitute for doctors.

EPILEPSY ASSOCIATIONS AND SUPPORT GROUPS

The EFA provides important resources at both the local and the national level (see Chapter 31). Local affiliates of the EFA and other epilepsy support groups provide essential services for many persons with epilepsy. These groups are sometimes directed by a social worker or may have social workers and counselors on the staff. Depending on the specific group, services include support-group meetings to discuss social and related issues, lectures on health issues, referrals for vocational rehabilitation, lectures to schoolchildren and school nurses on epilepsy, and assistance with referrals to pediatricians, neurologists, epileptologsts, and specialized epilepsy centers.

Individual doctors and health care workers at comprehensive epilepsy centers often work together with local epilepsy associations. Patients benefit when the resources of the medical centers and epilepsy associations are pooled.

SPECIALTY MEMBERS OF THE HEALTH CARE TEAM

The health care team is defined by the needs of the patient. In comprehensive epilepsy centers, consultation with a neuropsychologist and psychiatrist is common, especially by patients considered for surgical therapy. Specialists in vocational rehabilitation, physical therapy, occupational therapy, music therapy, speech therapy, or special education may prove important for selected patients.

The Neuropsychologist

Neuropsychologists assess various aspects of intellectual and behavioral function. The neuropsychologist typically administers a battery of tests that helps to identify relative strengths and weaknesses in areas such as thinking, reasoning, memory, language, perception, motor ability, and behavior. For example, memory, which may be a problem for persons with epilepsy, can be carefully studied by the neuropsychologist. These tests are essential in the assessment for epilepsy surgery, but they are also helpful for showing evidence of improvement or deterioration in certain intellectual functions of persons with epilepsy.

The neuropsychologist can also help define the effects of the injury to the brain from head trauma, stroke, or tumor. With a better understanding of the problems and personal dynamics of the patient, the doctor can formulate a more effective treatment plan. Neuropsychologists also perform therapy or other interventions for intellectual or behavioral problems and private psychotherapy for emotional problems related to brain disorders.

For patients considering epilepsy surgery, the neuropsychologist is often directly involved in performing the intracarotid sodium amobarbital test (see Chapter 11) and electrical stimulation of the brain to map areas of intellectual functions, such as speech and understanding spoken or written language.

The Psychiatrist

People often have negative feelings about psychiatrists, mainly because of stigmas associated with behavioral disorders and misconceptions about the nature of psychiatric care. Psychiatrists do more than simply listen to people. They use a variety of therapies, ranging from counseling and psychotherapy to prescribing medications.

Psychological and psychiatric problems are common in the general population. Some of these problems, such as depression and anxiety, appear to be more common among persons with epilepsy. Depression may be caused by medications, especially barbiturates. It may also be caused by psychosocial problems, such as loss of a job or a loved one, especially in someone who is dependent on that job or person for support. The psychiatrist can help to identify the problem, determine its cause, and recommend treatment. In some cases, for example, relief from the depression is obtained by adjusting the antiepileptic drugs, adding an antidepressant drug, or counseling for social and medical problems.

If "chemistry" is important in the doctor-patient relationship, it is essential in the psychiatrist-patient relationship. If the patient has a behavioral problem and is not comfortable with a particular psychiatrist, he or she should consider seeing another one rather than ignoring the problem. Because the psychiatrist may need to prescribe an antidepressant or recommend reducing the dosage of an existing drug, good communication between him or her and the primary doctor treating the epilepsy is also essential.

The Physical Therapist

Physical therapists help people with disorders of movement, coordination, or sensation to become more physically able. The movement disorders may be related to problems involving the brain, spinal cord, nerves, or muscles. Mobility and coordination can be enhanced through various programs of stretching, exercise, and skills development. Most individuals with epilepsy do not require physical therapy. However, for those with limited mobility or other physical disorders, physical therapists can provide important assistance.

The Speech Therapist

Speech therapists assist people with speech and language disorders. The disorders include problems with language functions due to brain dysfunction and problems with speech expression due to brain, spinal cord, nerve, or muscle disorders. Speech therapists assess the nature of the problem and recommend a program of therapy, which varies considerably depending on the problems and the approach of the specific therapist.

The Vocational Rehabilitation Counselor

Vocational rehabilitation counselors assist people with disabilities to obtain skills needed for employment. Specialized programs, some of which are sponsored by state or community agencies, may be available to facilitate this process (see Chapter 26). The therapist can help in a variety of ways, such as assessing skills and interests and recommending areas that seem worthwhile to pursue. They teach people how to accommodate and overcome aspects of the disability, improve work habits, train for specific job functions, develop more effective interviewing skills, and seek and obtain employment.

Vocational counselors work with people to help develop skills through training that will enable them to find work. The counselor first assesses a person's interests, their current knowledge and skills, and their potential in certain areas. A person may benefit from several counseling sessions to identify employment agencies or prepare a résumé. In other cases, a vocational rehabilitation program may be helpful. Such programs provide in-depth assessment and training.

The advice and training recommended by vocational rehabilitation counselors can be essential for obtaining a job. One young man who was seizure-free after epilepsy surgery at our center had difficulty obtaining a job in the printing industry, although he had worked in this area for more than 7 years. After a brief vocational rehabilitation program that included training with computers, he successfully found a job in printing and was promoted twice in the year; his expertise with computers, together with his background in printing, paid off.

THE COMPREHENSIVE EPILEPSY CENTER

Epilepsy centers are valuable resources for any person with definite or suspected epilepsy who has unresolved problems related to the disorder. Patients may be referred to a comprehensive epilepsy center for a single outpatient visit for an assessment of the current diagnosis and therapy, or for more long-term followup and treatment (see Chapter 32).

CHAPTER 8

Making the Diagnosis of Epilepsy

Although the diagnosis of epilepsy is usually straightforward, other disorders can cause sudden changes in behavior and may be confused with epilepsy. The correct diagnosis depends on an accurate description of the events occurring before, during, and after the attack. It is essential that the patient, or a witness to the seizure, give the doctor as much information as possible about the episode. If certain details are vague, the doctor should be told. No matter how accurate and complete the information, however, some episodes remain difficult even for experts to diagnose correctly.

CONDITIONS CONFUSED WITH EPILEPSY

Many medical, neurological, and psychiatric disorders can mimic seizures. Before recommending treatment, the doctor wants to be sure that the diagnosis is correct. A detailed discussion of the conditions that can be confused with epilepsy is beyond the scope of this book. Only a few of the disorders that are most often mistaken for an epileptic seizure are presented here. Chapter 14 discusses some conditions occurring only in children that can be confused with seizures.

Fainting

Fainting (syncope) occurs when the brain does not receive enough blood, oxygen, or sugar. Fainting, a brief loss of consciousness, is common, and is usually of no consequence in young people. Most often the person is standing and complains of dizziness, lightheadedness, or abdominal discomfort, turns pale, begins to sweat, and then falls to the ground. The body may stiffen slightly, and the arms or legs may jerk several times. An incorrect diagnosis of a seizure may be made when the doctor hears that someone suddenly lost consciousness, fell down, and then had jerking movements.

In rare cases of fainting, especially if the person is young and is kept in a standing or sitting position by a well-meaning bystander, a full-blown seizure can occur after the faint. In most cases of fainting, the loss of consciousness lasts less than 1 minute, and the person is fully alert within 10 to 30 seconds after awakening. Falling to the floor is a natural remedy for the faint. Many faints result from the heart's inability to pump blood up to the brain, so when the person is lying down, the heart is at the same level as the brain, and blood flows more easily to the head.

Many disorders can cause fainting. Orthostatic hypotension, or position-related lowering of the blood pressure, is a common disorder in which a person faints shortly after arising from a lying or sitting position. Fainting can occur almost immediately upon standing or after several minutes. All persons are subject to orthostatic hypotension after prolonged bedrest. Perhaps the most common instance of orthostatic hypotension is the lightheadedness that occurs when someone gets out of bed quickly after awakening.

Hypoglycemia

Hypoglycemia is one of the most overdiagnosed disorders in the United States. It does occur as a serious medical problem in some people, most often those with diabetes who take too much insulin. An endocrine tumor of the pancreas is another, but extremely rare, cause of hypoglycemia. Hypoglycemia can cause symptoms of dizziness, lightheadedness, fainting, and even tonic-clonic (grand mal) seizures.

Unfortunately, hypoglycemia is a common and popular diagnosis that is often made without strong supporting evidence. The diagnosis of hypoglycemia is often based on the results of a glucose tolerance test. For this test, the patient drinks a high-sugar-content drink, and the changes in blood sugar (glucose) are measured for the next several hours. After an initial rise in blood sugar, insulin, a hormone made by the pancreas, is released into the bloodstream to compensate for the rise and to lower the blood sugar level. In many healthy people, this rebound lowering of the blood sugar level extends beyond the "normal" lower limits, just as the initial rise in blood sugar level extended beyond the "normal" upper limits. Experts in endocrinology have found that the results of this test are often overinterpreted as abnormal. The diagnosis of hypoglycemia is supported by a low blood-sugar level when symptoms of hypoglycemia are present and relief of symptoms is obtained with foods containing sugar or carbohydrates.

Sleep Attacks

In sleep attacks, a person has an irresistible urge to sleep and suddenly dozes off, usually for only minutes. Upon awakening, he or she feels refreshed. Sleep attack may be a symptom of narcolepsy, a sleep disorder. These attacks usually occur during boring conditions, but can occur in dangerous settings such as driving. Patients with narcolepsy may also suffer sudden loss of muscle tone, causing something to drop from the hand, the head to nod, or the body to fall, when they experience strong emotions such as vigorous laughing or crying.

Panic Attacks

Panic attacks are episodes of profound fear and anxiety, often associated with increased heart rate, hyperventilation, shortness of breath, sweating, nausea, chest discomfort, and other bodily (autonomic) symptoms. Certain settings may precipitate panic attacks. Doctors may incorrectly suspect that the person is suffering from partial seizures, because simple partial seizures may have autonomic and emotional symptoms such as fear or anxiety. In contrast with seizures, which begin suddenly, the panic attacks often build up gradually and last longer than 5 minutes.

Psychogenic Seizures

Psychogenic (nonepileptic) seizures resemble epileptic seizures. The degree of resemblance varies considerably, but psychogenic attacks result from usually subconscious mental activity and not from abnormal brain electrical activity. Doctors consider most of these episodes psychological in nature, but not purposely produced. The person is usually unaware that the attacks are not "epileptic." Psychogenic seizures are common, and in many cases, years of therapy for epileptic seizures are spent in vain until the correct diagnosis is made. Approximately 20% of patients with psychogenic seizures also have epileptic seizures and require different treatment for each disorder.

Psychogenic seizures are most common in adolescents and adults but can also occur in children and the elderly. These episodes have been more widely recognized during the past several decades. In comprehensive epilepsy centers, where video-electroencephalogram (EEG) monitoring is performed, approximately 20% of referred patients are found to have psychogenic seizures.

Psychogenic seizures most often imitate complex partial or tonic-clonic seizures. Because doctors rarely witness an attack, the diagnosis is often delayed. Family members report episodes in which the patient stiffens and jerks, and doctors are immediately drawn toward the diagnosis of epilepsy. In studying these attacks, doctors have identified certain features that suggest nonepileptic or psychogenic seizures. These features are wild movements such as thrashing or rolling from side to side; screaming, crying, and moaning during the attack; jerking or stiffening of all extremities but with preserved consciousness; stiffening and jerking of the extremities but with immediate resumption of normal alertness after the attack (tiredness or confusion typically occurs after a tonic-clonic seizure); altered behavior that waxes and wanes (the jerking or the inability to respond to questions comes and goes); and prolonged episodes, lasting longer than 5 minutes. Any one of these features, however, does not confirm the diagnosis of a psychogenic attack. Epileptic seizures may occasionally include one or more of these behaviors.

The diagnosis of psychogenic seizures is most often made with video-EEG monitoring. Doctors often try to have a family member or friend observe the recorded attack to ensure that it is identical or nearly identical to the usual episodes. Certain tests may be safely used to help provoke a psychogenic seizure.

The treatment of psychogenic seizures varies. In many cases, when the doctor tells the person that the attacks are psychological, they stop. Psychogenic seizures are not necessarily an indication of a serious psychiatric disorder, but the problem needs to be addressed and, in many cases, treated. The prognosis for control of these episodes and for the patient's psychological well-being is very good in most cases. Counseling with a psychologist, psychiatrist, or clinical social worker for a limited time after the diagnosis is often helpful.

THE MEDICAL HISTORY

The medical history is the foundation of the diagnosis. It is essential that the doctor be given all information about the seizure, because most doctors never witness a patient's actual attack. The following questions may be asked:

Before the attack:
> Was there lack of sleep or unusual stress?
> Was there any recent illness?
> Had the person taken any medications or drugs, including over-the-counter drugs, alcohol, or illegal drugs?
> What was the person doing immediately before the attack: lying, sitting, standing, getting up from a lying position, heavy exercise?

During the attack:
> How did it begin?
> Was there a warning?

Were there abnormal movements of the eyes, mouth, face, head, arms, or legs?

Was the person able to talk and respond appropriately?

Was there loss of urine or feces?

Was the tongue or inside of the cheeks bitten?

After the attack:

Was the person confused or tired?

Was speech normal?

Was there a headache?

One of the most valuable pieces of information a doctor has is an accurate description of the typical attack from an eyewitness. It is worthwhile having witnesses accompany the patient to the doctor's office, or having the doctor or nurse speak with them about their observations. Ask them to write down a detailed description of what they saw because memories fade with time. Save these notes, as they may be helpful to another doctor.

It is also helpful for patients to review their background with family members. Was their birth difficult or traumatic? Did they have any seizures with high fevers in infancy or early childhood? Did they ever have a head injury? If so, did they lose consciousness after the injury? If consciousness was lost, how long did it last and were they taken to a hospital? Did they ever have meningitis, an infection of the membranes around the brain and spinal cord (bacterial meningitis is life threatening, viral meningitis is relatively mild), or encephalitis, a serious viral infection of the brain? Has anyone in the family had epilepsy or any other neurological disorder, or a disorder associated with loss of consciousness?

THE PHYSICAL EXAMINATION

Because seizures may result from medical disorders, doctors consider the physical examination an important part of the first consultation. The physical examination, together with laboratory studies, can tell the doctor whether or not the liver, kidney, and other organ systems are functioning properly. For persons who have seizures and medical disorders such as hyperthyroidism or kidney disease, the neurologist may let the primary physician know about the seizures for several reasons. First, the primary physician may have insights as to the cause of the seizures. Second, if an antiepileptic drug is recommended, the doctors need to discuss the possibility that it will interact with medication taken for the medical disorder.

THE NEUROLOGICAL EXAMINATION

Identifying whether there is an area of brain dysfunction is the essence of the neurological examination. The neurologist will question the patient about mental functions such as the ability to remember words, calculate, and name objects, and will then systematically assess his or her neurological function through tests of motor (muscle) and sensory functions, reflexes, walking, and coordination.

Doctors usually first perform a brief screening neurological examination, particularly in someone who is able to give the medical history. In some cases, a more detailed examination is required to define patterns of weakness or sensory loss. For persons with obvious language or intellectual disorders, a detailed neuropsychological assessment may be performed to help define the deficits and suggest cognitive or speech therapy.

A brief screening examination is also often done during follow-up visits to see if there is any change in neurological function. If the patient has slurred speech, impaired concentration, difficulty walking a straight line with heels touching the toes, jerking eye movements when the eyes are directed toward the left or right side, or trembling when the arms are outstretched, the dosage of antiepileptic drug may need to be reduced. Follow-up examinations are usually quite brief. After the initial examination, the doctor is only looking for minor changes that may be present, especially if there are no new complaints. Therefore, the doctor's time is often better spent listening than examining.

THE EEG

The EEG is the most specific test for diagnosing epilepsy, because it records the electrical activity of the brain. Electrodes are applied to the patient's scalp with paste to hold them in place. The electrodes are connected by wires to an electrical box, which in turn is connected to an EEG machine (Fig. 10). The EEG machine records the brain's electrical activity on paper as a series of squiggles called traces (Fig. 11); each trace corresponds to a different region of the brain. The wires can only record electrical activity; they do not deliver any electrical current to the scalp.

The EEG shows well-defined patterns of normal or abnormal brain electrical activity. Abnormal patterns may be either nonspecific or specific. "Nonspecific" refers to patterns that may be seen in a number of different conditions; for example, certain waves may be seen after head trauma, stroke, brain tumor, or seizures. "Slowing," in which the rhythm of the brain waves is slower than the rhythm that would be expected for the pa-

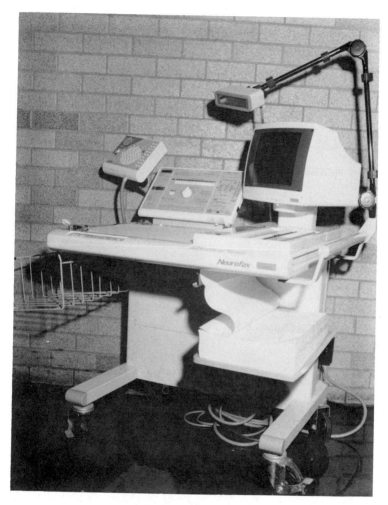

FIGURE 10. An EEG machine.

tient's age, is a nonspecific pattern. "Specific" refers to patterns that indicate a tendency toward seizures, as in "epilepsy waves" (spikes, sharp waves, and spike-and-wave discharges). Spikes and sharp waves occurring in a local area of the brain, such as the left temporal lobe, are markers of partial epilepsy (Fig. 12). Spike-and-wave discharges occurring in a widespread area over both cerebral hemispheres, and beginning simultaneously over both hemispheres, are markers of primary generalized epilepsy (Fig. 13). In some cases, actual seizures may be recorded during the EEG, particularly in chil-

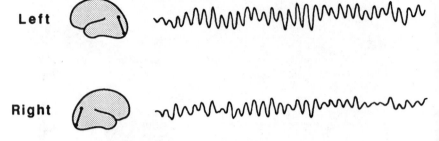

FIGURE 11. EEG traces from a person without epilepsy at rest.

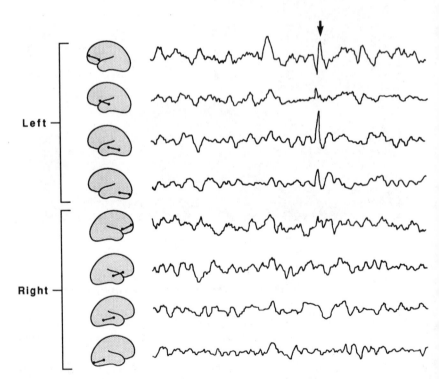

FIGURE 12. EEG traces of spikes and sharp waves (epilepsy waves) from the left temporal lobe of a person with partial epilepsy; traces from the right temporal lobe are normal.

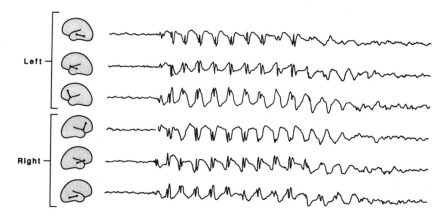

Left

Right

FIGURE 13. EEG traces of spike-and-wave discharges from a person with primary generalized epilepsy.

dren with absence seizures who are asked to breath deeply (hyperventilate) during the test.

A person with epilepsy may have a normal EEG. An EEG usually records the brain activity occurring between seizures, which is called interictal activity ("ictal" means seizure). The interictal activity may be normal if the brain activity is truly normal during the recording session or if the areas of abnormality are deep in the brain and "outside the reach" of EEG electrodes on the scalp. Several things can be done to increase the chances of finding an abnormality on the EEG: the EEG can be recorded during wakefulness and sleep (sometimes a sleeping pill can be used), after sleep deprivation (lack of sleep can cause epilepsy waves on the EEG), with 3 to 5 minutes of deep breathing (hyperventilation), with flashing lights, with special electrodes, or for prolonged periods.

The EEG is a safe and painless procedure. The actual recording usually lasts only 20 to 40 minutes, but the time needed to prepare for it often takes 40 to 50 minutes. Thus, the EEG procedure usually takes 1 hour to 1½ hours. The test is performed by an EEG technologist (see Chapter 7). The patient can help by washing his or her hair the night before the test, but he or she should avoid using conditioners, hair creams, sprays, or styling gels.

Routine EEG

The routine EEG is the most common test for epilepsy. The EEG technologist first measures the patient's head so that the electrodes, which are small, metal, cup-shaped disks attached to wires, can be placed in the correct position. The wax crayon used to mark the points on the scalp can be easily washed off later. Next, the technologist applies the electrodes, usually using a paste that holds them in place for several hours. The technologist often scrubs each position on the scalp with a mild abrasive cream before applying the electrodes. This will help improve the quality of the recording. The electrodes only record the brain waves. They do not stimulate the head with electricity, and pose no danger to the patient. The EEG machine then records the brain waves on paper as a series of squiggly lines called traces. The use of computerized, paperless EEGs will probably become more common during the next decade.

The patient may fall asleep briefly during a routine EEG, because the room is quiet and often dimly lit. That is fine and is often helpful, because an EEG obtained during both wakefulness and sleep may provide extra information. During the EEG, the technologist may ask patients to open and close their eyes several times, to breath rapidly or deeply, and may also shine flashing lights into their eyes (photic stimulation). Patients who have a medical problem, such as asthma or heart disease, that makes it unsafe to hyperventilate should tell the EEG technologist or the doctor. In some cases, the doctor may ask the patient to stay up the entire night before the EEG is performed. This sleep deprivation can increase the likelihood that epilepsy waves will be recorded.

Obtaining an EEG in children is usually easy, but it can pose a significant challenge. In babies, it is helpful to time the EEG around naps. Electrodes can be applied while the mother holds the child; a bottle may help to calm the baby. Then the baby is allowed to sleep naturally. In some babies and young children, sedation is required to allow the technologist to apply the electrodes and to record sleep activity. Children have difficulty lying still during EEG recordings, and the doctors who interpret these studies must separate the waves caused by movement and muscle activity from the brain waves.

After the EEG recording is done, the technologist will remove the electrodes from the patient's scalp, and the patient is free to go home and wash the paste out of his or her hair. The paste is lanolin- or water-based, so it can be easily washed off. The doctor usually reads the EEG after the test is completed and the patient has left.

EEG with Special Electrodes

Depending on the information the doctor is trying to obtain, the use of special electrodes may be needed. Sphenoidal electrodes (see Chapter 11) are most often used during video-EEG monitoring studies on patients in the hospital (inpatients), but they may be used during studies on patients outside the hospital (outpatients).

In some cases, nasopharyngeal electrodes are used to record electrical activity from deep parts of the temporal and frontal lobes. These electrodes are plastic tubes with a wire inside, ending as a blunt metal tip. The electrodes are inserted through the nose and the metal tip is situated in the upper back part of the nose (the nasopharynx). As with other electrodes, nasopharyngeal electrodes are usually placed by the EEG technologist. There may be some discomfort while the electrodes are inserted and less discomfort while they are left in place during the study for approximately 20 to 30 minutes. Nasopharyngeal electrodes have been used less frequently during the past decade, because regular electrodes placed in front of and slightly above the ears can often provide the same information with no discomfort to the patient.

Ambulatory EEG

The brain's electrical activity fluctuates from second to second. The routine EEG provides a 20- to 40-minute sample of brain electrical activity, which is often sufficient. In some cases, however, the recording is normal or shows only minor, nonspecific findings. In such cases, a more prolonged recording that includes long periods of wakefulness and sleep is desired. For example, in some people, epilepsy waves may occur only once every 3 or 4 hours or only after 1 hour of sleep, and a routine EEG will almost always be normal.

The EEG can be recorded for 24 hours with a special recorder that is slightly larger than a small portable cassette player. This recorder permits a person to go about his or her normal routine while the EEG is recorded (Fig. 14). Because the electrodes must stay on the head for a longer time than in a routine EEG, a special glue called collodion is often used to keep them in place. The technologist can easily remove them with acetone or similar solutions. For persons with a full head of hair, the electrodes, which are less numerous than those used in a routine EEG, can be fairly well camouflaged. Even so, many persons prefer not to go to work or school with the electrodes on their scalp and the cassette recorder on their waist, with the wires running under or outside their shirt.

If the patient scratches his or her head, which may get itchy because of the electrodes, it can appear as abnormal activity on the EEG. Therefore, the patient is usually asked to keep a diary of his or her activities during the day. Most recorders have an "event" button for patients to press if they experience any of the symptoms for which they are being tested, such as episodes of feeling "spacy" or confused. A family member should press the button if the patient is unable to do it.

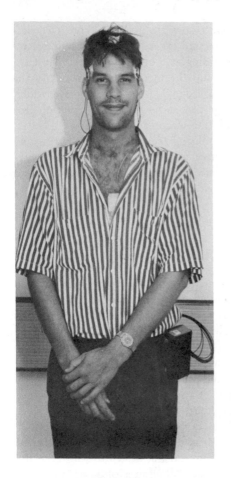

FIGURE 14. Recording the 24-hour ambulatory EEG. The cassette-type recorder, attached to the patient's belt, records the EEG signals from the electrodes on the patient's scalp while he pursues his daily activities.

Video-EEG Monitoring

Our understanding of epilepsy has been greatly advanced by video-EEG monitoring, which allows prolonged simultaneous recording of the patient's behavior and the EEG. The video and EEG images are usually presented on a split screen, permitting precise correlation between seizure activity in the brain and the patient's behavior during seizures (Fig. 15). Video-EEG recordings can be done on inpatients or outpatients. The electrodes used for video-EEG recording must also be glued to the scalp with collodion.

Inpatient monitoring allows the doctor to reduce and, in some cases, discontinue antiepileptic drugs safely under close supervision. Video-EEG is most helpful in determining whether spells with unusual features are actually epileptic, identifying the type of epileptic seizures, and pinpointing

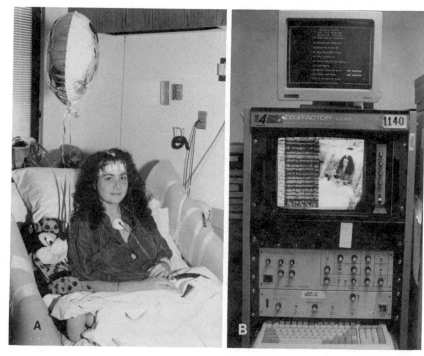

FIGURE 15. Video-EEG monitoring (*A*) A patient being monitored; a video camera (not shown) records the patient's activities, including any seizures that occur, and the EEG signals from the electrodes on her head are transmitted to an adjoining monitor. (*B*) The patient's seizure and EEG are recorded simultaneously and shown as a split-screen display on a television monitor.

the region of the brain from which the seizures begin. The last is a critical step in the assessment of a patient for possible epilepsy surgery.

A patient who is going to have video-EEG monitoring should bring clothing to the hospital that can be buttoned, not pullovers. The patient should also bring reading materials and things to keep busy, as a prolonged hospital stay for monitoring can be boring.

NEUROIMAGING OF THE BRAIN

Neuroimaging provides pictures of the brain. The most commonly used neuroimaging tests obtained in persons with epilepsy are computed tomography (CT) and magnetic resonance imaging (MRI) of the head. These tests produce pictures, or scans, of the brain. Like a photograph that shows the surface features of the face, CT or MRI of the head shows the anatomy of the skin, nose, mouth, skull, and brain. Doctors obtain a CT or MRI scan to determine if there is an abnormality in the structure of the brain such as excess spinal fluid (hydrocephalus), scar tissue, or a tangle of blood vessels (vascular malformation) that may be causing the epilepsy.

There are no absolute rules on which persons with epilepsy should be studied with a CT or MRI scan. In general, a CT or MRI scan should be obtained when a child or adult has had one or more seizures for which the cause is unknown. There are several important exceptions to this rule. First, if the cause of the seizures is known but has the potential to change, such as a benign tumor or a vascular malformation, or if the cause is suspected but indefinite, such as a mild or moderate head injury occurring a year before the first seizure, a CT or MRI scan should be considered. If someone has a benign tumor or other brain abnormality, follow-up scans may be indicated. Second, if a person has had epilepsy for more than a decade and has normal results on the neurological examination, some doctors do not recommend a CT or MRI scan, but others will, because the treatment may depend on the findings. If a patient with partial seizures previously had a normal CT scan but the seizures persist, an MRI scan may provide additional, helpful information. For patients with certain well-defined epilepsy syndromes such as absence seizures, juvenile myoclonic epilepsy, or benign rolandic epilepsy, many doctors will not order a CT or MRI scan, because the results are almost always normal or unrelated to epilepsy.

Other neuroimaging methods include single-photon emission computed tomography (SPECT) and positron emission tomography (PET). SPECT shows images of how much blood flows through different parts of the brain. PET shows images of how much sugar (glucose) or oxygen is metabolized, or used up, by various areas of the brain. Whereas CT and MRI show the brain's structure, or how it looks, SPECT and PET show its function, or how it works.

Computed Tomography

CT was first introduced in the United States in the early 1970s and has revolutionized the practice of neurology and neurosurgery. CT scans expose the patient to radiation, although the amount is low and the procedure is safe, even if it needs to be repeated several times over the years. The scanner is a large machine, but the patient's head is not in as confined a space as with MRI. Those who experience claustrophobia usually do not have problems with CT, but they may with MRI. The CT is normal in the majority of persons with epilepsy (Fig. 16). Brain abnormalities that might be de-

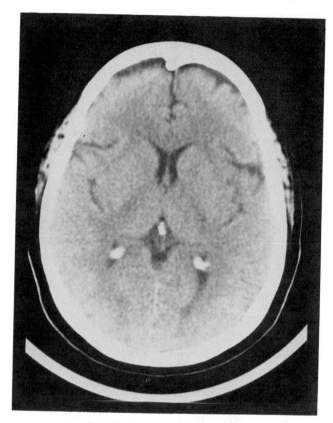

FIGURE 16. CT scan of the brain.

tected are atrophy (a decrease in brain substance), scar tissue, abnormal blood vessels or spinal fluid circulation, or tumors.

Magnetic Resonance Imaging

MRI was first introduced in the United States in the early 1980s and has further revolutionized the practice of neurology and neurosurgery. MRI is the most important neuroimaging test in epilepsy, because it shows even more details of the brain's structure than CT. The MRI does not use x-rays, but rather uses a powerful magnet that changes the spin on atomic particles that are normally part of the body, and then measures the changes in the magnetic field as the particles resume their previous course. The

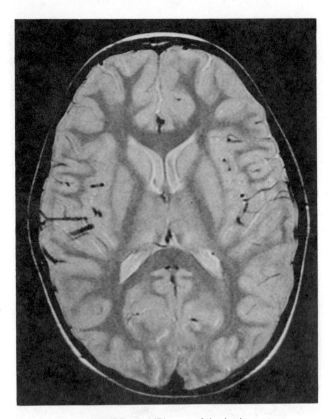

FIGURE 17. MRI scan of the brain.

patient does not feel anything. The images are a remarkably accurate representation of the brain's structure (Fig. 17). MRI is extremely helpful for identifying brain scar tissue, small brain tumors, and changes in the brain's white matter.

Although the MRI is safe and painless, most MRI machines require that the person's head and upper body be placed in a very confined space. Persons with claustrophobia (fear of small places), and many who never knew they were claustrophobic, may become frightened and uncooperative when they see the confinement required for the test. In such cases, medications for relaxation can be administered (children often require medications to put them to sleep), or a newer type of scanner that is not so confining can be used.

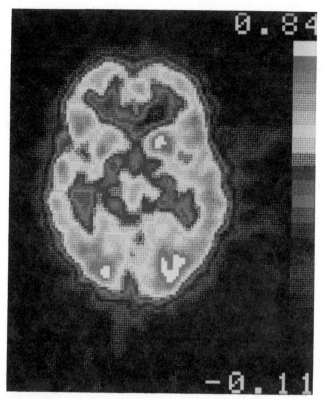

FIGURE 18. PET scan of the brain. PET scans use different colors (not shown) to reveal how well various areas of the brain metabolize oxygen or sugar (glucose). This metabolism is related to brain function. In this scan, for instance, a difference is apparent between the functioning of the right and left temporal and parietal lobes.

Single-Photon Emission Computed Tomography

SPECT shows the blood flow in the brain. A safe, very low strength radioactive compound is injected into the patient's arm, and the particles emitted by the compound are measured. The more blood that flows through a certain area, the more particles are emitted. This test is readily available in most hospitals, but its use as a *routine* test in patients with epilepsy is unjustified. SPECT scans obtained between seizures, or interictally, may show changes in brain blood flow; decreased flow is sometimes found in the area from which seizures arise, but the findings may be misleading. In patients undergoing assessment for epilepsy surgery, SPECT scans obtained during or immediately after a seizure may be more helpful than interictal scans in identifying the brain area from which the seizures arise.

Positron Emission Tomography

PET, which shows the brain's metabolism of oxygen or sugar (glucose), also requires the injection of a very low dose of a radioactive compound. This test is safe and helpful in identifying the area from which partial seizures arise, and may be performed in the period between seizures, the interictal period. PET scans (Fig. 18) are expensive, and currently there are problems with reimbursement by many insurance carriers. Localizing the seizure focus for epilepsy surgery is the most clearly defined clinical use of PET, and many insurance carriers are now reimbursing for this use when it is medically justified.

Ultrasonography

Although most people think of ultrasound as a test to observe the development of babies in the womb, it is also used to diagnose medical and neurological disorders. Ultrasonography may identify brain abnormalities in babies with neurological disorders, including seizures. Because ultrasonography uses only sound waves, it is very safe and can be performed easily in either a newborn intensive care unit or in an outpatient setting. The skull of the newborn has areas where the bones have not yet come together. These areas (fontanelles) permit the sound waves access to study the brain.

Ultrasonography can detect excessive spinal fluid (hydrocephalus) or blood (hemorrhage) in the brain. In some cases, a CT or MRI scan is obtained after ultrasonography to study the abnormality further, or if the ultrasonography test results are normal, to search for abnormalities that the test may have missed.

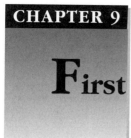

CHAPTER 9

First Aid for Seizures

A tonic-clonic seizure is frightening, but a single, brief seizure is rarely dangerous to the person having the seizure, and never dangerous to anyone else, except possibly a baby the person may be caring for. If the person has a definite history of tonic-clonic seizures, it is rarely necessary to visit the emergency room or doctor's office after a seizure unless there is evidence or suspicion of an injury. If this is the person's first tonic-clonic seizure, however, a prompt consultation with a doctor is essential. A person with epilepsy should wear a medical-alert bracelet or necklace that gives the telephone numbers of the doctor, the pharmacist, and the person to call in case of an emergency. It can help avoid unnecessary actions or costs if a seizure occurs in a public place. The doctor or pharmacist usually knows where these items can be obtained.

Prolonged, continuous, or repetitive tonic-clonic seizures deserve an urgent call for help. The patient is best transported to a medical facility by ambulance, as he or she may need oxygen, and a convulsion in a family member's car can be dangerous for everyone involved. How long does a seizure have to last to warrant a call for help? There is no absolute answer. This issue is worth discussing with the doctor. In general, if the actual convulsion lasts more than 5 to 10 minutes, or if the need for assistance is uncertain, it is best to call for help.

GENERALIZED TONIC-CLONIC SEIZURES

Generalized tonic-clonic (grand mal) seizures are convulsive seizures. They are frightening to watch. The person loses consciousness, falls, stiffens (tonic portion of the seizure), and jerks (clonic portion of the seizure). Although the convulsive seizure appears painful, the person is not conscious during the seizure and, therefore, is unaware of what is happening. After the seizure, however, there may be discomfort caused by tongue biting, muscle soreness, and bruises from falling. The attack is often followed by confusion and tiredness, in what is called the postictal period. The seizure usually lasts less than 4 minutes, but the time can seem like an eternity to family members or friends who are watching it.

Seizures may cause bruises, cuts, sprains, or a bitten tongue, but rarely cause broken or dislocated bones or other more serious problems. For those who are at risk of tonic-clonic seizures, first-aid guidelines should be known to persons with whom they spend a good amount of time. The following are some first-aid guidelines for a tonic-clonic seizure:

- Stay calm. Anxiety and fear are not helpful. Easy to say, hard to do.
- Help the person lie down, and place something soft under the head and neck. Keep the person, especially the head, away from sharp or hard objects such as the corner of a table.
- Roll the person on his or her side with the head and mouth angled toward the ground so that any excessive saliva or fluids will not accidentally be swallowed or inhaled. This position will also prevent the tongue from falling back and blocking the airway.
- Loosen all tight clothing by unfastening top shirt buttons, belts, and skirt or pant buttons. Remove any eyeglasses or tight neck chains. Do not worry about contact lenses. The eye can be easily scratched by trying to remove the small lens during a tonic-clonic seizure.
- Do not hold the person down; you may cause a bone dislocation or get injured yourself.
- Do not put anything in the person's mouth. The tongue cannot be swallowed during a seizure. A finger or object can be bitten off, and the person can choke on the fragment remaining in the mouth. The muscles for chewing are very strong.
- After the seizure is over, do not try to restrain the person; he or she may be confused, and restraint may provoke agitation and a violent reaction. Try to keep the person in a safe environment. Walking around is permissible, unless the person is near a street, stairs, or other potentially dangerous place.
- Avoid giving the person pills, beverages, or food until he or she is fully alert.
- Stay with the person until he or she is fully alert and oriented. Be careful. The person may say he or she is fine, but still be quite confused. Ask a series of questions that require more than a yes or no answer; for example, ask "What is your address?" and "What is the date?"
- If this is the person's first tonic-clonic seizure, or if the seizure lasts longer than 5 minutes, call an ambulance.

- During and after the seizure, keep onlookers away. One or two people can be responsible for first aid. Additional people often add confusion. Further, it is embarrassing for the person to awaken to a crowd of people.

After the seizure, the person may complain of discomfort in the mouth from tongue or cheek biting, or in the back related to the muscular contractions or a fall. Acetaminophen (Tylenol) is helpful for minor pains. In the case of severe back pain, the person should be seen by a doctor, because there is the possibility of a fracture, which is usually treated conservatively with rest. Fever may occur after a seizure. In most instances, the rise in temperature results from the muscle activity and the effects of the seizure. When the fever is unusually high (over 102°F), persists more than 6 hours, or develops more than 3 hours after a seizure, it is wise to consult with a doctor. In some cases, during the seizure, secretions pass down the respiratory tract and cause pneumonia.

COMPLEX PARTIAL SEIZURES

Complex partial seizures (temporal lobe seizures or psychomotor seizures) are called "complex" because they cause an impairment of consciousness and "partial" because they begin in a restricted region of the brain. Most complex partial seizures are associated with some automatic behaviors, termed automatisms (see Chapter 3).

The chance of bodily injury during a complex partial seizure is small. Single and brief complex partial seizures do not damage the brain. We do not know whether prolonged or repetitive complex partial seizures cause brain injury, but even mild problems, such as slight but persistent memory losses, are rare.

During a complex partial seizure, the person usually becomes motionless and stares or makes automatic movements such as fumbling movements of the hands. When someone has a complex partial seizure, speak quietly and in a reassuring manner, because some persons have only partial impairment of consciousness and can react to emotional or physical stimulation. Do not yell at the person, or restrain him or her unless absolutely necessary, which is rare. The most important aspect of first aid during a complex partial seizure is to keep the person safe from harm. For example, burns can occur when someone unknowingly touches or falls on a hot object. During and after some complex partial seizures, the person may walk or, in rare cases, run. When this occurs where there is dangerous equipment, on a busy city street, near train tracks, or near high places such as a construction site, there is a potential for serious injury.

Other behaviors during complex partial seizures may cause concern, but are not dangerous to the patient or other people. These include screaming, kicking, running, ripping up papers, disrobing, sexual-like movements, and, rarely, masturbation. If someone is known to have unusual automatisms, he or she should be led in a quiet and reassuring manner, not forcibly, out of public places, such as an office or store. In individual cases, specific strategies can be used to minimize the embarrassing effects of unusual complex partial seizures.

The greatest danger of an unexpected seizure occurs when the person is driving a car or operating dangerous equipment. These situations are best avoided by persons with seizures that impair consciousness or control of movement. In some cases, potentially dangerous equipment can be used safely if adequate precautions are taken.

First aid for someone having a complex partial seizure is simple: keep the person away from dangerous situations, but use restraints only if it is necessary for his or her safety.

CHAPTER 10

Antiepileptic Drug Therapy

Antiepileptic drugs are the principal therapy for epilepsy. Choosing the correct drug depends on making an accurate diagnosis of epilepsy. In addition, discussions between the patient and the doctor about the pros and cons of the different drugs can influence drug choice. For example, relevant issues include how often the medication has to be taken (most patients prefer once or twice a day rather than three or four times), the drug's adverse effects, the drug's cost, and the potential risks for the baby if a woman becomes pregnant while taking the drug.

Although antiepileptic drugs effectively control seizures in most people, they do not cure epilepsy. People often remark, "These drugs don't really treat or cure the epilepsy but just control the condition. They are like Band-Aids." There is a large element of truth in that statement. If scar tissue or an abnormal group of blood vessels in the brain causes seizures, antiepileptic drugs will surely not repair these structural problems. These medications suppress the seizures but do not "fix" the basic problem. However, the longer someone is seizure-free while taking medications, the better the chances he or she will remain seizure-free when the medications are stopped.

TIME REQUIRED FOR ANTIEPILEPTIC DRUGS TO WORK

A medication that is taken by mouth has to pass through the stomach and is absorbed in the small intestine. Once absorbed, it passes to the liver, where a fraction of the drug is metabolized, or broken down, and then passes into the bloodstream, eventually, in the case of antiepileptic drugs, reaching the brain. Most drugs are metabolized by the liver but some are mainly excreted in an unchanged form by the kidneys.

If a certain dosage of medication is taken, it will reach a peak, or maximum level, in the blood 30 minutes to 6 hours later. The time between taking the medication and reaching the peak level depends on the specific drug and its form (liquid, tablet, capsule, slow-release form), and, in some cases, the food consumed before taking it. The pharmacology of selected antiepileptic drugs when used in monotherapy (one-drug therapy) is summarized in Table 2.

The time required for the drug's concentration in the blood to become half the peak level is referred to as the drug's *half-life.* Some drugs, such as carbamazepine and valproate, have a relatively short half-life; some, such as

TABLE 2. **CHARACTERISTICS OF SELECTED ANTIEPILEPTIC DRUGS WHEN USED ALONE**

Drug	Daily Dose (mg/kg of Patient's Weight)	Time to Peak Blood Level (hours)	Therapeutic Blood Levels (μg/mL)	Half-life (hours)	Equilibrium Period (Days)
Carbamazepine[a]	10–25	2–12	5–12	8–25	2–6[b]
Clonazepam[c]	0.05–0.2[d] 0.1–0.25[e]	1–4	20–80 (ng/mL)	15–40	3–10
Ethosuximide[c]	15–60	1–4	50–100	25–70[f]	5–18
Felbamate[c]	15–60	1–4	?(25–100)	14–20	4–7
Gabapentin[c]	10–30	2–4	?(2–4)	5–7	2–5
Lamotrigine[c]	5–10	2–4	0.5–3.0	7–60[g]	9–20
Phenobarbital	4–10[d] 1.5–5[e]	2–12	12–40	40–140	10–30
Phenytoin	5–10	4–8	10–20	12–48	4–17
Primidone	2–5 10–20	5–18	5–10	2–6	
Valproate[c]	10–60	2–8 1–3[h]	50–140	8–16	1–4

[a]Active metabolites (see Appendix 1 for definition).
[b]Autoinduction of liver enzymes (see Appendix 1 for definition) results in a progressive decline of blood carbamazepine levels 1 to 10 weeks after the drug is started; therefore, a steady-state blood level obtained at week 6 may be lower than one obtained at the end of week 1.
[c]In general, when these drugs are coadministered with carbamazepine, phenobarbital, phenytoin, or primidone, their blood level is lower and their half-life is shorter.
[d]Dose for young children.
[e]Dose for older children and adults.
[f]Half-life is higher in adults than in children.
[g]Valproate prolongs the half-life of lamotrigine.
[h]After oral dose of valproic acid syrup (Depakene).

phenytoin, have an intermediate half-life, and some, such as phenobarbital, have a long half-life. The goal with antiepileptic drugs is to maintain a relatively constant level in the blood. Drugs with longer half-lives have more stable blood levels and need to be taken less frequently. Theoretically, phenobarbital could be given every other day. However, patients tend to forget to take their medication if they do not take it every day, and adverse effects are more likely to occur after taking a single large dose every other day. Drugs with short half-lives, on the other hand, are ideally taken several times a day to prevent adverse effects during periods of high blood levels and seizures during periods of low levels.

Steady state (equilibrium) refers to the condition in a person who is taking a constant amount of medication and whose blood drug levels are fairly constant. In most cases, it takes fives times longer than the half-life of the drug to attain equilibrium. Defined another way, there is a steady state when the amount of drug taken and the amount of drug being metabolized and excreted are equal.

Even when someone has been on a drug for a long time, and the blood levels of the drug are in equilibrium, the levels will fluctuate over the course of the day. Depending on the rate of absorption of the drug and the factors that influence the absorption rate (for example, taking some drugs after meals slows absorption), there will be peaks in the blood level within hours after the drug is taken and troughs (low points) shortly before or immediately after a dose is taken, especially if there is a long interval between doses. Fluctuations between the peak level and the trough level depend mainly on the half-life of the drug (drugs with short half-lives have greater fluctuations) and the number of times the medication is taken daily (frequent doses of drugs with short half-lives tend to stabilize the levels, minimizing the fluctuations between peak and trough levels). *Dose-related adverse effects* are more likely to occur at times of peak levels. A seizure is more likely to occur at times of trough levels.

Drugs are fully effective when their blood levels have reached a steady state. However, for some drugs, such as carbamazepine, the liver will break down the drug more rapidly after someone has been taking it for several weeks. Therefore, a carbamazepine level measured 6 weeks after the start of therapy is often lower than a level measured 3 weeks after the start of therapy. This effect, known as *autoinduction*, a process in which a drug induces an increase in its own metabolism, stabilizes by 8 to 12 weeks after the start of therapy.

Although antiepileptic drugs work well for most persons in low to moderate doses, some persons do not tolerate the medications, or their seizures cannot be controlled even with high doses of one or more drugs. Therefore, antiepileptic drug therapy must be individualized.

PRINCIPLES AND GOALS OF DRUG THERAPY

The goals of antiepileptic drug therapy are very simple: no seizures, no adverse effects. In many persons, those goals can be easily reached, but in many others the balance between seizure control and adverse effects is delicate. This is why communication between the doctor and patient is critical. Some patients err in accepting troublesome adverse effects because of a fear that the doctor will reduce the medication and a seizure will occur or because of a belief that the adverse effects of medication are a necessary evil. When a patient complains of abdominal discomfort and nausea, depression, lack of energy, or feeling "spaced out" while taking low doses of a medication and is found to have a low or "therapeutic" blood level of the drug, the doctor may incorrectly conclude that the complaints are psychological or related to the seizures. Unfortunately, some persons are extremely sensitive to medications and may have troublesome adverse effects even though their blood drug levels are low. On the other hand, some persons tend to blame every minor problem on a new drug. Open discussions between the patient and the doctor about what to expect, what is tolerable, what is experienced, and the impact of both adverse effects and seizures on the quality of life is the best way to manage drug therapy.

Changes in medications should be done systematically and be limited to one drug at a time whenever possible. This strategy makes it possible to establish a relationship between a change and an effect such as improved seizure control or reduction of an adverse effect.

The vast majority of antiepileptic drugs are not addictive. Many patients fear that once they start taking a medication, they will become "hooked." There is no basis for this fear. The benzodiazepines are the only antiepileptic drugs with addictive potential. The only benzodiazepines that are commonly used as antiepileptic drugs are clonazepam and clorazepate. (See color illustrations immediately following the Contents section.) These drugs can be successfully discontinued, but it must be done gradually to avoid seizures. Addiction to the benzodiazepines in persons with epilepsy is extremely rare. More often, as the drugs are gradually tapered, some persons experience mild and unpleasant withdrawal symptoms such as rapid heart rate, sweating, and anxiety.

FIRST SEIZURES—TO TREAT OR NOT TO TREAT?

A first seizure can be terrifying. At the time, it may seem to change the person's life permanently. Knowledge and understanding of epilepsy will remove much of the fear concerning the risk of having another seizure and allay the anxiety and feelings of vulnerability that arise with the loss of control and unpredictability of a seizure. Other concerns are related to the diagnosis of epilepsy and the real and perceived stigma associated with it, the possibility of physical injury, the possible loss of driving privileges, employment issues, embarrassment, and the effects of antiepileptic drugs on the patient and on the fetus in women of childbearing age. The fact is, however, that the vast majority of persons who have a single seizure do extremely well.

This discussion of first seizures applies only to tonic-clonic (convulsive) seizures. As a rule, when a single absence seizure is reported and confirmed by the typical electroencephalogram (EEG) pattern, the child usually has had many other staring spells, and treatment is usually recommended. Similarly, with partial seizures, a person may commonly have had several partial seizures, but one relatively prominent episode (or a convulsion) has finally brought him or her to the doctor. If the diagnosis of a partial seizure is uncertain and the neuroimaging and EEG studies are normal or do not show findings suggestive of epilepsy, most doctors would not prescribe antiepileptic drugs. If a partial seizure has definitely occurred, most doctors recommend treatment because there is a high probability of recurrence. The exception is with benign rolandic epilepsy, in which case some experts recommend treatment and others do not (see Chapter 4).

There is no simple answer as to whether to treat or not treat a single generalized tonic-clonic seizure. The chance of seizure recurrence after a single seizure varies from 16% to 61%, depending on the patient and the circumstances surrounding the seizure. A person may not require treatment if the results of the neurological examination and neuroimaging studies are normal, provocative factors such as sleep deprivation or excessive alcohol intake can be eliminated, the EEG is normal, the seizure occurred during sleep, and there is no family history of epilepsy. Nevertheless, some decisions about treatment are more difficult than others. A 10-year-old child with a single nocturnal seizure who has normal neurological examination results and a normal magnetic resonance imaging (MRI) scan and EEG should probably not receive medication. However, a 30-year-old saleswoman who has a single daytime convulsion and abundant epilepsy activity on the EEG and conforms with most of the guidelines for a decision not to treat, but who supports two children and drives hundreds of miles each week should probably be treated. Most patients fall between these two extremes. The decision should be based on the chances of another seizure occurring, the patient's lifestyle, the adverse effects of the medications, and the plan for discontinuing medications if seizures do not recur after a period of time.

Selecting a conservative plan for treating the seizures with antiepileptic drugs creates another set of difficult questions. Can the person drive immediately after medications are started, after therapeutic blood drug levels are reached, or after a period of time, such as 3 to 12 months? Assuming the seizures do not recur during treatment, how long should treatment last? Can driving resume when the medications are tapered off and discontinued? Many of these are legal questions, and the laws and regulations vary in each state.

PRIMARY ANTIEPILEPTIC DRUGS

For each type of seizure, one or more drugs are recommended as a first-line, or *primary*, treatment (Table 3). A drug is considered a primary treatment based on its effectiveness in controlling seizures and its profile of adverse effects. Because some medications are relatively specific for certain seizure types and can actually worsen other seizure types, correct seizure classification is essential (see Table 1). In prescribing antiepileptic drugs, doctors usually start with only a single drug, beginning with a low dose and increasing it slowly unless the patient's condition requires a more rapid build-up. The correct dosage is based on how well the patient is doing (Are seizures controlled? Are there adverse effects?) not on the amount of drug in the patient's blood.

In most patients, a single primary antiepileptic drug provides the best balance between seizure control and adverse effects. Unfortunately, some patients are treated with three or more antiepileptic drugs, at moderate doses, and they continue to have both seizures and troublesome adverse effects. This usually is not the best possible therapy. If seizures recur while a patient is taking a single medication that causes no adverse effects, it is usually best to increase the dose until seizures are controlled or adverse effects develop. A rapid increase in the dose can cause adverse effects and unnecessarily lead the patient and doctor to feel that the extreme fatigue, inability to concentrate, feeling like a "zombie," or other problems are inevitable effects of the drug. With many drugs, the key to patient tolerance is a *gradual* increase in the dosage.

Antiepileptic drugs vary considerably in how they work, how long they remain in the blood (half-life), and how they should be taken. It is important that patients not experiment with varying the schedule of their medications without first discussing the proposed changes with the doctor. Because some medications such as carbamazepine and valproate have relatively short half-lives, they almost always have to be taken more than once

TABLE 3. PRIMARY AND SECONDARY ANTIEPILEPTIC DRUGS* FOR DIFFERENT TYPES OF SEIZURES

Seizure Type	Primary Drug	Secondary Drug
Primary Generalized Seizures		
Absence seizures (typical and atypical)	Ethosuximide, valproate	Clonazepam
Myoclonic seizures	Valproate	Acetazolamide, clonazepam, mephobarbital, phenobarbital, primidone
Tonic-clonic seizures	Phenytoin, valproate	Carbamazepine, mephobarbital, phenobarbital, primidone
Atonic seizures	Felbamate, valproate	Clonazepam, phenobarbital
Partial Seizures		
Simple and complex partial seizures	Carbamazepine, phenytoin	Felbamate, gabapentin, lamotrigine, mephobarbital, phenobarbital, primidone, valproate
Secondary generalized tonic-clonic seizures	Carbamazepine, phenytoin	Felbamate, gabapentin, lamotrigine, mephobarbital, phenobarbital, primidone, valproate

*Drugs are listed in alphabetical order, not in order of preferred use.

a day. There are two reasons for spreading medications out over the day: improved seizure control and reduction of dose-related adverse effects.

In an ideal world, medication would be given only once a day and released in the body slowly. Unfortunately, steady-release antiepileptic drugs are not widely available, and we must work with the drugs we have. This means that it is often necessary to take a drug two to four times a day to prevent breakthrough seizures from low blood drug levels many hours after the last dose, or adverse effects from high blood drug levels, often within hours of a dose. Adverse effects are also common when a person forgets a dose and doubles up on the medication or takes two doses close together.

The schedule for taking medication should be flexible and adapted to the patient's lifestyle. In most cases, it is easy for the doctor and patient to work out a schedule that is convenient, minimizes adverse effects, and controls seizures. There are several common problems associated with taking antiepileptic drugs, such as forgetting a dose. For example, the patient may oversleep and, in the rush to get to work or school on time, forget the morning medication, or he or she may simply fall asleep before taking the bedtime dose. The doctor can advise the patient on what to do if a dose of medication is forgotten. With long-acting drugs such as phenytoin and phenobarbital, it is usually fine to take the medication as soon as the missed dose is remembered, and then continue on with the usual schedule. With shorter-acting drugs, it is important to make up the missed dose as soon as possible, because blood drug levels will decline rather quickly. However, two doses should not be taken too close together, as adverse effects are likely to occur. Medications with short half-lives, such as carbamazepine and valproate, should be taken after meals and at bedtime to avoid nausea, tiredness, or visual problems.

SECONDARY ANTIEPILEPTIC DRUGS

The development of a rash, a serious reduction in the number of white blood cells (which fight infection), or other problems may force the doctor to stop the primary antiepileptic drugs. In these cases, as well as those in which the primary medications fail to control seizures, a *secondary* drug (see Table 3) may be added to the regimen or used alone. When a medication is added to another medication, it is sometimes referred to as *adjunct therapy*. Although some drugs are called secondary because they tend to have fewer good and more bad effects than the primary drugs, secondary drugs can be extremely effective in certain instances and are well tolerated by some patients.

ADVERSE EFFECTS OF ANTIEPILEPTIC DRUGS

Doctors and patients with epilepsy see medical care from different perspectives. The doctor would like to see the patient regularly, have the patient take medication regularly, and have the patient's seizures well controlled. The patient would like never to see a doctor, never to take a pill, and have the seizures go away. In general, the patient finds taking pills is even worse than seeing a doctor.

Aside from their inconvenience and expense, antiepileptic drugs also cause adverse effects (Table 4). However, most persons can take a single

TABLE 4. MAJOR ADVERSE EFFECTS OF COMMONLY USED ANTIEPILEPTIC DRUGS

Drug	Dose-Related Adverse Effects*	Rare Idiosyncratic Adverse Effects	Long-Term Adverse Effects
Carbamazepine	Nausea, vomiting, blurred or double vision, tiredness, dizziness, unsteadiness, memory problems, slurred speech, low sodium (hyponatremia), rash,[†] fever[†]	Very low white blood-cell count (WBC) or complete blood-cell count (CBC), liver damage, severe rash, hypersensitivity reaction	Low sodium, heart block (a blockage of electrical impulses in the heart)
Clonazepam	Tiredness, dizziness, unsteadiness, hyperactivity, irritability, drooling (children), nausea, loss of appetite	None	None
Ethosuximide	Nausea and vomiting, loss of appetite, weight loss, behavioral changes, tiredness, dizziness, earache	Very low white blood-cell count (WBC) or complete blood-cell count (CBC)	None
Phenobarbital, mephobarbital, and primidone	Tiredness, depression, hyperactivity, dizziness, memory problems, impotence, slurred speech, nausea, anemia, rash,[†] fever,[†] low calcium levels and bone loss	Liver damage, severe rash, hypersensitivity reaction	Soft tissue growths, rheumatological disorders (frozen shoulder, stiffening of fingers)
Phenytoin	Tiredness, dizziness, memory problems, rash, fever, gum overgrowth, growth of facial hair, anemia, acne, slurred speech, low calcium levels and bone loss	Liver damage, severe rash,[†] hypersensitivity reaction, behavioral changes	Nerve damage, possible cerebellar damage
Valproate	Nausea, vomiting, tiredness, weight gain, hair loss, tremor	Liver damage, very low platelet count, pancreatic inflammation, hearing loss, behavioral changes	Hair loss, hair texture change, menstrual irregularities, weight gain

*Some of the adverse effects (very low blood-cell or platelet counts, liver damage, hypersensitivity reactions, severe rash, pancreatic inflammation) are serious and potentially fatal.
[†]Rash and fever are common (3%–6% of patients) but not related to the dosage.

antiepileptic drug, when the dosage is properly adjusted, with only slight, well-tolerated adverse effects.

Before starting to take a medication, the patient should ask the doctor what to expect. During the first weeks of taking an antiepileptic drug, the patient may experience some fatigue, abdominal discomfort, dizziness, or blurred vision. If the medication is started at a low dosage and increased slowly, and the patient is aware of what to expect, he or she can usually tolerate the adverse effects, which will probably stop after several weeks or months, as tolerance develops.

The adverse effects may be related or unrelated to the dosage and blood level of the drug. They may be minor or severe, short-lasting and reversible, or long-lasting and potentially irreversible. Unpredictable adverse effects unrelated to the dosage or blood drug level are called *idiosyncratic*. Idiosyncratic adverse effects of antiepileptic drugs include rash, inflammation of the liver or pancreas, and a serious reduction in the number of white blood cells. If a rash develops after a new medication is prescribed, the doctor should be contacted immediately. Although rashes are usually rather trivial and may be unrelated to the drug, or begin to resolve shortly after the medication is discontinued, they may, in rare cases, progress to a life-threatening condition. In persons taking more than one drug, the one that was most recently started has probably caused the rash, although rashes may also be caused by viruses, bacteria, allergic reactions, and insect bites. In addition, persons who have excessive bleeding, abdominal pain and tenderness, hair loss, fever, unusual infections, or other unusual symptoms while taking a drug should promptly inform the doctor.

Dose-related adverse effects are more common than idiosyncratic effects. When the dosage of an antiepileptic drug is increased, the blood level of the drug may become too high for the person to tolerate and troublesome effects, called *toxicity*, will occur. It is often difficult to predict the exact dosage or blood level of a drug that will cause toxicity in a given person.

The overwhelming majority of medication adverse effects, including toxicity, are neither dangerous nor permanent. The doctor can usually alleviate abdominal discomfort, blurred vision, headache, or fatigue by lowering the dose, or, when necessary, stopping the medication altogether. These are short-term effects related to the amount of medication. Some other adverse effects of the medication can be serious. Some of the more serious risks are rashes that cause peeling of the skin, infection resulting from a low white blood-cell count, serious bleeding resulting from a low platelet count, and liver damage. Thankfully, life-threatening problems are extremely rare. Fewer than 2 people in 150,000 who take antiepileptic drugs will die as a result; the chance of dying in a motor vehicle accident is much

TABLE 5. ANTIEPILEPTIC DRUGS THAT MAY AGGRAVATE SEIZURES

Drug	Seizure Type Affected
Carbamazepine	Absence, myoclonic
Clonazepam	None
Ethosuximide	Myoclonic, tonic-clonic
Felbamate	None
Gabapentin	None
Lamotrigine	None
Phenobarbital	None
Phenytoin	Absence, myoclonic, tonic-clonic*
Primidone	None
Valproate	None

*Tonic-clonic seizures may become worse when the blood phenytoin level exceeds 45 µg per mL.

greater. In almost all cases, when a doctor recommends treatment, the benefits of antiepileptic drugs clearly outweigh the risks.

Almost all adverse effects of antiepileptic drugs are short-lasting. People often ask, "If I stay on this medication for 5 or 10 years, isn't it going to chew up my liver and insides?" The answer is no. Liver function can be easily monitored with blood tests, and if a problem develops, it is reversible in more than 99% of patients when the medication is stopped. That is also true for almost all other kinds of adverse effects. Long-lasting adverse effects, such as nerve damage from phenytoin, are uncommon.

In rare cases, antiepileptic drugs can actually worsen seizures (Table 5). Further, seizures may be more frequent when a person is tired, and in this case, antiepileptic drugs that cause sedation may occasionally aggravate seizures.

BLOOD TESTING AND MONITORING BLOOD LEVELS OF ANTIEPILEPTIC DRUGS

Blood tests should be done before the start of any antiepileptic drug so that they can be compared with later blood tests. The blood tests include measurements of electrolyte levels (chemicals in the blood such as sodium and potassium), liver and kidney function tests and blood-cell counts, and monitoring of antiepileptic drug levels. The frequency of testing varies considerably from doctor to doctor. In general, it is wise to have one or more blood tests done within several months of starting a new drug. The frequency with which subsequent blood tests need to be done depends on the specific drug. For patients who have been on the same drug for more than a year, and when the results of the routine laboratory studies have been normal or unchanged, it is reasonable to have testing done once a year or less often. If new problems arise, such as pain in the upper abdomen, or if seizures increase, blood tests may need to be rechecked.

During the past decade, there has been a trend toward monitoring blood levels of antiepileptic drugs less frequently. If the patient is feeling well and is seizure-free, the value of monitoring the blood drug level is questionable. For example, consider the case of a patient with well-controlled seizures whose blood drug level is not in the arbitrary "therapeutic range." Should the dosage be increased to raise the blood drug level? No, the doctor will usually be satisfied with good seizure control and treat the patient, not the blood level of the drug. In some cases, however, attaining a therapeutic blood drug level is critical.

ANTIEPILEPTIC DRUGS AND BIRTH CONTROL PILLS

Most women with epilepsy can take birth control pills without affecting their seizure control. Most women who start taking birth control pills will have no change in seizure control, some will have a slight improvement, and others will have a slight worsening. Some antiepileptic drugs increase the breakdown, or metabolism, of estrogen by the liver and, therefore, reduce the effectiveness of birth control pills. Carbamazepine, phenytoin, phenobarbital, and primidone make birth control pills less effective. If a sexually active woman is taking birth control pills and one of these antiepileptic drugs, she should be aware that her chances of getting pregnant are increased.

Breakthrough bleeding between menstrual periods is a clue that the effectiveness of birth control pills is reduced. However, the absence of breakthrough bleeding does not indicate that the woman has adequate contraceptive protection and will not become pregnant. It is often necessary to increase the estrogen content of the pill while a woman is taking one of these antiepileptic drugs. In addition, if a woman wants to reduce the risk of pregnancy, it may be wise to add, or change to, another method of contraception such as a barrier device (diaphragm or condom) with spermicide.

ANTIEPILEPTIC DRUGS AND ALCOHOL

Persons with epilepsy are less likely than others to use or abuse alcohol. This largely reflects warnings from doctors and pharmacists to abstain from or limit the use of alcohol. Alcohol does not seriously alter the effectiveness of antiepileptic drugs, but persons who drink alcoholic beverages while taking them may become intoxicated quickly. Many of the antiepileptic drugs have dose-related adverse effects similar to the effect of alcohol, including slurred speech, unsteadiness, dizziness, and tiredness. This can be especially dangerous when someone who takes antiepileptic drugs has several drinks, becomes intoxicated, and has to drive, supervise small children, or operate dangerous equipment. Another danger occurs when someone taking high doses of phenobarbital or primidone drinks a very large amount of alcohol quickly. In this case, the person could lapse into a coma or die.

Persons with epilepsy should not consume more than two alcoholic beverages per occasion; such consumption can be followed by a withdrawal state during which time seizures are more likely to occur.

INTERACTIONS OF ANTIEPILEPTIC DRUGS

A doctor caring for a person with epilepsy should know about *all* of the drugs the person is taking. Drug interactions are common and can be dangerous. Antiepileptic drugs interact with each other (Table 6) and with other drugs (Table 7), and other drugs interact with antiepileptic drugs (Table 8). Interactions between two antiepileptic drugs vary—some combinations cause the levels of both drugs to fall, some cause one level to fall and one level to rise, and some cause unpredictable effects. Some antiepileptic drugs can lower or raise the blood levels of other types of drugs. For example, a person taking carbamazepine who has an infection for which a doctor prescribes erythromycin should not take the erythromycin unless the carbamazepine dose is lowered, because it can lead to a marked increase in the blood carbamazepine level and severe, but reversible, adverse effects. In another example, phenytoin and warfarin, a blood thinner or anticoagulant, can interact and alter the adverse effects and effectiveness of each other.

No list of drug interactions is all-inclusive, as doctors and pharmacists continue to learn of interactions between existing medications and new ones. Therefore, the doctor or dentist who prescribes medication for a person with epilepsy should be aware that he or she is taking an antiepileptic drug. Similarly, the pharmacist or doctor should know about the use of over-the-counter medications, some of which can alter antiepileptic drug levels, cause seizures in someone who has never had a seizure, or increase seizure frequency in a person with epilepsy (Table 9).

TABLE 6. **INTERACTIONS OF ANTIEPILEPTIC DRUGS**

Drug	Drug Affected
Acetazolamide	↑Phenobarbital
Carbamazepine	↓↑Phenytoin
	↓Primidone (↑phenobarbital)
	↓Valproate
	↓Felbamate
	↓Clonazepam
	↓Ethosuximide
	↓Methsuximide
Clonazepam	↓Carbamazepine
	↑Primidone
Ethosuximide	↓Carbamazepine
Felbamate	↓Carbamazepine
	↑Carbamazepine epoxide (active metabolite)
	↑Phenytoin
	↑Valproate
Gabapentin	None
Lamotrigine	None
Phenobarbital	↓Carbamazepine
	↓↑Phenytoin
	↓Valproate
Phenytoin	↓Carbamazepine
	↓Primidone (↑phenobarbital)
	↓Valproate
Primidone	↓Carbamazepine
	↓Clonazepam
Valproate	↓↑Carbamazepine (↑active metabolite)
	↑Ethosuximide
	↑Lamotrigine
	↑Phenobarbital
	↓Phenytoin (total)*
	↑Phenytoin (free)*

↑Blood level is increased. ↓Blood level is decreased.
*The effect of valproate on blood phenytoin levels is complex; a decrease in the total phenytoin level may be associated with an increase in the free phenytoin level (see Appendix 1). Therefore, as it is the free drug that reaches the brain, the adverse effects of phenytoin may increase despite a decrease in the total level, which is the level usually monitored.

DISCONTINUING ANTIEPILEPTIC DRUGS

Getting off antiepileptic drugs is the goal of most people with well-controlled seizures (see Chapter 16). Most doctors will consider discontinuing antiepileptic drugs after a seizure-free period of 2 to 4 years. If someone with only a single seizure has been seizure-free for 6 to 12 months

TABLE 7. INTERACTIONS OF ANTIEPILEPTIC DRUGS WITH OTHER DRUGS

Antiepileptic Drug	Other Drug Affected
Carbamazepine	↓Acetaminophen
	↓Alprazolam
	↑Clomipramine
	↓Dicumarol
	↓Doxycycline
	↓Haloperidol
	↓Steroid hormones*
	↓Theophylline
	↓Warfarin
Clonazepam	None
Ethosuximide	None
Phenobarbital and primidone	↓Chlorpromazine
	↓Cimetidine
	↓Cyclosporine
	↓Desipramine
	↓Lidocaine
	↓Quinidine
	↓Steroid hormones*
	↓Theophylline
	↓Warfarin
Phenytoin	↓Acetaminophen
	↓Amiodarone
	↓Cyclosporine
	↓Dicumarol
	↓Digoxin
	↓Disopyramide
	↓Doxycycline
	↓Lidocaine
	↓Metronidazole
	↓Mexiletine
	↓Nortriptyline
	↓Quinidine
	↓Steroid hormones*
	↓Theophylline
	↓Warfarin
Primidone	↓Cyclosporin
	↓Doxycycline
	↓Warfarin
Valproate	↑Antipyrine

↑Blood level is increased. ↓Blood level is decreased.
*Includes oral contraceptives, dexamethasone, and prednisone; decreases the effectiveness of oral contraceptives.

TABLE 8. INTERACTIONS OF OTHER DRUGS WITH ANTIEPILEPTIC DRUGS

Other Drug	Antiepileptic Drug Affected
Amiodarone	↑Phenytoin
Antacids	↓Phenytoin
	↑Valproate
Aspirin	↑Phenytoin (free level)
	↑Valproate
Chloramphenicol	↑Phenobarbital
	↑Phenytoin
Cimetidine	↑Carbamazepine
	↑Phenytoin
Cisplatin	↓Carbamazepine
Danazol	↑Carbamazepine
Diltiazem	↑Carbamazepine
Disulfiram	↑Phenytoin
Doxycycline	↓Carbamazepine
Erythromycin	↑Carbamazepine
Fluoxetine	↑Carbamazepine
Isoniazid	↑Carbamazepine
	↑Phenytoin
	↑Primidone
Metronidazole	↑Phenytoin
Nicotinamide	↑Carbamazepine
	↑Primidone
Oxacillin	↓Phenytoin
Phenylbutazone	↑Phenytoin (free level)
	↓Phenobarbital
Propoxyphene	↑Phenytoin
	↑Carbamazepine
Rifampin	↓Phenytoin
Sucralfate	↓Phenytoin
Sulfa drugs	↑Phenytoin
Theophylline	↓Carbamazepine
Verapamil	↑Carbamazepine
Warfarin	↑Phenytoin

↑Blood level is increased. ↓Blood level is decreased.

many doctors will also consider discontinuing the medication. In many cases, the medications can be gradually tapered and discontinued. Several predictors can help the doctor determine who is likely to remain seizure-free without medications: Seizures are unlikely to recur if the patient had few seizures before taking antiepileptic drugs, the seizures were easily controlled with a single medication, and the patient has normal results on the neurological examination and a normal EEG.

TABLE 9. SELECTED OVER-THE-COUNTER AND PRESCRIPTION DRUGS THAT CAN AFFECT SEIZURES OR ANTIEPILEPTIC DRUGS*

Aspirin-Containing Products[†]

Alka-Seltzer Extra Strength
Alka-Seltzer Plus
Anacin Tablets and Caplets
Arthritis Pain Formula Caplets
Ascriptin Tablets and Caplets
Azdone Tablets[‡]
BC Cold Powder, BC Powder
Bayer Aspirin Tablets and Caplets
Bayer Children's Chewable Aspirin Tablets
Bufferin Tablets and Caplets
Ecotrin Tablets and Caplets
Empirin Aspirin Tablets
Equagesic Tablets[‡]
4-Way Cold Tablets
Fiorinal Tablets and Caplets[‡]
Norgesic Tablets[‡]
St. Joseph Adult Chewable Aspirin Caplets

Cold, Flu, and Allergy Preparations

Alka-Seltzer Plus
Bayer Children's Cold Tablets
Benadryl
Benylin
Children's Tylenol Cold Chewable Tablets and Liquid
Comtrex Caplets and Liquid
Contac Caplets, Tablets, and Liquid
Coricidin-D
Coricidin-D Demilets Tablets for Children
Coryban-D Tablets
Deconex
Dehist
Dimetapp Tablets, Caplets, and Elixir
4-Way Cold Tablets
Histabid Duracap
Naldecon Children's Syrup
Noraminic
Oraminic
Ornade Capsules
Sinarest Tablets
Sine-off Sinus Medicine
Sinubid
Spec-T Decongestant Lozenges
St. Joseph Cold Tablets for Children
Sucrets Cold Formula Lozenges
Triaminic Tablets, Chewables

Diet Pills

Acutrim Appetite Suppressant Tablets
Control Maximum Strength
Dexatrim Capsules, Caplets, and Tablets
Prolamine
Westrim

Sleeping Pills

Compoz
Nytol
Sleep-eze 3
Sominex

---

*The use of these drugs may increase the risk of seizures or gastrointestinal bleeding or cause an increase or decrease in the blood level of some antiepileptic drugs.
[†]Low to moderate doses of aspirin (less than 1500 mg per day) are generally very safe for people with epilepsy taking antiepileptic drugs. High doses of aspirin should only be taken after discussion with a doctor.
[‡]Prescription drugs.

For certain types of seizures, such as benign rolandic epilepsy, it can be predicted with a high degree of certainty that after age 16 years, seizures will not recur. By contrast, the seizures in juvenile myoclonic epilepsy are often well controlled by valproate but are very likely to recur if the medication is stopped.

GENERIC VERSUS BRAND-NAME DRUGS

Brand-name drugs are manufactured by major pharmaceutical companies (see color pictures) and are more expensive than generic drugs. Although generic drugs may be manufactured by large pharmaceutical companies, they are often made by smaller companies, and it may be difficult to find out who manufactures the drugs distributed by a specific pharmacy. There is a general trend in medicine toward the use of generic drugs because they are less expensive. For antiepileptic drugs, however, the generics are often not equivalent to the brand-name preparations. The major difference between generic and brand-name medication is not the quality of the drug itself, but rather the consistency in the amount of medication and the way in which it is made. The manufacturing process can affect how much of the drug is absorbed and the rate at which it is absorbed. The absorption of brand-name drugs is usually quite consistent, but in generic antiepileptic drugs, the absorption tends to be more variable. Therefore, in some patients, using generic drugs is associated with fluctuating blood drug levels, leading to an increase in seizure frequency when the levels are low and an increase in adverse effects when the blood levels are high.

Although there are some good, reliable generic drug products, it is often difficult to know exactly which manufacturer makes the generic drugs that a person receives. Many pharmacies use a distributor, who will buy in large amounts from any company that has a drug available or is the least expensive. When the suppliers change, the formulation of the drug may change. Because of these unpredictable situations, most neurologists recommend brand-name epilepsy drugs only.

Most doctors, and also the Epilepsy Foundation of America (EFA), recommend that switching between different manufacturers' products should be avoided, because the possible differences in absorption and other factors may affect seizure control or cause adverse effects. These problems are most likely to occur in persons who have had trouble achieving seizure control or who have had problems with medication adverse effects. If a person is switched to a generic drug, he or she should be told, and the doctor notified so that any additional tests that may be required can be ordered. Once seizure control is established, every effort should be made to keep taking the same manufacturer's product, whether it is a generic or brand name. If a person is on a generic drug, it is important that he or she be assured that the manufacturer of the drug will not change. Changing preparations between different manufacturers poses the greatest risk of increased seizures or adverse effects. Patients should always check their antiepileptic drugs before leaving the pharmacy and question the pharmacist if the pills look different.

An interesting aside to the generic issue is that some patients who develop a rash while taking Tegretol (the brand name for carbamazepine) may not be allergic to the drug, but rather to the red dye used in making it. These patients may wish to use a generic preparation, or the lower-strength children's Tegretol chewable tablet, which is white, not red.

REDUCING THE COST OF ANTIEPILEPTIC DRUGS

Antiepileptic drugs are expensive, but there are several ways to cut their costs. When applying for health insurance, if there is a choice between different policies, the subscriber should find out if there is a prescription plan and, if so, how the plan works. It may be useful to compare the possible increased costs of a health care plan that includes partial or complete coverage for medications to the costs of the drugs, as well as the other benefits.

Before purchasing medication, it may be wise to shop around. There may be considerable differences in the price of prescriptions between pharmacies in the same town. It might also pay to shop in some nearby towns. Large pharmacies or chain stores often offer lower prices, and some pharmacies offer discounts for the purchase of larger quantities.

Pharmacy services are also available. For example, membership in the EFA also includes access to the American Association of Retired Persons pharmacy. There are other mail-order pharmacies such as Prescription Delivery Systems (800-441-8976), Preferred Rx of Ohio (800-843-7038), and Athena (800-528-4362). Local EFA affiliates, as well as other patients, also may have information on obtaining medications at lower prices.

RECENTLY APPROVED ANTIEPILEPTIC DRUGS

After a 15-year gap, the Food and Drug Administration (FDA) recently approved three new antiepileptic drugs: felbamate, gabapentin, and lamotrigine (see color pictures). In addition, several other drugs will be considered during the next few years. The exact position of these new drugs in the treatment of epilepsy will require further study. Felbamate, gabapentin, and lamotrigine, as well as other drugs that may be approved during the

1990s, appear to be effective, safe, and well-tolerated. Whether these drugs will become first-line or second-line drugs depends on how they compare with other drugs in carefully designed studies. So far, no studies comparing these drugs with more commonly used drugs have been performed.

All three of these new drugs have undergone extensive testing in animals, volunteers, and people with epilepsy. Some people have better seizure control and fewer medication adverse effects while taking these new drugs as opposed to the existing drugs. However, these new drugs are not miracle drugs. Only a few people whose seizures could not be fully controlled on the existing drugs have achieved full control of their seizures while taking the new drugs. These drugs, like all existing drugs, do have some adverse effects. Both their effectiveness in controlling seizures and their tendency to cause adverse effects vary considerably from one person to another. Just as epilepsy affects individuals in different ways, the treatment of epilepsy also affects individuals in different ways.

Felbamate

Felbamate is chemically unrelated to any of the existing antiepileptic drugs. It appears to work by blocking the action of excitatory neurotransmitters in the brain. These are substances in the brain that cause the cells to fire electrical signals (see Chapter 2). It has been developed through testing done only in the United States. In animal models of seizures, the drug has an unusually good safety profile and is effective for both partial and generalized seizures. Further, the effectiveness does not diminish over time. The safety profile in people with epilepsy has also been quite favorable, especially when it is used alone (monotherapy).

Felbamate is effective in treating partial and secondarily generalized tonic-clonic seizures. It is also effective for the Lennox-Gastaut syndrome. Children with this serious form of epilepsy had a significant decrease in seizure frequency, and the parents' overall rating of the patients' quality of life improved. Family members and patients often noted an increased level of attention and motivation, but some of the improvement may be related to the discontinuation of multiple and sedating medications. Preliminary studies suggest that felbamate is also beneficial for primary generalized epilepsy. However, additional testing will be needed to confirm these observations. Felbamate is indicated for both monotherapy and adjunct (add-on) therapy.

Felbamate has a half-life of approximately 17 hours. Despite its long half-life, at the higher dosages, it needs to be taken three times a day (and in some cases, four times a day) because of adverse effects with twice-a-day dosing. However, at lower dosages, twice-a-day dosing is possible. Although felbamate may be better tolerated when taken after meals, its absorption is not altered by food intake. Common adverse effects include nausea, decreased appetite, weight loss, and insomnia. Less-frequent problems are headache, vomiting, and irritability. Most of these adverse effects are dose-related and lessen with time and when felbamate is used alone (monotherapy).

Most adults with epilepsy tolerate a dose of 3600 milligrams per day, which was the highest dose used in the investigational trials. Felbamate has not seriously affected the liver or kidneys in any person treated thus far. A slight reduction in the number of white blood cells, similar to that commonly occurring with carbamazepine and phenytoin, can occur with felbamate. Felbamate can interact with several other antiepileptic drugs (see Table 6). It is unknown if felbamate alters the effectiveness of oral contraceptives.

Felbamate is available as an elixir for children (600 milligrams per 5 milliliters [teaspoon]) and in 400-milligram and 600-milligram tablets.

Gabapentin

Gabapentin was developed in both the United States and Europe. Gabapentin is also unrelated to any of the existing antiepileptic drugs. It is an amino acid that is chemically related to gamma-aminobutyric acid (GABA), a naturally occurring inhibitory neurotransmitter (see Chapter 2). Although its chemical relationship to GABA suggests that it works by affecting this neurotransmitter system, the exact way in which it works remains uncertain. Animal models of seizures suggest that gabapentin has the potential for effectiveness against both partial and generalized seizures, although clinical studies suggest that it is not effective in treating absence seizures.

Gabapentin is effective for complex partial and secondarily generalized tonic-clonic seizures. Its half-life is approximately 6 hours. Because of its short half-life, it usually needs to be taken three times a day. Gabapentin is very well tolerated, and most adverse effects, such as tiredness, improve after several weeks. Tiredness is most common when the dose is more than 600 milligrams per day, although most subjects tolerate doses of 1200 milligrams or more. Other adverse effects include dizziness, unsteadiness, and weight gain.

Studies suggest that gabapentin does not injure the liver, kidneys, or blood cells. Gabapentin has the advantage of not having serious interactions with other antiepileptic drugs. This is important, as it is indicated for adjunct therapy. Its absence of interactions (see Table 6) indicates that gabapentin probably would not decrease the effectiveness of oral contraceptives.

Gabapentin is available as a 100-milligram, 300-milligram, and 400-milligram pill.

Lamotrigine

Lamotrigine was developed in Europe and first marketed in England and other European and South American countries. It is unrelated to any of the existing antiepileptic drugs. Lamotrigine appears to prevent the release of neurotransmitters that excite nerve cells in the brain (see Chapter 2).

Lamotrigine has been used to treat complex partial and secondarily generalized tonic-clonic seizures. It also may be useful for treating typical absence and atonic seizures. Preliminary studies suggest that lamotrigine can be helpful in treating patients with Lennox-Gastaut syndrome. From available information, the effectiveness of lamotrigine does not appear to diminish over time. Its half-life is approximately 30 hours. Adverse effects of lamotrigine occur infrequently and include double vision, dizziness, unsteadiness, headache, tiredness, and rash. Lamotrigine does not appear to alter blood tests of the liver or kidneys or blood cell functions. Lamotrigine has no serious interactions with other antiepileptic drugs (see Table 6).

Lamotrigine is available in 100-milligram, 150-milligram, and 200-milligram pills.

INVESTIGATIONAL ANTIEPILEPTIC DRUGS

Some persons do not enjoy a good quality of life when taking antiepileptic drugs. Either their seizures are not fully controlled or they suffer from troublesome adverse effects of the drugs, or both. More than a dozen antiepileptic drugs are now in various stages of development or testing, many of which are being used in Europe, Canada, and other countries. The patients enrolled in the trials have seizures that are uncontrolled by the existing medications. If the existing, proven drugs were now tested in patients with uncontrolled seizures (who have, by definition, failed to respond to the best available drugs), their well-proved efficacy might not be found. Newer designs in drug studies are helping to solve this problem.

Some of the drugs discussed below are now being considered by the FDA for marketing in the United States, and others will be considered in the near future. The information provided here is, therefore, subject to change.

Persons with difficult-to-control seizures or troublesome adverse effects from the currently available antiepileptic drugs may want to consider trying one of the investigational or experimental drugs. Almost all antiepileptic drug studies are being performed at comprehensive epilepsy centers. The best way of finding out about new drug studies is to call or write nearby comprehensive epilepsy centers. A list of these specialized centers can be obtained from the national EFA or local EFA affiliates (see Appendix 3).

All drug studies must be approved by an institutional review board or ethics committee at each hospital or medical center. This review process helps to guarantee that the study carefully considers the relative risks and benefits to the patients enrolled and that they are clearly explained in a consent form. The study must be fully explained to the patient, who must carefully read and understand the consent form before signing it. For children, a parent or legal guardian must sign the consent form. The doctor in charge of the study, called the principal investigator, and the hospital's patient advocate should be available to answer any questions that arise once the study has begun.

A patient who considers entering a drug study but decides not to participate should have no fears that the doctor will be upset or withhold other therapies that he or she would otherwise recommend.

Flunarizine

Flunarizine belongs to the class of drugs known as calcium channel blockers and acts to block the entry of calcium into cells. Calcium is an important element in the regulation of electrical activity of nerve cells in the brain and other cells in the body in which electrical activity is important, such as the heart muscle. Calcium also controls the release of neurotransmitters from nerve cells in the brain. Calcium channel blockers are commonly used to treat high blood pressure, heart problems, and other medical disorders.

Flunarizine has been studied mainly in partial seizures, with positive results reported in more than a third of the patients. It has also been used to treat primary generalized seizures, but the data are too preliminary for any conclusions.

Flunarizine has a half-life of 2 to 3 weeks. Drowsiness and weight gain are its most common adverse effects.

Oxcarbazepine

Oxcarbazepine, as its name suggests, is closely related chemically to carbamazepine. It is now marketed in Europe. When compared with carbamazepine, oxcarbazepine appears equally effective for controlling complex partial seizures and primary and secondarily generalized tonic-clonic seizures, but it may be tolerated slightly better. It is less likely to cause a rash than carbamazepine. In patients who had a rash while taking carbamazepine, approximately a quarter will have a rash when later treated with oxcarbazepine. Oxcarbazepine's most common adverse effects are tiredness, dizziness, headache, and unsteadiness. Its half-life is approximately 6 hours.

Tiagabine

Tiagabine blocks the uptake by cells of the inhibitory neurotransmitter GABA and thereby prolongs its action. Preliminary studies have shown that tiagabine is safe and well tolerated and useful for treating partial and secondary generalized tonic-clonic seizures, but additional studies are needed to fully define its safety and effectiveness.

Vigabatrin

Vigabatrin was developed and is now marketed in Europe. It is unrelated to any of the existing antiepileptic drugs. Vigabatrin, a derivative of the inhibitory neurotransmitter GABA, has been used mainly to treat complex partial and secondarily generalized tonic-clonic seizures. It also has been used to treat infantile spasms and seizures in patients with the Lennox-Gastaut syndrome. Its half-life is 4 to 7 hours. However, vigabatrin's effect continues for at least 6 days after the last dose. Therefore, the effectiveness of vigabatrin does not fluctuate when the medication is taken only once or twice a day.

Vigabatrin is usually well tolerated. Drowsiness and fatigue are the most common adverse effects; others include irritability and nervousness, dizziness, headache, and confusion. Microscopic structural changes observed in the brains of animals treated with very high doses of vigabatrin have not been found in humans treated with standard doses of the drug, and most experts believe that these changes do not occur in humans.

Zonisamide

Zonisamide was developed in Japan and is now marketed there. It is unrelated to any of the existing antiepileptic drugs. Zonisamide has been used to treat simple and complex partial seizures, primary and secondarily generalized tonic-clonic seizures, tonic seizures, atypical absence seizures, and certain types of progressive myoclonic epilepsy (the variant called Baltic myoclonic epilepsy). Kidney stones were observed in some patients taking zonisamide, leading to suspension of clinical trials in the United States and Europe, which have been resumed. Other adverse effects include drowsiness, unsteadiness, loss of appetite, stomach discomfort, headache, and rash. The half-life is approximately 30 hours.

INTRAVENOUS GAMMA GLOBULIN

Gamma globulin is composed of antibodies derived from human blood. Antibodies are chemicals that help to fight bacteria, viruses, and other foreign "invaders." Although gamma globulin has been used for decades to bolster the immune system (the body's defense against infection and foreign substances), its use has recently been expanded to children with difficult-to-control forms of epilepsy. Only a limited number of studies have been completed, and the results are preliminary. Although some children have had a dramatic response to this therapy, many others have had no significant reduction in seizures. The effectiveness of gamma globulin for epilepsy remains to be proven.

The gamma globulin is given as an intravenous infusion, usually initiated in the hospital. By giving the infusion in the hospital, the nurses and doctors can watch closely for any type of allergic or other reaction and treat the child promptly if such a reaction occurs. The chances of a serious allergic reaction are small. The child then returns every 2 to 6 weeks for an additional infusion, which may be done as an outpatient or inpatient. The length of therapy varies, and in most cases in which there is a beneficial response, the improvement can be seen within the first few months of treatment.

Many parents ask whether a child can get the human immunodeficiency virus (HIV), which causes the acquired immunodeficiency syndrome, or AIDS, from gamma globulin. Because the HIV is destroyed during the process of preparing gamma globulin, there have been no documented cases of HIV infection from gamma globulin, even before the blood pool was routinely screened for this virus.

Intravenous gamma globulin is expensive. The issues of insurance coverage and expense should be addressed ahead of time.

CHAPTER 11

Surgical Therapy for Epilepsy

When seizures cannot be controlled by medications or control can be achieved only at the cost of severe and unacceptable adverse effects, surgery is an alternative. Surgical therapy for epilepsy has been used for more than a century, but the past two decades have seen a dramatic rise in its use, reflecting in part an increased awareness by both doctors and patients that it is an effective alternative to medical therapy. As with other surgical procedures, however, the benefits must be carefully weighed against the risks. Further, there is no guarantee that the surgery will be successful in controlling the seizures.

Patients with partial epilepsy who are considered for surgical therapy have difficult-to-control seizures that have not responded to aggressive treatment with antiepileptic drugs. As epilepsy surgery has become more widely established, the definition of difficult-to-control seizures has been adjusted. Surgery is now being performed on patients whose seizures have been uncontrolled for only 1 or 2 years. In general, the patient should be treated with at least two single drugs and with a combination of two or more drugs before surgery is considered. Medication trials must be adequate, that is, the drugs should be gradually increased to the maximally tolerated dose. In many epilepsy centers, other standard or investigational drugs are tried before surgery is considered.

Traditionally, surgery to control epileptic seizures has been done more than a decade after the seizures begin. There is some evidence, however, that the earlier the surgery is performed, the better the outcome. A person who has failed to respond to several adequate medication trials is unlikely to achieve complete seizure control by medical therapy. In such cases, the risks and benefits of surgery should be carefully weighed against the costs that continued seizures and high doses of medication impose on intellectual, psychological, social, educational, employment, and other aspects of life. If the epilepsy is unresponsive to medications and has severely troublesome consequences, surgery should be considered sooner rather than later.

Epilepsy surgery may be beneficial to persons who have seizures associated with benign brain tumors, malformations of blood vessels (arteriovenous malformations, venous angiomas, cavernous angiomas), and strokes. The surgery may be done either to control the seizures or to remove the abnormality in the brain. For example, in a child who has a stroke shortly after birth and has intractable seizures, the goal of surgery would be to control the seizures. In contrast, in a woman with a benign brain tumor and seizures, the primary goal would be to remove the tumor, with control of seizures remaining a secondary issue.

In the case of benign tumors and vascular malformations, simple removal of the abnormal tissue may successfully control the seizures. In many cases, however, it is the area adjacent to the abnormal tissue that is irritated and that serves as the origin of the seizures. Removing the abnormal tissue may or may not lead to improvement or complete control of the seizures. Occasionally, the structural abnormality may have little to do with intractable seizures. For example, certain cysts of the brain (arachnoid cysts) rarely cause seizures that cannot be controlled with medications. When an arachnoid cyst is associated with intractable seizures, removing the cyst is unlikely to control the seizures unless the cyst is large and exerts pressure on the brain.

There are two main types of surgery for epilepsy. The first, and by far the most common, removes the area of the brain that causes seizures; this is called resective surgery. It is performed in cases of partial epilepsy, with or without secondarily generalized tonic-clonic seizures. Patients often imagine that the area that causes seizures is tiny, for example, the size of a pea. In the vast majority of cases, however, the area is much larger (e.g., 1.5 to 3 inches in length and 1 to 1.5 inches in width). Examples of resective surgery are temporal and frontal lobectomy.

The second, less common type of epilepsy surgery is the interruption of nerve pathways along which seizure impulses spread. An example is corpus callosotomy, where no brain tissue is removed, but the large fiber bundle connecting the hemispheres of the brain is severed. Another example is functional hemispherectomy, where one of the hemispheres of the brain is disconnected from the rest of the brain. Candidates for this type of surgery are patients with partial and generalized seizures.

A third type of epilepsy surgery, called multiple subpial transections, is currently under investigation. This procedure may be helpful when the seizures begin in areas of the brain that are vital to functions such as language, movement, or sensation.

EXPECTATIONS AND CONSEQUENCES OF EPILEPSY SURGERY

Patients will have many fears and questions about their epilepsy surgery. Doctors, nurses, psychologists, and social workers can answer questions about the risks, complications, recovery period, and other medical details. In addition, it is often helpful and reassuring to speak with someone else who has had a similar surgical procedure.

Epilepsy surgery is major neurosurgery, and some risk is associated with it. The recovery period is rather long. A patient once asked me, "Is this (epilepsy surgery) an inpatient or outpatient type of surgery?" Epilepsy surgery requires a hospital stay of 6 to 8 days or longer after the surgery, and in some cases, the stay lasts 2 weeks or longer. There is some mild, temporary discomfort afterward. After being discharged from the hospital, the patient returns home to rest for several weeks and can usually resume normal activities 3 to 8 weeks after the operation.

The actual procedures vary according to the types of operations, which are described later. The patient is usually under general anesthesia. Sometimes patients are kept awake while the vital areas of the brain, such as those that control language and movement, are mapped with mild electrical stimulation. In such cases, a local anesthetic is used, and the surgery can be performed painlessly, as the brain is not sensitive to pain. Further, new short-acting anesthetics allow the patient to sleep during the initial and final portions of the surgery and only need to be awake during the mapping procedure.

It is critical to establish realistic expectations before the surgery. Some persons are completely free of seizures after surgery, and in many others the frequency or intensity of the seizures is markedly reduced. Some patients continue to have auras or infrequent complex partial seizures. In some cases, there may be no improvement in seizure control. Most persons who do become seizure-free after surgery must continue to take antiepileptic drugs, so the surgery is not a complete cure for epilepsy.

Strange as it may seem, becoming seizure-free after epilepsy surgery can be stressful and require a major adjustment. Seizure control may create greater pressure to work and to assume new responsibilities, and it may change relationships and other people's expectations. In addition, the surgery may cause memory lapses or other disorders even though the seizures are fully controlled. Such problems usually improve with time. Some people feel depressed by all these changes and may need a great deal of encouragement during this period.

Perhaps the greatest setback after epilepsy surgery is the occurrence of a seizure after a period of freedom from seizures. It can seem as though just when epilepsy is moving further into the background of one's life, it reappears. Emotionally, the recurrence of seizures can be devastating, but it does not mean that seizure control cannot be restored. In many cases, the seizures are caused by missed medications, a serious infection, childbirth, or other problems, and seizure control returns after the cause is eliminated. In other cases, a single breakthrough seizure occurs for no identifiable reason. In most other cases, intermittent seizures occur, but less frequently than before the surgery. In general, the longer the interval of seizure freedom after surgery, the greater the chances are of never having another seizure.

PREOPERATIVE ASSESSMENT

The first step in deciding whether someone should have epilepsy surgery is to make sure that the seizures are medically refractory, or uncontrollable with antiepileptic drugs. A patient may have been treated with numerous medications but not with high dosages of a single drug, which may be more effective than two or more drugs used at low dosages. Other persons may never have been treated with particular drugs or combinations of drugs that might be effective. Most patients with difficult-to-control seizures have been treated with two or more drugs in separate trials and in various combinations, and have been treated unsuccessfully for at least 2 years. If the seizures are frequent, relatively short trials of medications can reveal the failure of medical therapy. If the seizures are infrequent, a longer trial of medication is needed to determine that the therapy is ineffective. Therefore, it is important for epilepsy surgery candidates to have a complete record of the antiepileptic drugs that have been tried, including the maximal dosages, blood drug levels, and adverse effects. When a patient has seizures associated with a blood vessel malformation, benign tumor, or other structural lesion, proof of medically refractory seizures is not as important as it is in other patients with epilepsy.

After a patient's seizures are confirmed to be medically refractory, studies are performed before epilepsy surgery to identify the area of the brain from which the seizures arise and the areas that control vital functions such as language, memory, movement, and sensation. Doctors hope to find that the seizures arise from an area that is not vital for intellectual or other important functions. Some areas of the brain can be removed without any observable or measurable changes in intellect, personality, or mood. The removal of other areas may be associated with slight deterioration or, in some cases, actual improvement in memory or other vital functions.

Noninvasive Studies

The preoperative assessment begins with a series of consultations and noninvasive tests. Noninvasive tests are ones that do not invade the body or require a surgical procedure and, in general, involve minimal or no risk. The assessment includes electroencephalogram (EEG) recording and video-EEG monitoring to record epilepsy waves between and during seizures; neuropsychological studies to assess cognitive (intellectual) strengths and weaknesses, which can help to predict the area from which the seizures arise, as well as possible complications of the surgery; consultations with psychologists, nurses, and social workers to assess the patient's emotional well-being and social supports and to identify problems that should be addressed before the surgery; and neuroimaging studies [computed tomography (CT), magnetic resonance imaging (MRI), SPECT, or PET] to identify abnormalities in the area from which the seizures arise.

Invasive Studies

The preoperative tests may also include invasive tests. Invasive tests are ones that invade the body. Technically, the insertion of a needle into a vein to draw blood is an invasive procedure, but it is so common and safe that it is not considered invasive. In general, invasive studies are associated with some risk, but the risk varies dramatically with the different types of tests and procedures.

Sphenoidal Electrodes

Recording the EEG with sphenoidal electrodes is routinely done in many epilepsy centers. The electrodes are inserted into the cheeks with a needle to record brain electrical activity from regions deep within the temporal and frontal lobes. Some doctors use local anesthesia before inserting the electrodes, but others find that the injection of anesthesia hurts more than the needle. The needle is immediately withdrawn after insertion, leaving in place a thin wire that is bare at the tip. The patient feels some discomfort during the insertion and for several hours afterward, particularly when yawning or chewing.

The risks of using sphenoidal electrodes are rare and almost always minor. A small amount of bleeding may occur during the needle insertion, but it is rarely a problem. Other risks include the possibility of infection or of a tiny piece of the bare wire remaining in the cheek.

Foramen Ovale Electrodes

The foramen ovale is an opening in the skull near the temporal lobe. Electrodes can be inserted into this opening to provide recordings of electrical activity of the lower and middle portions of the temporal lobe, an area from which seizures often arise. These electrodes are intermediate between sphenoidal and subdural or depth electrodes in the information they provide, their invasiveness, and their risk of complications. Overall, the foramen ovale electrodes are well tolerated, and in selected cases can provide important information about the origin of the seizures. One of the problems with them is that they record information from a very limited area of the brain. Therefore, the actual area from which the seizures arise may be missed.

Subdural and Depth Electrodes

Subdural and depth electrodes are used to record electrical activity directly from the brain, and they are often used to map precisely the area from which seizures arise. The dura mater is one of the membranes covering the brain, and the word subdural means that the electrodes are placed on the brain underneath the dura mater. The need to use subdural or depth electrodes depends on the findings from the noninvasive studies and the intracarotid sodium amobarbital test, described later. For example, if the routine scalp-recorded EEG, video-EEG recording, neuropsychological testing, PET scan, and amobarbital test all point to the same area of the brain as the focus of the seizures, most epilepsy centers will proceed without using invasive electrodes. If the information is inconsistent or indefinite, however, subdural or depth electrodes are often used. For example, the neuropsychological tests and PET scan may suggest an abnormality in the left temporal lobe, but the video-EEG may suggest that seizures begin in the right temporal area.

With the use of subdural electrodes, the brain can be stimulated electrically for mapping of brain areas involved in language, movement, and other important functions. Seizures can occur with the electrodes in place, and care must be used to protect the patient, and therefore the electrodes, during and after the seizures. In many centers, invasive electrodes are used in an intensive care unit or similar setting. Invasive electrodes may be left in place for several days to weeks depending on the specific case and how quickly seizures occur after the electrodes are placed.

Subdural electrodes (Fig. 19) consist of a series of metal electrodes embedded in plastic and arranged as a strip or a large grid. Subdural electrodes have the advantages of covering a large area of the outer surface of the brain and recording directly from the brain, without interference from the scalp

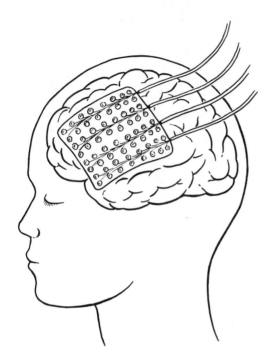

FIGURE 19. Subdural electrodes implanted in the brain.

and skull. An operation is required for placement of the electrodes. They are positioned directly on the brain, but do not penetrate it. In some cases, several strips of electrodes can be inserted through a small hole drilled in the skull called a "burr hole." In other cases, a large section of the skull is removed, the electrodes are put in place, and the skull is replaced. If the skull section is not immediately replaced, it is kept sterile and frozen, and the electrodes are covered with the dura mater (the thick membrane that covers the brain), the scalp, and a surgical dressing. After the testing is completed, the piece of the skull that was removed is then replaced. Some discomfort is associated with the placement of subdural electrodes. The greater the number of electrodes that are used (especially the grids), in general, the greater the headache that occurs during the first few days after the operation. Medicine can be given for pain relief.

The mapping procedures performed with subdural electrodes involve stimulation of the brain with mild electrical currents to temporarily activate or shut down certain brain areas. For example, activation of the left motor cortex controlling movement in the right thumb can cause a series of jerks in this finger, or stimulation of language areas in the temporal or frontal lobes can cause a person who is counting to suddenly stop speaking. The mapping procedure is almost always painless.

The major risks of subdural electrodes are infection, bleeding, and brain swelling. Depending on the number of electrodes used, the patient may have a moderate to severe headache for several days after the operation.

Depth electrodes (Fig. 20) are thin, wirelike plastic tubes with metal contact points spread out along their length. In contrast with subdural and other invasive electrodes, depth electrodes are placed directly into the brain. They do not require an operation with a large opening in the skull, as is needed to place a grid of subdural electrodes. The depth electrodes are inserted through burr holes drilled in the skull. The patient is usually awake during placement of the electrodes but may be sleeping. The placement of depth electrodes can be painful. The pain is related to the exact procedure that is used. In some centers, the electrodes are placed using a frame that attaches to the skull. The attachment of this frame, which allows a computer to assist in calculating the exact course of the electrodes in the brain, can be painful. The pain associated with depth electrodes is usually mild or moderate and lasts only hours, or occasionally, several days. Medicine can reduce the pain.

Depth electrodes provide the best recordings of seizures arising in deep areas of the brain, but they also carry some additional risks, especially bleeding within the brain. They are less likely than subdural electrodes to cause infection or brain swelling.

Intracarotid Sodium Amobarbital Test

In the intracarotid sodium amobarbital test, also called the Wada test, memory and language functions are tested by putting one cerebral hemisphere to sleep with amobarbital, a short-acting anesthetic agent, and studying what functions are preserved in the other hemisphere. The test begins with an angiogram, a test that examines the flow of a dye through the blood vessels. A thin plastic tube (catheter) is introduced through an artery in the inner portion of the upper thigh. A local anesthetic is given to numb the area, and a needle is then inserted into the artery. The tube is threaded through the needle, and the needle is removed. There is some mild discomfort during the local anesthesia, but the remainder of the test is painless. The tube is guided up to the carotid artery in the neck. A small amount of contrast dye is injected through the tube into the artery, and x-rays are taken to study the flow of blood in the brain. Some warmth or flashing lights may be experienced with the injection of the dye. Next, the radiologist injects the amobarbital, which quite literally puts almost half of the brain to sleep for several minutes.

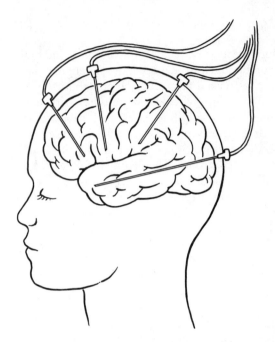

FIGURE 20. Depth electrodes implanted in the brain.

Immediately after the amobarbital injection, tests are given to see how well language and memory are working with half of the brain sleeping. This provides information on the functions of the cerebral hemisphere that is sleeping and the hemisphere that is awake. The same procedure is usually repeated on the opposite side after a delay (most centers wait 30 to 60 minutes, and some wait a day) to ensure that the patient's level of alertness has returned to normal.

Like any other test involving a cerebral angiogram, this test has an extremely low risk of causing a stroke. The risk is greatest, but still quite low, in older people with atherosclerosis ("hardening of the arteries").

SURGICAL PROCEDURES

Temporal Lobectomy

Removal of a portion of the temporal lobe (temporal lobectomy) is the most common and most successful type of epilepsy surgery. In most cases, a modest portion of the brain is removed, measuring approximately 2.5 inches in length (Fig. 21). The temporal lobes are important in memory and emotion. In addition, the upper and back part of the "language-dominant"

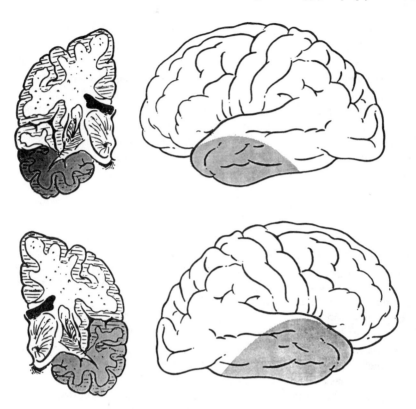

FIGURE 21. Brain tissue removed (*shaded areas*) in a standard temporal lobectomy of the left (*top*) or right (*bottom*) hemisphere. (Cross-sectional views, looking from the front, are on the left side of the figure, and side views are on the right.) A smaller amount of tissue is removed from the left hemisphere than from the right hemisphere, because, in most people, the left temporal lobe contains the area that is vital for language comprehension.

temporal lobe, which is on the left in nearly all right-handed people and most left-handed people, is vital for language comprehension. The preoperative assessment ensures that removal of the area causing seizures will not disrupt memory or language functions. However, when surgery is performed on the side of the brain dominant for language functions, usually the left side, there is often a slight reduction in memory functions after the operation. In contrast, after right-sided (nondominant) temporal lobectomy, memory functions often improve slightly. Persons with frequent seizures who achieve complete or nearly complete seizure control after surgery often have a mild improvement in memory functions. This is especially true for those who have troublesome memory problems after individual seizures or clusters of seizures.

The success rate for seizure control in temporal lobectomy is variable: 55% to 70% of patients are free of seizures that impair consciousness or cause abnormal movements, but auras can persist in some; 20% to 25% of patients have some seizures but are significantly improved (greater than 85% reduction of complex partial and tonic-clonic seizures); and 10% to 15% of patients have no worthwhile improvement. Therefore, more than 85% of patients enjoy a marked improvement in seizure control. Most of them are on less medication after surgery. Approximately 10% to 20% of persons who are seizure-free are able eventually to discontinue antiepileptic drugs.

The risk of a major complication such as a stroke, with weakness on the opposite side of the body, is about 1% to 2% in temporal lobectomy. If the surgery extends to the back part of the temporal lobe, there is an additional risk of superior quadrantanopsia, or loss of vision in the upper quarter of space on the side opposite that of the surgery (Fig. 22). For example, if in a temporal lobectomy on the right side, the surgeon needs to extend the area of removal toward the back part of the temporal lobe, a defect in vision in the left upper quarter of space is possible. Luckily, this impairment has no real effect on everyday living; affected persons are usually unaware of it. They are able to read, drive, and perform tasks requiring extremely precise visual accuracy, assuming that their vision was excellent before surgery. In rare cases (fewer than 1 in 200 patients who have temporal lobectomy), the visual loss is more severe and includes an entire half of the visual world on the side opposite from the one that was operated on. This impairment, called homonymous hemianopsia, causes functional problems and interferes with reading and driving. Mild memory impairment is common after left temporal lobectomy, and mild memory improvement is common after right temporal lobectomy. The risk of death from temporal lobectomy is less than 1 in 400 patients.

A common-sense question often asked by patients is, "If you are taking out a piece of my brain, won't I be a different person?" The answer is no.

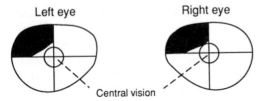

Left eye **Right eye**

Central vision

FIGURE 22. Superior quandrantanopsia. The patient's central vision is preserved; only the peripheral vision (to the sides) is affected, and most people are unaware of it. In most cases, only a portion of this area is affected.

In the vast majority of patients, personality, mood, and overall behavior are not disrupted or changed by temporal lobectomy. Part of the explanation is that many areas of the brain are redundant; that is, other parts can perform similar functions. Further, some parts of the brain, such as the front (anterior) portions of the temporal lobe and most of the right temporal lobe, are referred to as "silent areas." This means that if these areas are removed or damaged, as in a stroke, for example, changes are minimal or undetectable. In addition, areas that are removed in epilepsy surgery are areas that are not functioning properly, and in some cases, do not function at all. One of the pioneers of epilepsy surgery, Wilder Penfield, suggested that the area of the brain from which seizures arise is "nociferous," meaning harmful. Therefore, the area from which seizures arise is associated with problems in the functions normally served by that area, and the epileptic region can also impair functions of other brain areas. This is in contrast to a stroke, in which the problems are due to the injury to the affected area. The concept of nociferous areas may explain the improvement in memory and other cognitive functions in some patients after epilepsy surgery. In most cases, the area of brain that is removed is abnormal; it usually functions poorly, and when examined under the microscope, shows evidence of scarring.

Frontal Lobectomy

The frontal lobes comprise approximately one third of the cerebral hemisphere (see Fig. 1). This large area is often injured in head trauma and is involved in other brain disorders such as a stroke or tumor. Partial seizures often arise in the frontal lobes. A frontal lobe is the second most common brain area—after the temporal lobe—from which a portion is removed to treat epilepsy.

The back part of the frontal lobes (primary motor cortex) controls movement (see Fig. 1) and cannot be removed without causing severe weakness in muscles on the opposite side. The area just in front of the primary motor cortex is called the motor association cortex. This area also has motor functions and communicates between the primary motor cortex and other areas of the brain. The motor association cortex can be removed without causing any weakness. The top part of the motor association cortex, which extends to the most middle part of the frontal lobes (between the eyes), is called the supplementary motor area. This area is a relatively common place for seizures to arise.

The remaining parts of the frontal lobes are important in personality and behavior. The dramatic personality changes that occur after the destruction or removal of large portions of both frontal lobes (frontal lobotomy) very rarely occur in frontal lobectomy, because the operation is always confined to one side, and the area removed is usually much smaller than the areas removed in frontal lobotomy. It is possible, however, that mild behavioral changes will develop after frontal lobectomy (and less often, after temporal lobectomy).

The frontal lobes pose a greater challenge in determining the area from which seizures arise. The large size of the frontal lobes makes it difficult to record electrical activity from numerous regions. If depth electrodes are used, only a tiny fraction of the area is sampled. Subdural electrodes are able to sample a greater area, but they require a large grid, which means that only one side can be studied. Regardless of the technique used, it can be difficult to record activity from certain frontal areas.

The success rates for frontal lobectomy are not as good as those for temporal lobectomy: 30% to 50% of patients are free of seizures that impair consciousness or cause abnormal movements; an additional 20% to 40% of patients are markedly improved (greater than 90% reduction of complex partial and tonic-clonic seizures); and 20% to 30% of patients have no worthwhile improvement. The risk of major complications, such as a stroke, is about 2%. The risk of mild behavioral changes is higher than with temporal lobectomy. Behavioral changes associated with frontal lobe impairment are often difficult to measure and define. Personality, motivation, ability to plan and to follow up on a multistep process, social graces, and demeanor are among the behaviors that the frontal lobes help to serve. Some persons with seizures beginning in the frontal lobes may have some mild changes in these behaviors before the surgery.

Parietal and Occipital Lobectomies

Surgery to remove part of the parietal or occipital lobes, which are located in the back of the brain (see Fig. 1), is most often done when a structural abnormality is identified on the CT or MRI scan. The success rate in controlling seizures is higher when a structural abnormality is present. Other studies, such as invasive electrode recordings, may reveal that seizures come from one of these areas.

The successes and risks of parietal and occipital lobectomies are similar to those of frontal lobectomy. Since neither of these lobes controls movement, however, the risk of weakness is lower, whereas the risk of loss of touch or visual sensation is greater. On the dominant (usually left) side, the parietal lobe is important in language functions. On the nondominant (usually right) side, the parietal lobe is important for spatial perception and ability to focus attention toward the left side of space. The occipital lobes are essential for vision. The left occipital lobe receives information about vision in the right half of space and vice versa.

Corpus Callosotomy

Corpus callosotomy cuts the large fiber bundle (corpus callosum; see Fig. 1B) that connects the two hemispheres of the brain. In contrast with lobectomy, corpus callosotomy does not involve removal of brain tissue. In most cases, the operation involves cutting the front two thirds of the callosum in the hope that the operation will markedly reduce the seizure frequency. In some cases, a second operation is performed to cut the remaining back third. Corpus callosotomy is most effective for atonic, tonic-clonic, and tonic seizures. Seizure frequency is reduced by an average of 70% to 80% after partial callosotomy and 80% to 90% after complete callosotomy. Partial seizures are often unchanged, but they may be improved or worsened. In many cases, especially after partial callosotomy, seizures are less frequent but persist.

Complications of corpus callosotomy are slightly greater than with frontal or temporal lobe resections. Behavioral, language, and other problems may affect neurological function and the quality of life, but serious problems are uncommon. Further, the potential risks of callosotomy must be weighed against its possible benefits, such as a reduction in the frequency of seizures that cause injury and other problems. The persons most susceptible to behavioral problems after callosotomy are those in whom language and motor dominance are controlled by different hemispheres; for example, the left side of the brain controls language, but in left-handed persons, the right side of the brain controls motor actions. Some of the problems resulting from callosotomy are caused by injury to the frontal lobes during the operation. Since the corpus callosum is buried deep between the frontal lobes, the middle portions of these lobes must be separated, which poses some risk. Surgical advances may help to minimize this risk.

Hemispherectomy

The dramatic procedure of hemispherectomy originally involved the removal of one whole side of the brain. Now, it usually involves disconnecting one cerebral hemisphere from the rest of the brain, with removal of only a limited area (Fig. 23). It is only considered in patients, usually children, with severe epilepsy in whom seizures arise from only one side of the brain and in which that hemisphere functions poorly. Before surgery, these patients typically have severe weakness (paralysis) and loss of touch sensation and vision on the opposite side of the body. Therefore, the side of the brain that is to be disconnected is already functioning very poorly and is often impairing the functions of the other side of the brain.

If the operation is performed on young children, the opposite hemisphere may make up for the loss, as these children can learn to walk despite

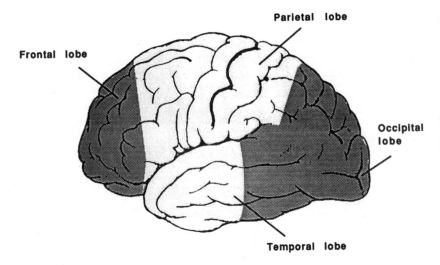

FIGURE 23. Outer surface (*side view*) of the left hemisphere, showing the area of brain removed (*light shading*) and the areas of brain disconnected from the opposite hemisphere (*dark shading*) in a hemispherectomy.

their paralysis. They will never have motor function or sensation in the hand, forearm, foot, and leg on the side opposite the operation. However, controlled movements are possible in the upper arm and thigh, thus permitting the person to walk. Physical therapy is often needed after hemispherectomy.

The results of hemispherectomy are quite good. More than 75% of the patients experience complete or nearly complete seizure control. If the patient has a progressive disorder, such as Rasmussen's syndrome, the prognosis for seizure control is less good.

Focal Resective Surgery for Infantile Spasms

Infantile spasms are classified as primary generalized seizures and are almost always associated with electrical abnormalities over both sides of the brain both during and between seizures. The spasms also involve muscles on both sides of the body in roughly equal fashion. These features suggest that infantile spasms could never be treated by any form of surgery that removes a limited portion of the brain. However, some patients with infantile spasms have a restricted area of decreased brain metabolism on the PET scan. When this area overlaps with the area of abnormality shown on the EEG, and the infantile spasms do not respond to medications, the patients may have a good response to surgical procedures that remove the abnormal portion of the brain. The abnormalities are usually found in the parietal, occipital, or temporal areas. Under microscopic examination, the abnormal brain areas that are removed often show cortical dysplasia, an abnormality in the pattern of brain cell development. Preliminary reports suggest that after the operation, the children's development and seizure control are greatly improved.

Multiple Subpial Transections

The novel procedure of multiple subpial transections was pioneered as an alternative to removal of brain tissue. It is used to control partial seizures originating in areas that cannot be safely removed. For example, if the seizure focus involves the dominant temporal-lobe language area (Wernicke's area) critical for comprehension, the removal of this area to control seizures would cause a devastating complication: the inability to understand spoken or written language. Similarly, if the primary motor area is part of the seizure focus, its removal would cause permanent weakness on the opposite side of the body.

The operation involves a series of shallow cuts (transections) into the cerebral cortex (Fig. 24). The transections are made only as deep as the gray matter, approximately a quarter of an inch deep. Because of the complex way in which the brain is organized, these cuts are thought to interrupt

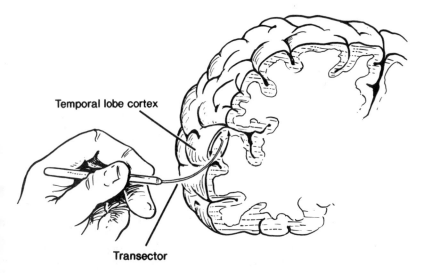

FIGURE 24. Multiple subpial transections of the brain.

some fibers that connect adjacent parts of the brain but do not appear to cause long-lasting impairment in the critical functions served by these areas.

There may be bleeding at the site of the transection, but the procedure has been generally well tolerated, with no major complications reported in the first 70 patients treated. Additional studies are needed to better define the risks and benefits of this procedure.

Stimulation of the Vagus Nerve

Electrical stimulation of the vagus nerve is a new, experimental technique for controlling seizures. The vagus nerve is part of the autonomic nervous system, which controls bodily functions that are not under voluntary control, such as heart rate. The vagus nerve passes from the brainstem through the neck and into the chest and abdomen. Preliminary studies suggest that stimulation of this nerve can, in some cases, help control seizures.

The stimulating device must be surgically implanted, and has a battery that lasts approximately 18 months. The risks of having the device implanted are low; approximately 1% of implants cause some damage to the nerve supplying some of the muscles in the voice box and can result in permanent hoarseness or a change in voice quality. In addition, when the vagus nerve is stimulated, approximately one-third of patients will have some change in their voice quality, which is reversible by reducing the amount of stimulation. The stimulator can be easily adjusted with a magnet held near the implanted device. For people with warnings (auras) before their seizures, activating the stimulator with the magnet when the warning occurs may help to abort the seizure.

Initial results with the vagus nerve stimulator are encouraging but preliminary. The device has not been shown to completely control seizures in persons with previously uncontrolled seizures, and it has not been able to replace medications in persons whose seizures are well controlled by antiepileptic drugs. Whether the vagus nerve stimulator will find a place in the treatment of epilepsy remains to be determined.

COST OF EPILEPSY SURGERY

Epilepsy surgery is expensive. Because of the complexities involved in the presurgical planning, it must be performed at a comprehensive epilepsy center that has a team experienced in epilepsy surgery. Strategies, philosophies, and costs differ among epilepsy centers, depending on the part of the country and the extent of the presurgical assessment. At some centers, for example, patients are monitored with video-EEG for prolonged periods; at others, the monitoring periods are shorter. In addition, if electrode implantation is used, the cost is much greater than if only a routine video-EEG is done. Overall, the cost of epilepsy surgery varies from $25,000 to more than $100,000. Patients should feel free to ask different centers about their average costs, outcomes, rates of complications, and other factors related to the surgery.

Health insurance plans usually cover epilepsy surgery. In cases in which the insurance companies deny coverage, it is often worthwhile to have both the patient and the doctor write to the insurance company. The doctor should provide documentation showing that epilepsy surgery is an established procedure for treating people with epilepsy in whom antiepileptic drugs do not control the seizures.

CHAPTER 12

Other Therapies for Epilepsy

For centuries, starvation and dehydration have been reported to improve seizure control. In addition, substances ranging from mistletoe to turpentine have all been claimed to be highly effective in treating epilepsy. In 1858, Sir Edward Henry Sieveking wrote, "There is scarcely a substance in the world, capable of passing through the gullet of man, that has not at one time or other enjoyed a reputation of being an anti-epileptic" (see Appendix 4). Aside from the dietary and medicinal therapies, the other therapies for control of epilepsy include the ancient practice of acupuncture and the relatively modern relaxation techniques.

DIETARY THERAPY

The Ketogenic Diet

Research in the 1930s showed that a ketogenic diet, consisting mostly of fats with little or no carbohydrate and a minimal amount of protein, reduced the frequency of seizures in more than half the children who followed it. The diet is named the ketogenic diet because a diet rich in fat causes a metabolic change in the body called ketosis. On the ketogenic diet, the body metabolizes its own protein, producing chemical substances called ketone bodies and uric acid. With the introduction of phenytoin in 1938, the ketogenic diet became a therapy of historical interest rather than practical use. During the past several decades, however, new studies have confirmed its therapeutic value in epilepsy.

Many doctors are uncomfortable prescribing the ketogenic diet, because they are unfamiliar with it, unsure of its risks and benefits, or unimpressed with its results. Therefore, the diet is most often used in epilepsy centers, which usually reserve it for children with extremely difficult-to-control seizures.

The ketogenic diet is often difficult to enforce, especially in older children and adults, because eating even small amounts of carbohydrates renders the diet ineffective. The diet is most often used in children between 1 and 5 years of age whose seizures cannot be controlled by antiepileptic drugs. The best results have been obtained in children with atonic, tonic, and myoclonic seizures, but virtually all types of seizures have been improved or controlled by this diet. Children younger than 1 year of age cannot maintain adequate ketosis to obtain the beneficial effects of the diet. In children older than 1 year of age, successful use of the ketogenic diet depends on the child's previous diet, adaptability, and motivation. After the age of 3 to 5 years, children in our society usually have been exposed to foods that they are unwilling to part with. Therefore, using the ketogenic diet in older children can be extremely difficult, if not impossible.

Starting and Stopping the Diet

The ketogenic diet should be used only under a doctor's supervision, usually with the help of a dietitian. In most cases, the diet is started while the child is in the hospital. During the first 2 or 3 days, the child is not allowed to eat anything and is permitted to drink only a certain amount of water or other fluids. The child's blood sugar level falls during this period of starvation. If the fall in blood sugar is too great, the child may become pale, sweaty, tremorous, irritable, confused, and unresponsive, or even have seizures, and will need some sugar or other carbohydrate supplementation. The blood sugar level can be safely monitored in the hospital.

After several days of starvation, the ketones in the blood and urine rise, and the diet is gradually introduced. The urinary ketones can be easily measured at home by the parents, using an indicator strip. The presence of urinary ketones indicates that the diet has achieved its metabolic goal of ketosis.

The diet consists primarily of foods high in fat, with the remaining 25% to 35% of the calories made up of protein foods. Examples of high-fat foods include mayonnaise, butter, and cream. The child is allowed only small portions of cheese, meat, fish, or poultry each day. Fruit is allowed in modest amounts. There is an alternative source of fat, known as MCT, which is an oil. The use of the MCT allows a slightly greater expansion of nonfat foods in the diet. However, some authorities find that MCT is not as beneficial in controlling seizures as other fat sources such as butter and cream.

Because sugar is prohibited in the diet, the parents must be careful about all types of children's medications, cough syrups, vitamins, toothpaste, and any other nonfoods or foods that may contain sugar. Even small amounts of sugar can reverse the effects of the diet and cause a seizure. Therefore, teachers, babysitters, grandparents, siblings, and others who may be with the child in the parents' absence must be knowledgeable about the dietary restrictions.

There are no absolute rules about the length of time someone should stay on the ketogenic diet. If the diet is well-tolerated and effective, the doctor will usually recommend continuing the diet for 1 to 3 years, after which the percentage of carbohydrate is gradually increased. Suddenly stopping the diet may cause a temporary increase in seizures, which is similar to the rebound effect that may occur after the abrupt discontinuation of antiepileptic drugs. After the diet, some children remain seizure-free without medications. Sometimes, however, the seizures will relapse, in which case they may be well controlled with medications that were ineffective before the diet.

Using Antiepileptic Drugs with the Diet

If a child is taking high dosages of several antiepileptic drugs, tapering of one drug is often started during the period of starvation. Barbiturates are often discontinued first, because they are the most sedative of the antiepileptic drugs; furthermore, their blood levels can rise when the diet is started even though the dosage is unchanged. If adequate ketosis is maintained, and seizure control improves, a further reduction in medications is often possible. In some cases, all medications can be tapered and stopped.

Potential Risks of the Diet

The long-term effects of a high-fat diet, even if it is used for only several years, are unknown. Many experts believe, however, that the potential risk is much less than the benefits of improved seizure control and reduced dosages of antiepileptic drugs for brain development and intellectual and social functions.

The most dangerous potential risk of the ketogenic diet is low blood sugar during the period of starvation. Other potential problems include a deficiency of the B vitamins, vitamin C, and calcium. It is often wise to supplement these nutrients (making sure the supplement does not contain sugar). Many parents worry about the potential effects of large amounts of dietary fat. We know that high-fat diets in adults can accelerate atherosclerosis, which contributes to heart attacks, stroke, and other disorders of blood vessels. However, there is no evidence that the ketogenic diet accelerates atherosclerosis in children or adolescents. Unfortunately, we cannot be sure that the diet has no long-term effects on the blood vessels. Weight gain is not usually a problem on this diet.

The ketogenic diet can cause a slight delay in a child's growth, which is usually compensated for when the diet is stopped. Children on the ketogenic diet also have a small risk of kidney stones, but the risk is minimized by adequate fluid intake.

Vitamins and Other Nutritional Supplements

Although many holistic and chiropractic books contain lists of vitamins, amino acids, and other nutritional supplements that are said to control seizures, there is little scientific support for such claims. Unconfirmed reports claim that vitamin E and dimethylglycine, an amino acid, reduce seizures in some patients (see Chapter 6). However, no experts in the treatment of epilepsy would recommend the routine use of these substances.

With the exception of the rare vitamin B_6 deficiency that causes seizures in the newborn, it is unknown if any vitamin or nutritional supplement is beneficial or detrimental to seizure control. Western medicine has not studied the role of nutrition in health as intensively as it deserves. However, most "authorities" who recommend nutritional therapy for epilepsy are doing so without solid evidence of its effectiveness.

ALTERNATIVE THERAPIES

The gaps in knowledge of doctors who practice Western medicine are matched by the spectrum of alternative health care, which ranges from spiritual to herbal to nutritional to behavioral. People with epilepsy whose seizures are not fully controlled or who experience troublesome adverse effects from medications may tire of these problems and look for help outside the traditional medical boundaries.

Although Western medicine can be criticized fairly for studying only those therapies and approaches that it chooses to recognize as being potentially effective, it can be praised for the care with which it assesses the effectiveness and safety of its treatments. It is difficult for the average person to appreciate the power of bias and placebo effects. Bias refers to the effects of prejudice and expectation. For example, someone who tests a product in which he or she has a financial interest may be biased. A placebo is a substance that has no effect of its own except for that associated with the power of suggestion. For example, when persons with chest pain caused by heart problems are given a placebo and told it will make them better, more than a quarter of them will report a definite beneficial effect.

When practitioners prescribe a treatment—be they medical doctors, holistic health specialists, or nutritionists—all want their therapy to be effective. In medicine, we have learned our lesson over and over—unless the effectiveness and safety of a therapy are demonstrated in controlled studies, beware. The best doctor's suspicions, hunches, and clinical experiences over several decades of practice are often dead wrong. Alternative therapies are rarely subjected to careful scrutiny, and certainly not to the rigor of a double-blind (that is, neither the doctor nor the patient knows if subjects are receiving the "active" drug) controlled study. For most alternative therapies, we unfortunately do not know if the therapy is helpful, harmful, or simply ineffective.

Relaxation Therapy and Biofeedback

The majority of adults with epilepsy believe that stress can provoke a seizure. Because stress can alter brain chemistry and electrical activity and disrupt normal sleep, it is possible that stress can worsen epilepsy in susceptible individuals. Stress can also cause a person to breathe rapidly, or hyperventilate. Some persons with epilepsy, especially those with absence seizures, are more likely to have seizures when they hyperventilate.

Relaxation therapy involves a variety of strategies designed to reduce stress and foster relaxation. Breathing maneuvers, hypnosis, and other techniques can be used in relaxation therapy. Biofeedback involves learning to control bodily functions that are usually not under voluntary control. One can learn to control these functions by providing information about them to conscious awareness. For example, the heart rate can be modified by listening to a beep every time one's heart beats and concentrating on lowering or raising the heart rate. Similarly, biofeedback can be used for relaxation by concentrating on lowering the tension in the facial muscles or breathing at a slower rate.

Almost all of us, including people with epilepsy, would benefit from more relaxation and less stress. Relaxation therapy and biofeedback can help reduce stress and control hyperventilation, thereby helping to improve seizure control in some persons. These procedures, however, will probably never make someone seizure-free. Unfortunately, because there has been little systematic study of these techniques in persons with epilepsy, their role in epilepsy therapy is unclear.

Self-Control of Seizures

Many persons with epilepsy have warnings of their seizures and have learned techniques to "fight off a seizure." The warnings take the form of an aura, or a simple partial seizure, that typically occurs seconds before a complex partial or tonic-clonic seizure. Warnings may involve premonitory symptoms that occur 20 minutes to several days before a seizure. Some patients and doctors have developed specific methods for stopping a seizure. One technique described in the 1800s was used by persons who would experience a tingling sensation or jerking movement in an arm or leg. The sensation rose toward the head and would be followed by a tonic-clonic seizure. The seizure could be stopped by vigorously rubbing or scratching the arm or leg, or tying a cloth tightly around it. Similarly, some patients with seizures beginning with a smell (olfactory aura) can stop their seizure from progressing by smelling an unrelated strong odor.

Premonitory symptoms include irritability, depression, fatigue, "not feeling right," or a headache. In patients who have well-defined premonitory symptoms, obtaining additional sleep or taking additional medication under a doctor's supervision can potentially help prevent a seizure from occurring.

Acupuncture

Acupuncture is used in China and by some practitioners in the West to treat seizures. There is no question that acupuncture can alter brain activity. Many surgical procedures can be performed using acupuncture instead of anesthetic drugs. The ways in which acupuncture works are poorly understood, and its usefulness in the treatment of epilepsy is unconfirmed.

Chiropractic Therapy

Some chiropractic teachings suggest that specific nutrients or forms of spinal manipulation can improve seizure control. There is no evidence to support these claims.

PART THREE

Epilepsy in Children

CHAPTER 13

Epilepsy in Infancy

A new child is a bundle of anticipation and expectations. Any illness that the child may have, including epilepsy, is traumatic to the parents and family. The stigma that some people still associate with seizures and epilepsy creates unique challenges. Seizures in a newborn almost always subside quickly but may recur as epilepsy in later childhood. The greatest challenge for the parents of a newborn with seizures is fear of the unknown. If the cause of the seizures is understood, the doctor will be better able to make predictions about the baby's development than if the cause is unknown. Even if no cause can be found, however, and all diagnostic studies are normal, there is an excellent chance that the baby will develop normally.

SEIZURES IN NEWBORNS

Jane was 2 days old and was on a respirator in the intensive care unit. I was so afraid she wouldn't live, or if she did, that there would be permanent brain damage. Then they told me that she was having seizures and needed to be treated with phenobarbital. It was all very frightening, but Janey is now 2 years old, has been off phenobarbital since the age of 6 months, and has not had any seizures since leaving the hospital at 2 weeks of age.

Seizures in newborns (babies in the first month of life) may appear as fragments of seizures that occur in children and adults. The seizures are fragmentary because the infant's brain is still developing and is unable to make the coordinated responses characteristic of a tonic-clonic seizure. The baby may have jerking or stiffening of a leg or arm that alternates from side to side, or the whole upper body may suddenly jerk forward, or both legs may jerk up toward the belly with the knees bent. The baby's facial expression, breathing, and heart rate may change. Impairment of responsiveness, which is critical in defining many types of seizures in children and adults, is difficult to assess in newborns. Parents may suspect that responsiveness is impaired when their voices are unable to attract the newborn's attention.

Even experts have difficulty in recognizing seizures in newborns. Neurologists are often told not to watch their own babies too closely, especially when they sleep, because even they may mistake normal gestures for seizures. Normal babies have many sudden, brief jerks, grimaces, stares, and mouth movements that might suggest epilepsy in an older child or adult. A diagnosis of epilepsy in an infant is supported by behavioral changes that are atypical of children of the same age (some parents videotape the suspected behavior at home for viewing by the doctor), repeated episodes that are identical in their behavioral features and duration, and episodes that are not brought on by changes in posture or activity.

The Moro reflex in babies is a perfectly normal response that can be easily mistaken for a seizure. When a baby is startled, such as by momentary removal of support of its head, a loud noise, or a bright light, its spine will stiffen, its arms and legs will extend outward from the body, and its fingers will fan out. The Moro reflex is present in its full form until age 3 months, and in a fragmentary form until age 5 months. Another example of normal behavior in infants that may be confused with seizures is jitters. Jitters are shivering movements or tremors and are not epileptic seizures. They are similar to the shivering that occurs with fever in older children and adults.

The electroencephalogram (EEG), which is normally so helpful in defining seizures, is more difficult to interpret in newborns. Although the normal and abnormal patterns of brain electrical activity in newborns are becoming more clearly defined, areas of uncertainty still exist, and only a few neurologists can expertly interpret newborn EEG patterns. To complicate the situation, some seizures seen in newborns are not associated with any specific seizure patterns on the EEG.

SEIZURES IN INFANTS

I just knew something was not right. My other children had sudden jerks when they were startled and sometimes when they slept, but Jessie's jerks happened while he was awake, just watching a mobile. The pediatrician said not to worry, but when his whole body stiffened, the doctor ordered an EEG, and it showed epilepsy waves.

Seizures in infants (babies age 2–12 months) are similar to those that occur in newborns. Because older infants are able to focus their attention briefly, parents and doctors are better able to identify impaired consciousness during seizures. Some seizures can be recognized by episodes of staring from which the infant cannot be distracted. Because all children daydream, it may be difficult to distract the healthiest of babies when their minds are focused on an object or a thought. Seizures cannot be diagnosed simply because the child appears to stare. During some staring spells, the infant may make sudden, involuntary movements or jerks or may have a sudden loss of muscle tone. With other seizures, he or she may make repetitive movements that appear purposeless or semipurposeful. At times, the seizure may be more violent, and the baby may fall, or its entire body may stiffen and jerk. Because breathing may be briefly interrupted or irregular, the baby's face may become pale or blue, but the seizure is almost never life-threatening.

The vast majority of seizures in infants last less than 5 minutes. When seizures, especially the first one or violent ones, last more than 5 minutes or occur in a series, the baby should be taken to an emergency room. The parents of an infant who has a definite diagnosis of epileptic seizures should be told when to call the doctor or to take the child to the doctor's office or a hospital if the seizures worsen.

EEG patterns in infants are more clearly defined than those in newborns. However, the normal range of variability is still quite large. The patterns seen during the waking and sleeping periods can vary considerably between healthy children of the same age, leading to problems with interpretation. Most seizures occurring in infancy are associated with EEG changes during the seizure.

Infantile spasms (West's syndrome) usually develop during infancy and last an average of 5 to 6 months with treatment (see Chapter 4). Adrenocorticotropic hormone (ACTH), a hormone that stimulates the body to make steroids, reduces or eliminates these seizures in many infants. A typical course of therapy lasts 3 months. The dosage is highest during the first week and then is usually lowered gradually over the next several months. The adverse effects of ACTH depend on the dose used, the duration of therapy, and the baby's sensitivity to the drug. Although rare allergic reactions may occur, all other adverse effects are produced by ACTH stimulating the infant's body to manufacture cortisol, a steroid hormone. The potential adverse effects of excessive cortisol include severe irritability, increased appetite, high blood pressure, redistribution of body fat to make the face and trunk fatter and the arms and legs thinner, metabolic changes that alter the blood concentrations of sodium and potassium, and increased risk of infection. However, the majority of babies with infantile spasms tolerate ACTH therapy fairly well and experience no serious adverse effects. In many cases, the baby will be given another medication after the spasms have stopped and the ACTH therapy has been completed.

Febrile seizures are tonic-clonic seizures that may occur in infants and young children when they have a high fever. They are discussed in detail in Chapter 4.

DIAGNOSIS OF NEWBORN AND INFANT SEIZURES

Doctors try to identify the cause of seizures in newborns and infants, although in many cases no cause can be found. Brain injuries causing seizures may be impossible to pinpoint, especially injuries occurring in the womb or those associated with only microscopic damage. For example, seizure disorders in infancy may result from viral infections in the mother during pregnancy that are undetectable with our current tests. However, the vast majority of pregnant women who have mild viral infections have perfectly healthy babies. Commonly recognized causes of epilepsy before the age of 1 year include fever, birth injury and trauma, birth defects resulting from abnormal brain development in the womb, genetic disorders, encephalitis (an infection of the brain), and meningitis (an infection of the membranes covering the brain).

Depending on the baby's medical history and examination, the doctor may order a variety of tests or procedures, including an ultrasound, computed tomography (CT) scan, or magnetic resonance imaging (MRI) of the head to examine the structure of the brain; an EEG to study the electrical activity of the brain; a variety of blood and urine tests to look for metabolic problems; chromosomal studies to look for genetic disorders; and a spinal tap (lumbar puncture) to search for evidence of infection or metabolic disorders. The lumbar puncture, which is done to obtain a sample of cerebrospinal fluid, is safe and not very painful; the baby's worst crying usually comes when the doctor cleans the skin with a cool antiseptic solution.

TREATMENT OF NEWBORN AND INFANT SEIZURES

Therapy for seizures in newborns and infants is determined by their cause and the type of seizure that occurred. In some cases, no therapy is needed because the seizure is an isolated event, as in a single seizure associated with a high fever. In other cases, replacement of a missing nutrient can stop further seizures, as in low blood sugar levels or a calcium or vitamin B_6 deficiency in a newborn.

Babies who have epilepsy usually require treatment with antiepileptic drugs. As in treating patients in any other age group, doctors try to balance the benefits of seizure control against the risks of adverse effects from the drugs. They sometimes prefer to keep the dosage low and let the baby have a brief seizure followed by several minutes of lethargy once a week, rather than use a high dosage that makes the baby seizure-free but always sedated, listless, and developmentally slow.

This raises an important question if a baby with epilepsy is also developmentally delayed: What is causing the delay—the seizures, the epilepsy waves found on the EEG, the medicines, or the underlying problem? This question is difficult to answer and may even be impossible to answer definitively because when one factor changes, it can alter the others. For example, lowering the dosage and the number of antiepileptic drugs reduces the adverse effects but may increase the epilepsy waves on the EEG and make the seizures worse. In babies with CT or MRI evidence of a brain abnormality, the structural problem is probably a major cause of developmental delay. Such babies, however, may be even more sensitive than usual to the effects of seizures and medications. Despite the difficulties, these questions should be addressed, and often there must be a trade-off to get the best results.

Pediatricians and family physicians often treat babies with seizures. Seizures are common in children under 1 year of age, and doctors who see many infants are usually familiar with epilepsy and its treatment. The pediatrician or family physician may refer the baby to a pediatric neurologist for a consultation or long-term care. In complex or difficult cases, referral to a pediatric epileptologist at a comprehensive epilepsy center is often helpful.

CHAPTER 14

Epilepsy in Childhood

All types of seizures occur in children, but they are slightly more likely to have primary generalized epilepsies than partial epilepsies, in contrast with adults, in whom partial epilepsies predominate. The various types of seizures are described in Chapter 3. Some special types of seizures or epilepsy syndromes begin or only occur in childhood. These disorders, discussed in Chapter 4, include febrile seizures, infantile spasms (West's syndrome), Lennox-Gastaut syndrome, absence seizures, juvenile myoclonic epilepsy, benign rolandic epilepsy, and reflex epilepsies.

Seizures in children have many causes (see Fig. 8). Common causes of childhood seizures or epilepsy include fever, metabolic disorders such as low blood sugar, head injury, infections of the brain and its coverings, lack of oxygen to the brain, hydrocephalus (excess water in the brain cavities), and disorders of brain development. Less common causes of childhood epilepsy include brain tumors or cysts and degenerative disorders. There is an important difference between something that causes seizures, such as a high fever in a young child, and something that causes epilepsy, such as a severe head injury.

The issue of immunizations as a cause of epilepsy remains controversial, although the overwhelming consensus of experts is that immunizations do not cause epilepsy. However, a seizure may occur within several days of an immunization, especially if it is followed by a fever. In such cases, the child probably had an innocent febrile seizure. When the child receives subsequent immunizations, the parents should ask the doctor about using acetaminophen (Tylenol) or ibuprofen (Advil, Motrin) before a fever develops and cool soaks or baths after a fever develops. Children who have a single seizure following an immunization can usually receive further immunizations.

Many childhood seizures are benign. That is, they are self-limited, meaning that they will end without treatment, and the child's development and intellect are usually normal. Other seizures are serious and often are associated with developmental delay or mental retardation and persistent seizures. The prognosis for seizures only partially depends on their cause. Consider the following example: two children are infected with the same bacteria and both have meningitis, an infection of the membranes covering the brain and spinal cord. One child is left with severe epilepsy, but the other child never has a seizure. There may be an explanation for the different outcomes. The bacterial infection in one child may have been more widespread, involving a sensitive area of the brain, whereas in the other child, the infection may have largely spared the surface of the brain. Alternatively, in one child the bacteria could have infected a vein and caused a small stroke, which then caused the epilepsy, or one child may have had a genetic (hereditary) predisposition to seizures, and the infection was enough to bring this trait to the surface.

All people are capable of having a seizure. It remains uncertain why some children have seizures after certain stimuli such as moderate head trauma and most others do not. "Seizure threshold" refers to the conditions necessary for the production of a seizure. In animals, the seizure threshold can be precisely defined by observing their response to certain chemicals or electrical stimulation. In human beings, the term "seizure threshold" is used in a more abstract sense. In persons who have a predisposition to seizures, the threshold is lower than in people who have a greater resistance, or higher threshold, against seizures. Genetic factors probably influence an individual's seizure threshold.

MAKING THE DIAGNOSIS OF EPILEPSY

A detailed and accurate history of a child's episodes is the most helpful tool for making the diagnosis of epilepsy (see Chapter 8). The doctor will want to know how the episode began and what happened. Did the spell begin suddenly, shortly after standing, or after an argument? Was consciousness lost or impaired? Was the episode associated with jerking movements, automatic chewing or hand movements, eye blinking, or loss of bladder control? Afterward, did the child go to sleep? Or act confused? How long did the episode last? It is best to time an episode with a watch, as a minute may seem like 5 minutes to an observer. This information will help the doctor to determine if the episodes were seizures, and if so, what type.

Obtaining an accurate description of seizure symptoms in children is an art. Symptoms are subjective, and only the person who experiences them can accurately describe them. In some cases, the symptoms can be readily identified. For example, the child whose face is suddenly filled with fright and who holds her belly and then begins to stare is most likely experiencing a partial seizure with an emotion of fear and abdominal discomfort. In many children, however, the symptoms cannot be deciphered from behavioral features, and one must rely on the child's report. Many children simply fail to report what they feel because of shyness, embarrassment, inability to put their feelings into words, inability to recognize the relationship of the symptom to a seizure, inability to recall the event, and other less obvious reasons. Simply asking such a child what he or she experiences may elicit nothing more than a shrug of the shoulders. When given a choice of possible symptoms, however, the child will often say that one or more occurred before the seizure. The challenge is then separating true from imaginary symptoms. Therefore, all children who are willing or able to talk about their symptoms should first be asked in a nonthreatening way if they feel anything before or during the episode, or if they ever have sudden, strange feelings separate from the episode, which could possibly be a simple partial seizure. If they answer no, inquiries should be made about specific types of symptoms.

CONDITIONS CONFUSED WITH CHILDHOOD SEIZURES

Not every event that involves jerking, staring, or impairment of consciousness is a seizure. All kinds of behavior can look like seizures, and it may take some time and many tests to sort out which, in fact, are true seizures.

Daydreaming

We all daydream, and children daydream more than adults. Daydreaming in children can be easily confused with absence or complex partial seizures, in which staring is a prominent and common feature. However, lip smacking, eye blinking, or alterations in muscle tone are common during seizures but not during daydreaming. Daydreaming can be stopped by calling the child's name, producing a startling noise, or gently touching the child's hand. Absence and complex partial seizures can only rarely be stopped by such means, although with atypical seizures, the child may be partially responsive. Absence seizures usually last less than 10 seconds, and complex partial seizures 30 seconds to 3 minutes. Daydreaming tends to occur when the child is tired or bored or is involved in monotonous activity, such as riding in the backseat of a car, but seizures can occur at any time. Another important distinguishing feature is the beginning of the attack. Seizures often begin abruptly. For example, in the middle of a sentence or while playing with a toy, the child may suddenly stop and stare. In contrast, daydreaming often represents the continuation of a natural pause in activity.

For example, a child may be reading and raise his or her head to reflect on a sentence and then daydream.

"Blue" Breath-Holding Spells

In the classic case of "blue" breath-holding spells, a young child cries intensely for a long time, holds her breath, and then loses consciousness and becomes limp. The child often turns bluish and may sweat profusely. The typical attack lasts 30 to 60 seconds. With more prolonged spells, the entire body may become rigid and jerk, as the lack of oxygen to the brain actually triggers a seizure.

When children cry vigorously, they may exhale and then pause before taking another breath. When the pause is unusually long, it is considered a breath-holding spell. Because of the way they affect the child, breath-holding spells may be confused with atonic, tonic, or tonic-clonic seizures. Distinguishing epileptic seizures from breath-holding spells is based mainly on the typical sequence of a physical or emotional upset, followed by crying and breath-holding, which helps the doctor determine that the spell was an episode of breath-holding, not epilepsy. Breath-holding spells usually begin between 6 and 18 months of age and stop before the child is 6 years old. About 25% of the patients have a family history of breath-holding spells.

In the majority of cases, breath-holding spells are caused by some minor upset such as a bump on the head, being scolded for running into the street, or being told not to play with a toy. This upset triggers the crying and breath holding. Prolonged breath holding produces a lack of oxygen in the brain and causes fainting, sometimes with a "seizure." Although the seizure looks just like an epileptic seizure, the child neither has, nor is likely to have, epilepsy. Furthermore, the lack of oxygen in breath-holding spells and the occasional seizure that follows do not cause brain injury.

The outlook for a child with breath-holding spells is excellent, and in most cases no treatment is needed. Parents may try to distract the child during the intense crying, as this can prevent the breath-holding spell. In children who are prone to prolonged vigorous crying tantrums, parents should try to ignore the behavior, thereby withholding the attention and concern that reinforces such behavior. In some cases, the help of a psychologist can be enlisted to modify the child's behavior.

Pallid Infantile Syncope

Syncope (**sin**-co-pee) is a faint. Pallid infantile syncope may be confused with atonic, tonic, or tonic-clonic seizures. In this nonepileptic disorder, which usually begins between 12 and 18 months of age and ends before age 6, the child suddenly becomes pale (pallid) and then faints. Other family members often have a history of similar spells, sometimes called "pallid breath-holding spells," in early childhood. In contrast with breath-holding spells, the episodes are not consistently preceded by intense crying. With more prolonged spells, the entire body may become rigid and jerk as the lack of oxygen to the brain triggers a seizure. The episodes may result from sensitivity of the vagus nerve, which controls the heart rate. The prognosis is excellent, and treatment is rarely needed, although for some patients doctors may prescribe small doses of atropine.

Other Forms of Syncope

Faints are common in children as well as adults. In many cases, other family members have a history of fainting. Painful situations such as having blood drawn can cause a faint. Some faints in children result from the depletion of fluids in the body (dehydration) caused by inadequate fluid intake or excessive fluid loss, as occurs, for example, with sweating or diarrhea. Excessive sun exposure can also cause faints. In other cases, heart disorders cause slowing of the heart beat or a decrease in the force of the heart's contractions, causing a faint. Faints are often preceded by lightheadedness or dizziness before consciousness is lost but are not normally followed by confusion or tiredness. Frequent episodes of fainting should be thoroughly investigated by a doctor.

Movement Disorders

Many nonepileptic movement disorders can be easily confused with tonic or motor seizures. Children with these disorders assume abnormal postures (parts of their body are in an unusual position, such as the fingers curled up as if in a cramp, or the foot turned inward) or make sudden unusual movements (such as eye blinking or jerks of a body part), and the attacks may begin suddenly, thus mimicking seizures. Most of these movement disorders occur spontaneously, but others are triggered by specific events such as eating (Sandifer's syndrome).

Tics are involuntary, repetitive, intermittent, brief movements. Although tics are purposeless, they may resemble purposeful movements. The most common tics in children are eye blinks, facial grimaces, shoulder shrugs, and head movements. The most severe form of tics occurs in Tourette's syndrome, which is also associated with vocal tics ranging from grunts and throat-clearing sounds to involuntary cursing and other embarrassing noises. Tics are not seizures.

Sleep jerks (benign nocturnal myoclonus) are brief, involuntary muscular contractions that occur as a person falls asleep. In some cases, they may awaken someone who is drifting off to sleep. Sleep jerks are common in healthy children and adults. These normal movements may be confused with myoclonic seizures.

TAKING MEDICATIONS

Hardly anybody likes taking medications. They are a hassle to remember, may be embarrassing to take, and disrupt other, more pleasant activities. When doctors recommend a treatment, they assume that the patient will follow their instructions. This may be a false assumption. Noncompliance, or failure to take medications as prescribed, is common. There are many reasons why patients do not follow the doctor's instructions. Perhaps the most important reason is that the patient and family are not involved in the treatment plan. They should be told about the possible choices of therapy, their benefits, and the common minor or troublesome adverse effects, as well as the rare but serious adverse effects, of antiepileptic drugs. Communication is the key to avoiding noncompliance.

Compliance is a problem in children. Young children often hate taking medications but can usually be coaxed. It may be necessary to crush the pills and put the powder in the child's favorite foods, or to give the child a small reward if he or she takes the pills. Even small children can understand the importance of taking their pills. Young children can be told that it will help keep them well. Older children can understand that they are taking their pills so they will not have seizures. Parents may want to use themselves as an example. They can show their children that they occasionally take an aspirin when they have a headache. They might take a vitamin so the children can emulate their behavior. Children love to imitate their parents. *Caution: Keep all medications out of the reach of young children.*

VIDEO GAMES AND EPILEPSY

Reports in newspapers and on television have heightened public awareness that playing video games can, in rare cases, trigger seizures, but there is no scientific evidence that video games can cause epilepsy. Playing video games is an extremely common pastime for many children, and they often play them for long periods of time. Because epilepsy is a common disorder of childhood, it is not surprising that some children coincidentally will have their seizures while playing video games. How often this happens, and to what extent, if any, the games trigger the seizures, is not known.

In some children who have epilepsy, stress, fatigue, or hyperventilation may trigger seizures during video games. Further, photosensitivity may be involved when seizures are directly associated with playing video games, because in photosensitive children, flashing lights or flickering images can trigger seizures or epilepsy waves on the electroencephalogram (EEG). Photosensitivity, however, occurs in only about 3% of people with epilepsy. Most children who have epilepsy are not photosensitive and should be able to play video games without ill effects.

Parents who are unsure whether a child who has epilepsy is also photosensitive should check with the doctor. Photosensitive children may be able to play some games quite safely but have problems with others. Medication can often prevent seizures caused by photosensitivity.

Although there is a natural tendency to fear that a child may have seizures triggered by playing video games, the overwhelming majority of children, with or without epilepsy, can play these games without any risk of seizures. Restricting a child from playing video games simply because he or she has epilepsy is not justified.

For parents who are concerned about the possible risk of seizures, it may be helpful to observe the child during the game and watch for brief episodes of blank staring in which the child seems momentarily frozen in place, rapid blinking or twitching of the mouth or face, jerking movements of other parts of the body, loss of attention, brief inability to talk or respond, or reports from the child that things look, sound, smell, or feel different than usual. Although the presence of one or more of these signs does not necessarily mean that a child has epilepsy or is photosensitive, a medical consultation is recommended.

The following suggestions on ways of reducing the risk of seizures in photosensitive children while watching television may be helpful with regard to video games as well:

- Play in a well-lighted room to reduce the contrast between the lighted screen and the surrounding area. Reducing the brightness of the screen may also be helpful.
- Keep as far back from the screen as possible.
- Use smaller screens in which it is more difficult to see the horizontal scan lines.
- Avoid playing for long periods.
- Take regular breaks, and look away from the screen every once in a while.

- Cover one eye while playing (an eye doctor may recommend alternating between the right eye and the left eye and the length of time each eye should be covered).
- Stop the game if strange or unusual feelings develop.
- Seek a medical consultation if a child has strange or uncomfortable sensations caused by light shimmering on water, sunlight flickering through the trees, flashing strobe lights, or any usual reaction to sudden or strong light.

CHAPTER 15

Epilepsy in Adolescence

Adolescence is the passage from childhood to adulthood. It is surrounded by the issues of rebellion, independence, heightened self-consciousness, experimentation, dating, driving, and concerns for the future. Adolescents and their parents share the highs and lows of this often stormy period, and communication between them is essential to temper the turbulence of adolescence. This is a challenge for both parents and children, as adolescence, almost by definition, brings parents and children into conflict. The intense emotions and feelings that come with adolescence are both positive and negative: parents are both heroes and villains, best friends and "police officers," and the source of great affection and frustration. The boundaries of the child's independence, which were tested in early childhood, are retested in adolescence.

The tidal waves of emotions on which adolescents often ride or by which they are consumed affect those around them. Emotions are infectious. Parents must maintain their perspective and must be sensitive to their child's insecurities, peer pressures, and need for support. The parents must communicate with their children about drugs, smoking, drinking, and sexually transmitted diseases, including infection with the human immunodeficiency virus (HIV), which causes the acquired immunodeficiency syndrome (AIDS). The key to communication is letting children know that they can feel comfortable talking with their parents. If the parents become too judgmental too quickly, they will harm the trust and openness between them and their children. The balance becomes difficult. Parents need to educate and let their feelings be known, but they should try to do it in a positive manner. If adolescents engage in dangerous or irresponsible activities and parents need to "read them the riot act," they should try to pause and not react in the midst of their own emotional storm. Adolescents often know when they have done something wrong and are embarrassed and frustrated by their actions.

Adolescence does not need any complicating factors, but epilepsy is just that. In a time of life marked by continuous adjustments to dramatic

164

physical, mental, and social changes, a medical disorder such as epilepsy can upset the tenuous balance. Adolescence is a period of heightened self-consciousness, with exaggerated concerns over physical and social image. Epilepsy, even if it is well controlled, can torment an adolescent—stimulating fears of isolation, ridicule, and possible humiliation. Restrictions on their activities can further accentuate differences from their peers. For children entering into adolescence with good self-esteem and a sense of independence, the impact of epilepsy can be minimal. For adolescents with low self-esteem, dependency, and behavioral difficulties, epilepsy can create and aggravate psychosocial problems. Caring for adolescents with epilepsy requires special patience and understanding.

Children with superior, average, or near-average intelligence whose epilepsy is well controlled are able to achieve independence during adolescence and adulthood. Children with more severe physical and mental problems confront a different situation as they mature. Parents of adolescents who cannot achieve independence in the community must begin to explore the options for their future living arrangements, employment possibilities, legal and financial security, and social and sexual adjustments.

PUBERTY

Puberty marks the transition from childhood to adolescence. The sex hormones estrogen and progesterone in girls and testosterone in boys, which were produced in small amounts during childhood, go into a mass-production phase during puberty. These hormones initiate the physical changes associated with puberty. Boys experience deepening of the voice and muscle growth, and girls have breast enlargement and an increase in body fat. Both sexes experience growth of the sex organs and body hair, and both usually have acne. Some breast enlargement is also common in boys during puberty. There is often a large growth spurt. These physical changes are the source of anxiety and adjustment. The age at which puberty begins varies considerably from one child to the next, and children who have early or late changes may be concerned or, in some cases, teased about the differences in their bodies as compared with those of their peers. Children may be too embarrassed to discuss their concerns with their parents.

The sex hormones affect not only the body but also the brain. Many of the sex hormones enter the brain and bind to receptors on nerve cells there. These hormones alter the activity of the brain. Changes in brain activity are related to changes in personality and mood. Just as hormones cause some women to experience emotional changes before their menstrual period begins, and abuse of steroid hormones related to testosterone causes some athletes to become irritable or aggressive, adolescents also undergo changes in behavior related to hormones. In fact, sometimes these hormonal changes bring out seizures for the first time.

For some children, seizures begin or stop around the time of puberty. Although this may be coincidental, the relation between epilepsy and puberty is probably a result of hormonal changes affecting the brain. Certain hormones such as estrogen may increase the likelihood of seizures. Further, many women report that seizures most often occur around the time of their menstrual period. However, this does not mean that birth control pills will make seizures more likely; studies have shown no such effect for the large majority of women.

Other brain changes that may be less directly related to hormones also occur during puberty. Early in adolescence, children gain greater fine motor control and begin to show more mature responses to complex problems. Their ability to think about abstract problems and moral issues is greater. Shortly after puberty, children are much better able to understand the consequences of certain behaviors in a theoretical sense; that is, they can understand the outcome of some behaviors without experiencing the outcome itself. For example, girls can understand that they may become pregnant as a consequence of sexual activity. This ability to consider the consequences of behavior has important implications for health matters such as epilepsy. At this point in their development, children are better able to participate in their own care.

The increased production and release of sex hormones into the bloodstream during puberty is not always a gradual, smooth process. The hormones may be released in large amounts over short periods of time. The changes in hormone levels can be associated with relatively rapid changes in personality, mood, and physical features, such as a new crop of pimples. The irritability, moodiness, and other personality changes associated with puberty and early adolescence are often due to hormonal changes. The child is not "bad" or "misbehaving," but simply experiencing natural changes as part of development.

Metabolic changes as well as the rapid changes in growth that accompany puberty may be unpredictable and can alter the blood levels of antiepileptic drugs. If seizure control worsens in an adolescent, the possibility of a decrease in the drug levels should be considered.

Puberty also brings about changes in psychosocial development. The early adolescent is active in three arenas: the peer group, family, and school. The peer group is often the main focus of the young adolescent's life. The bonds are usually strongest among members of the same sex, with a strong emphasis on conformity and joint activities. Early adolescence brings major changes in the family as the child seeks independence. Earlier relationships with parents and, less often, with brothers and sisters are disrupted. As the physical changes of puberty begin, the child often seeks greater privacy, especially with regard to the parent of the opposite sex. The adolescent's testing of parental limits is a conflict between the desire for parental guidance and the desire for autonomy. School life can also be affected by puberty. Children who undergo the changes of puberty earlier or later than their classmates may have more adjustment problems. Intellectual and behavioral maturation will also have an impact on school performance.

The maturity of children evolves during adolescence but often does so in an erratic fashion. Behaviors that demonstrate a remarkable degree of maturity are followed hours later or the next day by immature actions and reactions. Parents must be available to discuss questions and problems. They must be supportive of the child's independence while watching out for his or her safety and well-being. It is reasonable to raise gingerly some important issues that the child may be avoiding, but if he or she is uncomfortable with the discussion, it is best not to push.

TAKING MEDICATIONS

I know Steve doesn't take his medication regularly. I try to remind him every morning and every night. It's more than forgetting. By not taking his medications, he is saying, "I don't really have epilepsy." I hope he realizes that he won't be able to drive if he still has his occasional complex partial seizures.

The maturity that adolescence brings should make children more aware of the benefits of taking their antiepileptic drugs. For some adolescents, however, rebellion or denial dominates the scene, making them less likely to take their medications as prescribed. It is essential, therefore, that the reasons for taking the antiepileptic drugs that were taught during childhood be repeated during early adolescence. Adolescents are normally able to understand the consequences of taking or not taking the medications. Education about antiepileptic drugs can come from both the parents and the doctor, but the adolescent should be enlisted as an active partner in his or her treatment. Teenagers with epilepsy should be allowed to take greater responsibility for managing their care. It is often helpful for the adolescent and doctor to be alone for a portion of each visit or even the whole visit. This makes the adolescent feel more in control and more mature and helps to establish trust with the doctor and the parents.

One of the most powerful factors in securing a child's compliance is peer pressure. At the age of radical change, the desire for conformity is strong. Seizures can be embarrassing and cause fears of social isolation. Further, uncontrolled seizures may result in restrictions on certain activities such as driving. Adolescents should know that the longer they are free of seizures with medications, the better the chances are that they will be seizure-free without medications.

Measuring the level of antiepileptic drugs in the blood at regular intervals can tell the doctor and the parents if the adolescent is taking the medications as prescribed and can reinforce compliance. However, problems with drug absorption or metabolism, or a period of rapid growth in height and weight, can cause the levels to be low even though the drugs are taken regularly.

PARENT-CHILD RELATIONSHIPS

The nature of the relationships with his or her parents and peers will strongly influence the impact of epilepsy on the adolescent. Parents who have open communication and a strong basis of trust with their child before adolescence will have a much easier time relating to him or her during the difficult times ahead. For parents who have relationship problems with their child, counseling may be helpful. Parenting is never easy, and parenting of a child with epilepsy during adolescence can be especially difficult. Parents should not hesitate to ask for help. The help can come from a friend, family member, religious leader, social worker, psychologist, or psychiatrist.

Parents must set limits, such as restricting activities and setting curfews. Setting limits is difficult for parents and children. The concern for the child's safety must be balanced against his or her need for independence and peer group acceptance. All children face some risks. Minimizing the risks does not justify severe restriction of their activities. The parents' goal should be to help their child achieve a mature and independent state. Parents should encourage adolescents to "think things out," and to weigh the positives and negatives of their decisions. Parents should discuss strategies that can be used to reduce or eliminate negative factors. For example, if a child wants to go on a canoeing and camping trip, it may be safe if certain precautions are taken. The child can, therefore, experience the excitement and adventure of a new activity without the parents and can be included in the peer group. The parents' role should not be simply to protect their child from possible dangers, for the greatest danger may be bringing up a dependent child who has poor self-esteem.

PEER RELATIONSHIPS

The adolescent peer group strongly influences the behavior of its members. In early adolescence, there is a strong need to be part of a group and a need to conform. Although the bonds appear strong, the relationships are often shallow.

Parents should want their children to be socially active, but the friends they make are often not ideal in the parents' eyes. Friends should be responsible and mature and not encourage the child toward risky or trouble-making activities. If friends clearly push a child toward dangerous behaviors, then the parent must intervene. That does not mean forbidding the child from ever socializing with these friends, but it does mean that the child should understand why such behaviors are dangerous and must be avoided. A real problem arises when the undesirable behaviors of a friend or peer group are repeated and the child is pressured into participating.

Because acceptance by peers may be an even more important issue for adolescents with epilepsy, parents must be careful in how they react. Often, social isolation is a much more dangerous situation than the rebellious activities of adolescence. On the other hand, young people used to rejection can be particularly vulnerable when undesirable groups show a willingness to associate with them.

DRIVING

Driving a motor vehicle is one of the greatest acts of independence in our society. There is no other time in life when a certain birthday takes on such meaning as the age at which one can obtain a license to drive. Many people with epilepsy can drive, but there are obvious safety concerns (see Chapter 23).

In most states, a person with epilepsy must submit a letter or form from the doctor about his or her seizure disorder. Many states ask the doctor about compliance with medications. It is often helpful to remind adolescents that a favorable doctor's report depends on their taking the medications as prescribed.

As the age for driving approaches, it is often worthwhile to review the adolescent's medical care. If he or she has been seizure-free for several years, it may be wise to attempt to lower and eventually stop medications at least 6 months or a year before the driving age is reached. For those whose seizures remain poorly controlled, approaching the legal age for driving may prompt referral to an epilepsy center for reevaluation and possible changes in the treatment plan.

Adolescents with uncontrolled seizures cannot obtain a driver's license. Alternatives to driving include riding with friends, carpools, or public transportation. Lack of a driver's license should not stand in the way of social activities or holding a job, although it often does.

DATING

Dating is a natural activity, but it does not come naturally to most people. Adolescents are often uncomfortable or uneasy when they start to date, and having epilepsy can complicate an already complicated social situation. Anyone who is interested in dating someone should first try to get to know the person in school or a group setting. Although it is a good idea to discuss epilepsy with anyone who is being dated regularly, it is reasonable to wait until the relationship feels comfortable. The person should not be tested. For example, it is best not to make up "people you know with epilepsy" to see how the other person will react. If the discussion is open and honest, friends will be more willing to ask questions and share their feelings. When the seizures are not well controlled, it may be a good idea to discuss the epilepsy sooner rather than later. This situation can be awkward. It is best done in person, not over the telephone. However, it is wise to wait a bit before talking about epilepsy with new friends. Even if it seems necessary to tell them on the first date, it is best to wait for a good moment.

Every person who has asked someone for a date has known the fear of possible rejection. It underlies much of the anxiety and discomfort associated with dating. Someone with epilepsy has the added fear that he or she will be rejected because of the epilepsy. This fear is not completely unfounded. Some people who hear the word epilepsy become frightened. They may have little or no knowledge about epilepsy. Fear of the unknown is the greatest fear. People can be educated by someone who has the disorder. Their understanding of epilepsy and feelings about it will reflect the understanding and feelings of the person who lives with it.

Rejection is part of the dating game. No one is spared. People are attracted to others because of physical features and personality. The physical reasons may be more important at first, but the compatibility of personalities and the rapport that develops between people are what keep a couple together. People are rejected because their nose is too big, waist is too wide, eyes are too small, stature is too short, build is too muscular, or for countless other physical reasons. People are also rejected because they are too insecure, arrogant, obnoxious, lazy, selfish, or generous, or for many other personality traits. Most of the time, the reasons for rejection are not clearly defined in the mind of the person who is doing the rejecting. Although epilepsy is one of many possible reasons that someone may reject someone else, it is often not *the* reason. In addition, some people perceive rejection when it is not there; they expect it and so imagine it to exist. If the other person is already aware of the disorder before dating begins, the situation is much easier. In this case, there is less to explain, and less fear that epilepsy will "turn the other person off."

SEXUAL ACTIVITY

As one grows closer in a relationship, there is a natural tendency to want to hold hands, kiss, and have other intimate contact. There are no universal rules about when to kiss or engage in other intimate activities. Religious upbringing, the attitudes of parents, local society, peers, one's personal beliefs, and feelings about a certain person all influence these decisions. Friends provide the richest source of information about sex and about what other people are "doing." Unfortunately, adolescents, especially boys, often exaggerate their activities. This can lead their friends to have unrealistic expectations. There should be no rush to experience sexual intimacy. If there is pressure from friends to engage in sexual activities, they are being immature. It is not worth ruining a relationship trying to impress friends who themselves may not be all that experienced. For more information and discussions about dating and sex, it is helpful to talk with a trusted adult. This can be a parent, an older brother or sister, an uncle or aunt, a school counselor, or a nurse or doctor. If the person is uncomfortable talking about these topics, it is best to go to another adult who is more at ease.

When two people share a mutual attraction and desire for some intimate contact, sparks often fly. There is no reason to fear having a seizure during kissing or other intimate contact any more than at other times. However, intimate contact does not protect someone from a seizure. Therefore, if a person has uncontrolled seizures, it is possible that one will occur during intimate contact. Thus, a partner should know about the disorder and what to do if a seizure occurs.

Although the vast majority of persons with epilepsy are able to enjoy sexual feelings and activities, some have less interest in sexual activity than their peers. The libido, or interest in sexual activity, may be affected by high dosages of antiepileptic drugs, especially the barbiturates, or possibly by the epilepsy itself. In most instances, the person with epilepsy is not aware of a problem. Instead, it may be noticed by a parent or even a boyfriend or girlfriend. It may not be a problem, however, as people have a wide range of interest in intimate relationships and sexual activity. If it becomes an issue, it may be helpful to discuss it with a doctor. In some cases, changing medications or reducing the dosage can be helpful.

USE OF ALCOHOL AND ILLEGAL DRUGS

When adolescents use alcohol or illegal drugs, trouble is not far behind. Their immaturity and willingness to take chances often place adolescents who use alcohol and other drugs in particularly dangerous places, such as behind the wheel of a motor vehicle. Few adolescents understand the potential dangers of drugs. Those who have grown up in homes where alcohol and drugs were never abused have no idea what intoxication is, or what dangers these substances can bring. Those who have grown up in a home where drugs such as alcohol were abused may be more prone toward substance abuse.

The dangers of adolescent drug use should be clear to us all. Drinking contests continue to kill young people. Alcohol is the leading cause of motor vehicle accidents in the United States. Snorting cocaine and smoking crack can cause strokes, heart attacks, seizures, or death.

The rules concerning alcohol use and epilepsy apply to adolescents but with greater caution. In adults, one or two alcoholic beverages cause no meaningful changes in the blood levels of antiepileptic drugs or in seizure control. The problem with one or two drinks for adolescents, whether or not they have epilepsy, is that their understanding of alcohol and their ability to limit its intake is often inadequate. One or two drinks become three or four, intoxication clouds judgment, and serious problems can follow. Teenagers often will sleep off a hangover, and those with epilepsy may fail to take their bedtime and morning medications. Therefore, it is a good idea for all adolescents, especially those with epilepsy, to avoid alcohol or to use it only under adult supervision, such as having a glass of wine or a beer during dinner. Adolescents with epilepsy should know that alcohol abuse can worsen seizure control. In addition, the combination of antiepileptic drugs and alcohol can have a strong sedative effect, and when excessive amounts of alcohol are consumed, the combination can be dangerous.

Crack and cocaine can cause seizures in people who have never had one before. Although there are no studies of the effects of crack or cocaine on seizure control, there is an obvious risk that these substances would make the occurrence of seizures more likely. Seizures that occur with cocaine or crack use are much more dangerous, and can be fatal. This was clearly demonstrated by the case of Len Bias, a basketball star from the University of Maryland, who reportedly had seizures and died after using crack. Deadly seizures or heart attacks can occur after the first-time use of these substances. Crack and cocaine are associated with other serious health problems as well, and should be avoided at all costs.

Seizures can be caused or made worse by the use of uppers (amphetamines), downers (barbiturates, benzodiazepines), heroin, certain pain killers, LSD ("acid"), PCP ("angel dust"), or "ecstasy." The effects of these drugs on epilepsy are not known with certainty, but they can bring on seizures by causing the user to forget to take antiepileptic medications or to lose sleep. These drugs may also have direct and indirect (withdrawal) effects on the brain. The possession or selling of all these drugs is illegal, and the severe penalties for even casual association with them, coupled with their numerous health risks, make their use foolish and dangerous.

THINKING ABOUT A CAREER

Most people do not decide on their future career while in high school. Nevertheless, it is often helpful for adolescents with epilepsy to give some thought to the type of career they would like to pursue. Certain classes in high school or college can be aimed toward advancing the knowledge and skills required for an area of interest. These classes can be a helpful head start on a career. Guidance counselors and vocational counselors often are available in high school to discuss career plans.

Persons with well-controlled or infrequent seizures should have few or no limitations on possible careers, but those with uncontrolled seizures may face some career limitations. Adolescents should ask the doctor about their prognosis for seizure control. With new medications and other new therapies such as epilepsy surgery, it is likely that many persons with uncontrolled seizures will become seizure-free in the future.

PART-TIME EMPLOYMENT

Part-time work can be rewarding for adolescents who have epilepsy. In addition to the financial rewards, work can provide discipline, skills, education, and a sense of accomplishment and success. A part-time job is often an important step toward independence. A part-time job can be a way of getting some exposure to a career that the young person may be interested in pursuing. It can also provide an opportunity for future full-time work.

Adolescents can work before or after school, or during the summer. When working during the school semester, the student must balance schoolwork and job demands. A job should not interfere with a healthy personal life. Students who work too many hours often sacrifice sleep while trying to keep up with schoolwork and a social life. Loss of sleep or the stress of overwork can cause an increase in the frequency of seizures. It is important, therefore, to limit the number of hours worked.

CHAPTER 16

Outgrowing Epilepsy

Most children outgrow epilepsy. This simple and positive fact raises important questions: Which children should be treated? How much medication should they receive? How long should the antiepileptic drugs be used? In recent years, doctors have changed their minds about the use of antiepileptic drugs. Several decades ago, the prevailing attitude was that seizures must be stopped at all costs, and once seizures had been stopped, that the medications should be continued indefinitely. This approach reflected a conservative and, we now think, overly pessimistic outlook on life with epilepsy. The risks of seizures were overestimated; the adverse effects of medications were underestimated. Issues such as the quality of life, or how patients felt about the frequency and severity of seizures and the adverse effects of therapy, were never considered, and the natural course of epilepsy in children was rarely studied.

This outdated medical approach, favoring seizure control at all costs, was based on several assumptions that we now know are incorrect. All seizures were thought to cause permanent brain damage. Seizures were considered so shameful that it was worth almost any adverse effect of therapy to suppress them. Epilepsy was uniformly considered a lifelong disorder. Seizure disorders were thought to become worse after puberty. Once someone was near the age for driving, it was always considered unsafe to discontinue antiepileptic drugs. It was thought that persons with epilepsy usually do not get married and that women with epilepsy should not have children. Unfortunately, a few doctors still recommend that women with epilepsy should not have children, and a few others even go so far as to suggest that they should be sterilized. The stigma associated with epilepsy has lessened dramatically during the past quarter century, and many of these attitudes merely reflect an older frame of reference. The past several decades have witnessed a dramatic growth in our knowledge of the epilepsies. We are now familiar with the natural history of various seizure types and epileptic syndromes and understand more about the safety of discontinuing antiepileptic drugs.

STOPPING ANTIEPILEPTIC DRUGS

Most children who remain seizure-free while taking medications for 2 to 4 years can safely have their medications slowly tapered by their doctors, and eventually discontinued. The majority of these children will not have another seizure. During the past decade, there has been a trend toward discontinuing medication earlier rather than later, as the chances of staying seizure-free after 2 years of treatment are similar to those after 4 years. Among children who remain seizure-free while taking antiepileptic drugs for 2 years, approximately 75% will remain seizure-free after the medication is stopped.

The chances of a specific child remaining seizure-free if medications are stopped cannot be predicted with accuracy. No matter how good the odds, there is a chance that the seizures will recur, and no matter how bad the odds, there is a chance that the seizures will not recur. Many cases fall between the extremes, making the decision more difficult. As a general rule, it is usually worthwhile to attempt to discontinue the medication after 2 years. When the child has two or more risk factors for seizure recurrence, it is reasonable to continue the medications for 4 years before attempting to withdraw them.

Favorable signs for remaining seizure-free are a diagnosis of idiopathic epilepsy, that is, when there is no identifiable cause for the seizures, normal development and neurological function, the absence of epilepsy waves on the electroencephalogram (EEG), and seizures that are easily controlled with medication. When all of these conditions are met, the child has a better than 90% chance of remaining seizure-free after the medications are stopped.

Signs indicating less chance of remaining seizure-free without medications are a progressive brain disorder or brain damage such as a birth injury; viral infection of the brain; head injury, developmental delay, mental retardation, or other neurological abnormalities; the presence of epilepsy waves or moderate to severe slowing on the EEG; and seizures that are not easily controlled with antiepileptic drugs. When all of these factors are present, the chance of seizures recurring after medication is stopped is 50% or more. These are *average* risks, however.

The decision to taper and discontinue medications should be made by the doctor and the parents; if the child is old enough and understands the issue, his or her opinion is also valuable. Some times are better than others for stopping medication. For example, a girl who is on the school gymnastic team and who does difficult routines and dismounts on the uneven parallel bars probably should not begin tapering medications shortly before or during the gymnastic season. Driving is another consideration in timing medication withdrawal. It is a good idea, if possible, to stop medications at least a year before the teenager is eligible for a driver's license.

When all of these risks are considered, some parents and children may ask, "Why not simply continue to take the drugs, as they don't seem to be doing any harm?" If there is a moderate to high risk of seizure recurrence, and the medications have few adverse effects, the risks of stopping the drug may outweigh the benefits. However, there are some important benefits of stopping the medications that make it worthwhile considering their discontinuance.

Risks of Stopping Medication

I was frightened when the doctor recommended that we take Katie off the Tegretol. Of course, I wanted her off all medications, but even more, I wanted her seizure-free. We lowered the medication slowly. I slept poorly for months, thinking that any noise in the house was a seizure. She's been off medication for 3 years, and has had no seizures.

The most obvious danger of stopping the medications is the chance that seizures will recur. If the medications are stopped abruptly, there is a chance that a recurrent seizure will be more severe or prolonged than the previous seizures. When any drug is withdrawn, the body reacts and undergoes chemical, electrical, and hormonal changes that may cause problems.

Discontinuation of an antiepileptic medication can also cause a withdrawal reaction. The withdrawal of barbiturates (phenobarbital and primidone) and benzodiazepines (clonazepam, clorazepate, diazepam, and clobazam) are associated with the highest risk of a seizure or unpleasant symptoms such as anxiety, irritability, a racing heart, difficulty sleeping, sweating, abdominal pain, vomiting, and problems with concentration. All withdrawal symptoms are reduced, and in many cases eliminated, when the medication dosage is very slowly lowered. When antiepileptic medications are properly discontinued slowly, the risk of a withdrawal seizure is very small.

Rapid discontinuation of any antiepileptic drug can be dangerous and should only be done under a doctor's supervision. Abrupt withdrawal can cause status epilepticus, which may lead to broken bones, permanent neurological impairment, or even death.

When an antiepileptic drug is tapered or withdrawn, seizures may occur simply because the drug was needed to control them. Depending on the type and severity of the seizures, the medications may need to be restarted, although the child may remain seizure-free at a lower dose. Differentiating this type of seizure recurrence from a withdrawal seizure is important, because withdrawal seizures can be managed by a temporary increase in the dosage followed by more gradual tapering. Unfortunately, it is usually hard to know whether recurrent seizures are due to withdrawal of the drug or the need for medication.

If the medications are stopped, the child, family, and school need to be prepared for the possibility that a seizure could occur. If the child has been seizure-free for 2 years or more, people tend to forget to take precautions. During the tapering and at least 3 to 6 months after stopping the medications, the child is at a somewhat higher than usual risk for seizure recurrence, and simple precautions should be taken. For example, the child should not swim without supervision or climb to high places. Three quarters of seizure relapses occur within 1 year of stopping the medication.

If a seizure recurs after a period of freedom from seizures, it is an emotional setback for both the child and the family. Parents must be prepared for this possibility and discuss it with the child. When children or adults are aware that something is possible, they are much better able to handle it if it happens. Although children will often privately worry about the possibility of seizure recurrence, their fear diminishes with time.

A rare consequence of discontinuing the medication is the reemergence of difficult-to-control seizures or the development of intolerance to a medication that was previously well tolerated. Luckily, these situations are extremely uncommon.

Benefits of Stopping Medication

In the best of all worlds, when the medications are stopped, seizures will not recur, the child will feel better, show improved school performance and behavior, and enjoy the freedom of good health without medication. When a child has been taking a medication for more than 2 years, it can be difficult to estimate the effect that the drug has on the child's behavior. In many cases, although the medication was thought to have no adverse effect, the child's alertness, ability to concentrate, memory, ability to reason, and behavioral problems such as irritability and hyperactivity improve after the medication is stopped.

In a few persons, long exposure (usually more than 5 years) to a medication can cause problems such as soft-tissue growths, caused by phenobarbital, and nerve injury, caused by phenytoin. Finally, girls who continue taking medication and want to become pregnant later on in life will expose their babies to a higher-than-normal risk of birth defects. All of these problems can be avoided by stopping the medications as soon as possible.

LONG-TERM TREATMENT

Although most forms of childhood epilepsy are outgrown, some forms are associated with a high risk of recurrent seizures if the medications are stopped. If the EEG shows abundant epilepsy waves or epilepsy waves arising from multiple regions of the brain, the risk of seizures after stopping medications is high. Juvenile myoclonic epilepsy, for example, is associated with a high rate of seizure recurrence after medication is stopped. However, this epilepsy disorder varies dramatically in its severity, and some children may have only mild myoclonic jerks a few hours after awakening. In cases such as these, stopping the medication may be reasonable. In the Lennox-Gastaut syndrome and the progressive myoclonic epilepsies, the seizures are severe and difficult to control. If control is achieved, it is usually wise to continue the medication. In these cases, it is more reasonable to try to reduce the dosage of the medication slightly than to discontinue it.

CHAPTER 17

Intellectual and Behavioral Development

For parents, watching the growth and development of their child's mind and body is magical. That magic is unique for each child. Our society loves to compare things such as cars, houses, and unfortunately, children. Comparing the development of children is unwise, because it is a highly specific and individual process. Although there are yardsticks that help to define a range of developmental milestones in the general population, development is complex. A child must be viewed as an individual, not a statistic or a point on a graph. Delays in one area of development are often accompanied by precocious advances in other areas. There are no prizes for getting to a certain point first.

Most children with epilepsy are developmentally no different from children without epilepsy. However, children who have frequent or severe seizures that remain uncontrolled, who are being treated with large amounts of antiepileptic drugs, or who have other disorders of brain function may experience some delays in development.

Table 10 summarizes the major milestones in control of gross and fine movements (motor control), personal and social behavior, and language development in babies and young children. It gives a rough estimate of "average" development. It is important to remember that some children may attain specific skills somewhat later than indicated and grow up to be bright and well-coordinated adults.

If development is significantly delayed, parents should consult a pediatrician or pediatric neurologist about the cause of the delay and what it may mean for the future. In most cases, though, doctors cannot make precise predictions about a child's future development. In children with frequent seizures, who are often taking high dosages of one or more antiepileptic drugs, it can be difficult to determine whether the slow development is the result of a physical brain abnormality, seizures, or medications. In some children, development slows or stops when seizures become frequent

179

TABLE 10. **MILESTONES* IN THE DEVELOPMENT OF INFANTS AND CHILDREN**

Age (Months)	Gross Motor	Fine Motor	Personal-Social	Language
1	Strong suck	—	Smiles responsively	—
3	Rolls over, can pick up head while lying down	Briefly grasps rattle, puts hands together	Smiles spontaneously	Laughs, squeals
6	Sits with support with steady head	Reaches for object, begins to grasp with one hand (not two)	Feeds self cracker	Turns to voice
9	Sits well, pulls self to sitting position, crawls with arms	Grasps object between thumb and forefinger	Plays pat-a-cake and peek-a-boo	Imitates speech sounds, may say mama or dada
12	Stands alone, walks holding furniture or walls (cruises), may walk without support	Grasps small object (raisin) between thumb and forefinger	May drink from cup, may play ball, often shy	Says dada or mama (specific person)
15	Walks by self, toddles and falls	Scribbles with crayon, tower of two cubes	Drinks from cup, indicates wants without crying	Says one to three words other than mama and dada
18	Walks up or down stairs holding on, throws ball, walks backward	Removes shoes and socks, unzips clothes	Uses spoon well, imitates housework	Combines two words, points to one to three body parts and common objects
24	Walks up steps by self, bends over and picks up objects, runs	Turns knob, kicks ball	Washes hands, puts on some clothing, assists housework	Uses two- or three-word sentences, points to four or five body parts

TABLE 10. *(Continued)*

Age (Months)	Gross Motor	Fine Motor	Personal-Social	Language
30	Jumps with both feet, pedals tricycle, walks on tiptoes	Tower of four to eight cubes, dumps raisin from bottle	Puts on most clothing, uses spoon with little spilling, helps put away toys	Asks questions, knows full name, knows one to six colors
36	Stands on one foot, broad jumps, rides tricycle	Copies "0"	Dresses self except buttons, plays well with others	Recites nursery rhymes, asks "why," uses pronouns correctly
48	Hops on one foot, walks one foot per step on stairs	Copies "+" and square, picks longer of two lines	Buttons clothing, separates easily from mother, cooperates in play	Tells stories, understands opposites, counts three to four objects

*These milestones are usually attained at the ages shown, but children vary considerably in their development, and some children with average or superior motor and language functions in later childhood may lag in one or more of these early milestones.

or severe; when the seizures come under better control, their development improves.

Even children with severe cerebral palsy or mental retardation show development. The rate may be slow, the process laborious, but the gains are no less meaningful and exciting. In rare cases of degenerative disorders of childhood (or adulthood), development can regress. The child may lose some milestones previously attained, but the loss does not necessarily mean that he or she has a degenerative disorder.

JJ developed tonic-clonic seizures without fever at age 8 months. He was started on phenobarbital and did well for several months. Then tonic-clonic and myoclonic seizures developed and continued despite high dosages of phenobarbital. Carbamazepine and, later, valproate and phenytoin were added to the phenobarbital without any improvement. At age 14 months, he stopped attaining new developmental milestones. A magnetic resonance image (MRI) of the brain revealed areas of slightly delayed development. The pediatric neurologist started him on clonazepam, and the seizures lessened, but within 2 weeks his walking became unsteady, and he couldn't move his left leg as well as his right leg. A diagnosis of a degenerative disorder was incorrectly made, and the mother was given a dismal prognosis. Another neurologist was consulted. The clonazepam was gradually lowered, and he again walked normally. JJ, now 3 years old, is taking felbamate, and after a course of intravenous gamma globulin, has been-seizure-free for more than 6 months. His motor skills are excellent, and his language is improving.

EFFECTS OF SEIZURES AND ANTIEPILEPTIC DRUGS ON MENTAL FUNCTIONS

Single seizures do not permanently impair intellectual or behavioral functions. The long-term effects of numerous or recurrent seizures are still the subject of study. The current view is that most types of seizures do not have permanent effects on mental functions. This is especially true for absence and simple partial seizures. Children who have frequent complex partial seizures may have some mild memory impairment, but it has not been proved that the seizures actually cause the problem. Many of these children have scar tissue in the parts of the brain that are important for memory, and this scar tissue may be responsible for the memory difficulties as well as for the seizures.

Children who have frequent or prolonged tonic-clonic seizures tend to do less well on tests of intelligence and memory, which suggests that, if frequent or prolonged, this type of seizure may be harmful. In addition, a large number of tonic-clonic seizures (for example, more than 100 in a lifetime) or repeated episodes of status epilepticus are associated with some adverse effects on mental function. However, many children with this type of seizure disorder can also have associated brain disorders such as cerebral palsy. The intellectual problems can be caused by the underlying condition of the brain, and not just by the seizures. Children who have frequent atonic, tonic, and tonic-clonic seizures, who are prone to falling, should wear a protective helmet, because head injury (especially repeated episodes) also can impair intellectual function.

Antiepileptic drugs can impair intellectual performance and cause behavioral problems. However, among the primary antiepileptic drugs (see Table 3), these effects are usually slight, particularly when the drugs are given in the usual dosages. In studies comparing children's cognitive (intellectual) functions before and after the discontinuation of antiepileptic drugs, a wide spectrum of cognitive functions was not improved or only slightly improved after the drugs were stopped. However, the cognitive and behavioral effects of antiepileptic drugs are often dose-related. Therefore, children on high dosages of the drugs are more likely to have significant adverse mental effects. In addition, drugs affect children (and adults) individually. Although group averages may show no statistically significant difference, some individuals may experience real problems, even at low therapeutic blood drug levels.

> The first pediatric neurologist told me that phenobarbital was like water, that we would never know that Brenda was on it. He was wrong. She became cranky, hyperactive, slept poorly—she was a different child. We were told this would pass, but it only seemed to get worse as time went on. We felt like we had lost our child. If we had to choose between the seizures or the adverse effects, we would take the seizures. We eventually went for a second opinion, and she was changed to Tegretol. She had a rash 2 weeks later. Then she was put on Depakote. She has had no seizures, and we have our daughter back.

> The drugs never seemed to bother Allison. She has been on phenobarbital since she was 5 years old. When Dilantin was added to the phenobarbital, she still did well. We eventually got her off the phenobarbital, and now she is just on the Dilantin. She is in the top of her class and on the field hockey team.

Aside from the barbiturates, such as phenobarbital and primidone, and the benzodiazepines, such as clonazepam and clorazepate, there is no convincing evidence that one of the other major antiepileptic drugs is much more likely to cause cognitive or behavioral problems than another drug. The barbiturates and benzodiazepines are most likely to cause intellectual and behavioral problems. Their most common adverse effects are hyperactivity, irritability, decreased attention span, memory impairment, sleep alterations, aggressiveness, and mood changes, including depression. Children and adolescents who have a close family member with major depression (a serious depressive disorder) may be at special risk for becoming depressed when treated with a barbiturate. Nevertheless, barbiturates and benzodiazepines are useful in treating seizures and are well tolerated by many children.

As the dosage and blood levels of antiepileptic drugs increase, the adverse effects also increase. Excessive drowsiness and need for sleep, slowed thinking and movement, decreased initiative and motivation, memory lapses, and other cognitive deficits become more pronounced with higher blood levels. Combinations of antiepileptic drugs are also more likely to cause cognitive problems, as well as other adverse effects. When high doses or combinations of antiepileptic drugs are used, the doctor tries to strike a careful balance between the beneficial effects and the adverse effects of the therapy. The goal of treatment is freedom from seizures without adverse effects. In some cases, this goal cannot be attained, and the adverse effects of the seizures must be weighed against the adverse effects of the drugs. For example, the doctor probably would not choose to increase the dosage to the point of sedation or emotional and intellectual dulling in order to reduce complex partial seizures to one a month from three a month. The adverse effects would be present, in varying degrees, throughout each day of the child's life, whereas a complex partial seizure may be disruptive only 1 to 3 minutes during the seizure and perhaps 20 minutes during its aftereffects.

Difficult decisions about the use of antiepileptic drugs come when the adverse effects are subtle and intermittent. A description of the child's behavior, based on the parent's observations and supplemented by reports from teachers and others who are familiar with the child, is invaluable to the doctor. Careful documentation of the adverse effects and their relation to the time medications are taken is extremely important. The adverse effects and seizures can often be reduced by altering the medication schedule. For example, the medication can be given after meals to minimize adverse effects caused by rapid absorption of the drug. In other cases, more frequent but smaller doses can help to maintain more steady blood levels of the drug, thereby reducing adverse effects and improving seizure control. When adverse effects are bothersome in the daytime, or seizures are most likely to occur during sleep or shortly after awakening, the bedtime dose can be increased and the daytime doses decreased. Midday doses of medication during the school day should be avoided if possible, so that the child does not have to feel embarrassed by going to the nurse for medication.

When a child has taken antiepileptic drugs for years, it may be difficult to detect the adverse effects of the medication. It is often impossible to untangle the effects of the normal turmoil of youth, an underlying neurological disorder, the recurrent seizures, and the medications. Further, if the child has been on medications from an early age, it is impossible to know exactly what his or her behavior would be like without them. Even if the child has been seizure-free for years and is old enough to understand the question, "Does the medication make you tired or cause any other problems?", he or she often cannot remember what it was like to be free of medications and, therefore, cannot answer accurately. It is only after the medications are discontinued or changed that a difference can be appreciated, making everyone realize how the medication was affecting the child.

Some children with epilepsy have associated neurological disorders such as mental retardation. Although these disorders affect intellect and behavior, it is common to blame the antiepileptic drugs or seizures for the problems. In fact, children with associated neurological disorders may be more susceptible to the adverse effects of both seizures and antiepileptic drugs.

BUILDING SELF-ESTEEM IN CHILDREN WITH EPILEPSY

It seems strange that it took a social worker at the epilepsy center to make me realize what I had been doing. Doing everything for Tricia was making her more dependent on me—making her bed, helping her dress, clearing her dishes, always staying within a few feet in case she were to have a seizure, and everything else I was doing because I'm her mother and I love her. I never thought she could put her own sneakers on until she did it at the hospital. It is hard to let go, but exciting to see what Tricia can do.

Of all the things that parents can give children, the opportunity to develop self-esteem and self-confidence is among the most important. For children to develop, learn, and interact at school, and to grow successfully toward independence and adulthood, they must have a strong and positive sense of self. Building self-esteem requires a parent to be patient, to use educational discipline, to provide opportunities for children to do things independently, and to praise them for their initiatives and progress.

The parents of a child with epilepsy must first maintain their own self-esteem (see Chapter 19). Having a child with an illness, especially one that has been associated with negative attitudes, punctures and deflates the balloon of perfection that all parents like to imagine in their children. Before they can help their child to build his or her own self-esteem, the parents should reflect on their own feelings about the child's disorder. Even very young children can sense and understand their parents' feelings.

Parents must emphasize the positive and minimize the negative. They should focus on the things that the child can do and build on those achievements. Negative messages can limit self-esteem and motivation. Parents must not show their frustration at what the child cannot do, or compare their child negatively with brothers or sisters, relatives, or other children. Talking about "the problem" in front of the child is not good. This is not to say that parents should not discuss the epilepsy in a supportive fashion, but they should not focus on the child as a problem. Discussing financial problems and the burden of the medical care in front of the child should be avoided. The child's condition should not be used as an excuse for avoiding family activities. It is not a good practice to say, for example, "We'd love to come over for the party, but Judith's seizures have really been a problem lately, and I think we should stay home." Brothers and sisters should not be made the child's caretakers, thereby limiting their independence and activities, and causing their resentment. The child's condition must not be used as an excuse for limiting his or her participation in activities such as school clubs or scouts, as this will send the message to the child that the parents do not have confidence in him or her.

No parent is perfect. All parents get frustrated and say things and show emotions they later wish that they had not. Children are resilient. The important thing for parents is to recognize ways in which they can be more positive and encouraging to their child who has epilepsy. Parenting of children with special skills is an exceptional challenge, and resources are available for parents who need support (see Appendixes 3 and 4).

Encouraging Personal Responsibility

Children can understand epilepsy. That includes both children with and children without epilepsy. Children should be told about the condition in words they can understand. They should know why taking medication on time is important, why tests are done, and why certain activities may have to be restricted. Children usually understand more than adults give them credit for. The Epilepsy Foundation of America (EFA) has pamphlets for children that explain the disability in simple terms.

If possible, a child with epilepsy should know the name of the medication, the color of the pill, the dosage, and the schedule for taking the medication. Certainly an attentive parent can do everything needed to manage the condition and can make the child a passive participant in his or her care, but this should be resisted. The earlier that trust and knowledge are given to the child, the sooner the disorder will cease to be a disability.

Avoiding Overprotectiveness

There is a fine line between healthy caution and overprotection. Parents have a strong and natural tendency to direct their children's behavior. They want them to do the things they think are right and not to do the things they deem wrong or dangerous. For children with epilepsy and other related disorders, this tendency may become exaggerated, and parents may drift into being overprotective. They are often unaware of their directive behavior, or fiercely defend it. Doing everything for children and restricting their exposure to the usual challenges of childhood takes away independence, slows their social growth, and lowers their self-esteem. They see their peers maturing while they remain children.

Overprotectiveness can take many forms. In the extreme form, children may never be told they have epilepsy; they are given medications by their parents, who refuse to tell them why. They may try to figure out what the problem is by going to the public library and reading about medical disorders. There are still some children and even young adults who are largely confined to their rooms or their houses because of the parents' fear that they could be injured if they go out. Fortunately, mild overprotectiveness is much more common. Children are encouraged to do things and to take responsibility, but their parents are still too fearful of dangers and show their love by doing and restricting too much. Sometimes, less is better.

The excessively dependent child is in danger of becoming overly attached to the person who cares for him or her most of the time. Prolonged dependence and overattachment foster separation anxiety. This can make it difficult for the child to adjust later to play groups and school settings. In addition, it may leave the child vulnerable if the caretaker and child become separated. A clinging, overprotective parent does not produce a happy, secure child, but one who is anxious, dependent, and frightened of the rest of the world.

Children usually survive their parents. Most children will become independent long before their parents are gone. However, some children with severe epilepsy and associated neurological disorders remain dependent and will require some degree of supportive care throughout their lives. Because parents of these children will not be around forever, they must plan for the child eventually to live in some type of supportive environment, such as a residential home or "independent living center," as it is now called. Such planning should begin early, so the young person gets into the system while the parents are able to oversee the conditions and make sure the living arrangement meets their son's or daughter's medical and social needs. Parents who have cared lovingly for a severely affected child may feel reluctant to let go in this way, but when they do, they assure a smooth transition for the young adult. Regardless of the severity of the epilepsy or associated neurological and physical disorders, young people should be encouraged toward independence and self-care.

Encouraging Social Contacts

One of the most important parts of childhood is learning to relate, play, disagree, share, make friendships, and grow together—in other words, to socialize. Perhaps the greatest cost of overprotection and isolation is limited social contacts. No matter how loving and giving parents are, they can never replace the joys and lessons that children bring to each other. Although children can inflict the cruelest insults and most painful taunts and teasing, the parents must move beyond the fears of possible problems. Children, even those with epilepsy, need other children.

Parents should encourage their child's participation in activities with other children. These activities can range from play groups and play dates, where parents and children get together, to "mommy and me" classes for 18-to-36-month-olds; preschool programs; nursery and kindergarten classes; school classes; extracurricular activities such as sports, dancing, singing, or crafts; and, for older children, independently playing with other children after school and on weekends. Parents should emphasize the principle of inclusion, not exclusion. Epilepsy is not a reason for excluding a child from the social world of children. Although the parents may believe some activities are unsafe, it is often worthwhile speaking with the doctor and the child about such activities. In some cases, special precautions, including supervision by parents, can be used to make these activities safer.

Children with epilepsy may benefit from meeting, talking, and playing with other children who have epilepsy. Local EFA affiliates frequently offer camps, buddy systems, and other programs that provide ways for children with similar disorders to come into contact. For a child to learn that he or she is not alone can be enormously comforting; there is something special about a comrade. The chance to see someone else who has a similar problem can change a child's entire outlook on the disorder. If an area has no groups for children with epilepsy, a motivated parent is the perfect person to get one going. Parents can work with the pediatrician, neurologist, and local EFA office to help establish a group for children with epilepsy, or even a simple buddy system of two kids getting together regularly.

If a child wishes to join a group for children with epilepsy, the parents should inquire about the range of neurological and other handicaps among children in the group. Many groups have a mix of children, some who have had only one or two seizures and have normal physical and neurological development, and others who have severe cerebral palsy with multiple physical challenges and mental retardation. In such cases, the child should be told that the group includes other children with more serious problems and should be reassured that these difficulties are not what will happen to him or her.

Using Educational Discipline

Susie has always been impossible. She does what she wants, when she wants. Nothing worked—taking away her favorite toys or foods, sending her up to her room, or raising my voice. We wanted to give up. Then a friend with a child who has cerebral palsy and hyperactivity told me what she thought we were doing wrong. We were inconsistent, often giving in to her tantrums. We reacted to Susie with frustration, never really understanding her needs. It took a lot of hard work. Before Susie could change, we had to change. Now Susie's favorite book is *Clifford's Manners* (see Appendix 4).

Some parents of children with epilepsy often overindulge them and ignore bad behaviors as a way of "making up" for the epilepsy or because they fear that sterner punishment will cause more seizures. Although seizures can occasionally be brought on by emotional stress, there is no evidence that they are caused by educational discipline. Educational discipline means explaining why the child's behavior was wrong, and withholding something the child desires or using the technique of "time out," in which, for example, the child must go to the corner of the room and stand quietly for a minute or so because of bad behavior. There is ample evidence that an undisciplined child can face serious problems in learning to socialize in a healthy fashion with other children, to behave and learn at school, and to grow up to be an independent and well-functioning adult. If a child has epilepsy, the problems will be compounded by allowing the child to have and do whatever he or she wants.

Caring for children means some frustration. Even the best-natured child gets ornery, cranky, mischievous, jealous, angry, or even aggressive. Children reflect the emotions and behaviors of those around them. When a child requires discipline, it is often best to pause before reacting. Most children respond well to a quiet and calm explanation of why their behavior was wrong, or why they cannot have what they want. However, any child can challenge even superhuman patience at times.

For children with epilepsy, who have to deal with more problems than average, educational discipline is critical. Because of their seizures, medications, and in some cases, their associated neurological disorders, these children are more prone toward certain behavioral problems. The unwanted behavior can be prevented or controlled by taking the time to explain things, not by corporal punishment. If behavioral problems develop after a new medication is started or after the dosage is increased, the doctor should be told, because the medication may be causing or aggravating the problems.

MANAGING BEHAVIORAL PROBLEMS

The coexistence of a specific problem, such as irritability, and a specific disorder, such as epilepsy, does not prove that the disorder causes the problem. Nevertheless, behavioral problems are more common among children with epilepsy. As mentioned earlier, determining the cause of behavioral or intellectual disorders in children with epilepsy can be difficult. Parents may think their child is misbehaving when, in fact, the problems are caused by absence seizures, partial seizures, or other disorders such as tics. It is natural for parents to consider "not listening," for example, as misbehaving. When the behavior is accounted for by a diagnosis of epilepsy, parents may feel guilty for chastising the innocent child. Guilt, although equally natural, is neither justified nor productive.

Children with epilepsy have not only seizure-related problems—temporary disturbances occurring before, during, and after their seizures—but also, in some cases, other behavioral disorders that may or may not be related to the epilepsy.

Seizure-Related Problems

Although behavioral disorders preceding seizures by hours to days have been described by doctors for more than a century, there is still a scarcity of information about these problems. Many family members and older children with epilepsy describe changes in personality, mood, and other symptoms, such as a headache, that reliably precede a seizure by hours or days; these are called premonitory symptoms.

Behavioral problems are most often seen shortly after seizures, but they can also occur during seizures. During complex partial and absence seizures, children are inattentive and cannot understand or remember what is happening in the world around them. Some parents and teachers may feel that the child is not paying attention, is purposely ignoring what they say, or has a learning disability. During complex partial seizures, unusual automatisms can cause a child to act in an unusual manner—for example, laugh or cry for no apparent reason, scream, shout, kick, spit, run, make rocking movements, or partially undress. Such actions are easily confused with a behavioral disorder.

Simple partial seizures can cause a variety of symptoms that are upsetting for adults and bewildering or frightening for children. The symptoms include bodily sensations and discomforts; powerful emotions such as fear, anxiety, depression, or embarrassment for no apparent reason; feeling as if the mind and body are separating; strange thoughts suddenly racing through the mind; seeing objects and people get larger or smaller or appear distorted; seeing things that are not there (visual hallucinations); smelling things that are not there (olfactory hallucinations); and hearing things that are not there (auditory hallucinations). Many children have great difficulty describing these symptoms to their parents or the doctor. In many cases, they are only discovered when someone specifically asks about them. Even then, it may be hard to separate the willingness of some children to say "yes" to the questions from what they have actually experienced.

Temporary behavioral changes observed after seizures include confusion and tiredness, as occur in most children with complex partial and tonic-clonic seizures. Further, verbal or physical aggressiveness, or running away, may occur if the child is confronted or restrained after the seizure. These difficulties can often be avoided by speaking in a soft and comforting manner and avoiding restraint. The confusion that follows certain seizures may be mild but can cause difficulties with memory, understanding language (including parental instructions), and ability to do schoolwork. If a seizure goes unnoticed, the parents may think that the child has "misbehaved" when he or she fails to do as the parent has asked. However, children with epilepsy are like all other children: they often do not do (or do the exact opposite of) what their parents ask them to do. Therefore, parents should not blame every little thing on seizures and epilepsy. Kids with epilepsy usually misbehave simply because they are kids.

Other Behavioral Problems

The period between seizures is the time when children with epilepsy live most of their lives. Behavioral problems that may occur in this period often have a serious impact on them. In many cases, the epilepsy itself is probably unrelated to the problem behavior. The types of problems include learning disorders, difficulty with concentration (attention deficit), hyperactivity, and language and cognitive impairments, as well as anxiety, irritability, aggressive verbal or physical behavior, depression, mood swings, poor social skills, lack of motivation and energy, and inability to plan and organize behavior.

Learning Disorders

In children with learning disorders, there is a discrepancy between intellectual level and academic achievement; that is, intelligence outpaces achievement. A major cause of learning disorders is a neurological disorder. Children with epilepsy, by definition, have a neurological disorder and, therefore, have an increased risk of a learning disorder. However, although the rate of learning disorders is higher among children with epilepsy than among the general population, most children with epilepsy do not have learning disorders.

To learn is to absorb, remember, and apply information. It requires a complicated series of brain processes. The absorption process requires paying attention and perceiving (seeing and hearing the material). The memory process requires actively comparing the newly acquired information with previously learned information and recalling it when necessary. These are but a few of the many complex steps in the process of learning.

The learning process can be disrupted in many different ways. The most extensively studied learning disorder is dyslexia, a developmental reading disorder. (Alexia, an acquired disorder of reading, occurs, for example, after a stroke.) The cause of dyslexia is not understood, but it may result from some microscopic abnormality in the structure and functions of the left temporal and parietal lobes, areas of the brain known to be critical for reading and language comprehension. These are areas that are also prone to seizures.

Reading can be impaired by many things. Children who are unable to focus their attention for more than a few seconds will be unable to read. Poor vision that is not corrected can impair reading. Reading will also be impaired if there is a problem with sending visual information from the eye to the brain, with the areas of the brain that process visual information, or with the language areas of the brain. Reading can also be disrupted by abnormalities on the right side of the brain that allow someone to see only the right half of the page or the right half of individual words.

Reading is only one of many specific functions that can be impaired in persons who have learning problems. Some persons have problems with learning arithmetic, spoken information (because of impaired hearing or processing of sound by the brain), visual information other than reading, relating visual information to movement components (visuomotor disorders), or relating objects in space (disorders of visuospatial analysis).

A child who is suspected of having a learning disability should be evaluated by specialists such as school psychologists, neuropsychologists, or child study teams. Such services can be requested through the child's school (see Chapter 20). The evaluation can often identify the cause of a learning disorder. Testing should not be limited to measuring the intelligence quotient (IQ test), an achievement test, and measures of emotional function. A common scenario is that a child is found to have a normal IQ, substandard achievement, and some emotional difficulties. With a diagnosis of "behavioral disorder," the child is placed in a classroom for "children with behavioral disorders." To avoid misdiagnosis, neuropsychological testing must include assessment of language, memory, and other cognitive functions not assessed with an IQ test.

Seizures can affect academic performance and learning. Brief staring spells, whether they are absence seizures or complex partial seizures, can lead to missed information. When the seizures are frequent, the child can miss large amounts of information; the child is essentially "tuned out" and does not hear or absorb what is being taught. In the case of complex partial seizures, memory is often affected for minutes or longer after the seizure has ended. In the case of tonic-clonic seizures, memory can be affected for hours after the seizure has ended. Epilepsy, especially when it is severe or associated with other medical and neurological disorders, may require medical treatment or hospitalization that causes the child to miss school, which can affect learning. In some children, antiepileptic drugs can contribute to learning problems. In other cases, the ability to learn can be impaired temporarily by frequent small epilepsy waves on the EEG that do not cause obvious symptoms, by frequent minor seizures, or by occasional tonic-clonic seizures.

Attention Deficit Disorder

Just over a century ago, the American psychologist William James penned the following description of attention: "Everyone knows what attention is. It is the taking possession by the mind, in clear and vivid form, of one out of what seem several possible objects or trains of thought." Attention is the cornerstone on which intellectual functions rest. If we do not pay attention, we cannot efficiently understand, learn, or remember. We are all confronted by a swarm of sensations, feelings, and thoughts at any one moment. Only a small fraction of these reach our conscious awareness. Attention is the filtering process that allows us to focus on the important things. Without the complex attentional systems of our brains, our minds would be overwhelmed by the bombardment of images and sensations coming at us from the inside (our mind and body) and outside (our environment). We take for granted the amount of filtering out of unimportant information that our brains do every moment we are awake. The filtering system develops in children just as the systems that control fine movements and ability to learn abstract mathematic relationships also develop. A 3-year-old simply cannot sit quietly for 3 hours and read; his or her attentional system is too immature to filter out distractions such as the sound of the television or the sight of a friend.

Attention deficit disorder (ADD) is a common problem in schoolchildren and is characterized by the inability to maintain attention, poor concentration, distractibility, and impulsivity. These problems clearly exceed the normal behavior for the child's age and interfere with learning. They are usually noticed by teachers and parents. ADD usually begins before the age of 5 years and is more common in boys. Hyperactivity and ADD often exist in the same child, and both were once considered part of minimal brain dysfunction. The two disorders are separate, however, and one may occur without the other. ADD refers to cognitive behavior, whereas hyperactivity refers to motor behavior. Children with epilepsy may have higher rates of both ADD and hyperactivity.

The cause of ADD is unknown. Parents of some children report that consumption of sugar "sets them off" and "winds them up," reducing their attention span. Medical studies, however, have generally not found dietary restrictions to be effective, other than the possibility that eliminating foods with colorings and additives may improve 5% to 10% of cases. ADD may be a disorder of brain maturity or a chemical imbalance. The majority of children adapt to their ADD, although many continue to have attentional problems in adolescence and adulthood.

Medications can cause or accentuate attentional problems. Any drug that makes a person tired has the potential to impair attention. Among the medications used to treat epilepsy, phenobarbital and primidone are the most likely to impair attention and cause hyperactivity; the benzodiazepines (diazepam and clonazepam) can also have the same effect. If attentional problems develop or worsen after a drug is started or the dosage is increased, the doctor should be informed. In some cases, the problem may lessen within weeks or a few months; in other cases, the dosage may need to be reduced or the medication changed.

When ADD causes troublesome learning or social problems, medical therapy may be helpful. The drugs used to treat ADD are classified as stimulants because in adults they increase alertness and decrease the need for sleep. In children with ADD, however, the stimulants act in an opposite manner, leading to a more relaxed and focused state of mind. The drugs most commonly used are methylphenidate (Ritalin), dextroamphetamine (Dexedrine), and pemoline (Cylert). They can be used safely in children for prolonged periods, but their use must be carefully supervised by a doctor. Short-term use of these drugs may cause decreased appetite and weight loss, stomach discomfort, and difficulty sleeping. Their long-term use may lead to a slight decrease in growth, although this remains controversial. As the child grows older, gradual reduction of the medications should be considered, because ADD is often outgrown. In the overwhelming majority of children with epilepsy, drugs used to treat ADD and hyperactivity can be used safely.

Hyperactivity

Children are much more physically active than adults. A 4-year-old child, for example, is always moving and doing things. His or her arms and legs never seem to hold the same position for more than a few seconds. Children, by nature, are very active.

In some children, excessive movement, or hyperactivity, causes problems. The increased activity may take several forms, such as excessive fidgeting, an inability to stay seated for more than a minute, and running around endlessly. Hyperactivity causes problems because it prevents the child, usually a boy, from staying in one place for long. It is disruptive in both the classroom and at home and exhausting for teachers and parents.

As with ADD, an immaturity of the brain may contribute to the cause of hyperactivity. In general, all young children are more active than older children and adults. Therefore, hyperactivity may reflect relative immaturity of the brain. As the brain matures, the hyperactivity lessens.

Hyperactivity is slightly more common among children with epilepsy. It is also more common among children with tic disorders and mental retardation. The drugs that can improve ADD have the same desirable effects on hyperactivity.

Severe Language and Cognitive Impairments

Some children with epilepsy have severe language and cognitive deficits. Social and behavioral problems may further impair their intellectual development, because socializing is the primary process by which children obtain language skills. Most children react positively to a voice or smile, but to many children with severe developmental disabilities, these sounds and gestures can be threatening and confusing. Their reactions to stimuli are inappropriate, unpredictable, and sometimes destructive.

The parents' reaction to this situation is sympathy and pity, leading them to make their child's world as pleasant and comfortable as possible. Their attempt to foster trust and comfort may be successful, but often it is not. Some children may only communicate *on their own terms*. Fortunately, behavior management techniques are available to change the child's avoidance patterns and create new patterns of interaction, which can provide the child with a base of trust in our complicated world (see Appendix 4). For example, the child is presented with a simple social choice: either control his or her behavior or the adult will control it. Through time and effort, the child chooses self-control. Initially, a simple social world must be created. As the child improves, the social world is steadily and slowly made more complex.

In this behavioral management technique (which is one of many possible approaches), the first step in controlling the child's behavior is the establishment of routines that incorporate demands to adapt to variation. The initial routine must be simple, and demands must be minimal, but complied with. This means that the child must inhibit behavior that interferes with desired activities or attentiveness. For example, the child must lift up or put down his or her arms on command when getting dressed and undressed, sit in a chair with no self-stimulatory behaviors, or pick up objects on request. To maintain and increase the child's sense of stability, everything that is taught must be preserved even as new tasks are being added. The child must feel the comfort of practicing well-established skills while new demands are being introduced. These techniques are often difficult and time-consuming. Yet, if parents are consistent in incorporating them into the child's daily regimen, they will be successful in establishing key behavior patterns that will allow the development of cognitive and language skills.

CHAPTER 18

Telling Children and Others about Epilepsy

Epilepsy was once shrouded in secrecy. The word, like "cancer" or "leprosy," evoked fear and isolation. Those days are largely gone. The more the word "epilepsy" is used, the more children and adults understand what epilepsy is and is not, and the more an openness surrounds epilepsy, the more the vestiges of secrecy and fear about epilepsy will disappear.

TELLING CHILDREN ABOUT EPILEPSY

Children should be told about epilepsy. I recently met a woman who was never told about her disorder, which began at 6 years of age. She finally went to a library at age 20 to research her symptoms, and recognized that she had been treated for epilepsy but was never told about it. She was furious at her parents and doctors.

It is always a balancing act when deciding how much to tell children about epilepsy. The child must not be overwhelmed with words and ideas that are either incomprehensible or frightening. However, "protecting" the child by withholding the truth can be the worst choice of all. There is no chart of what to say to children at different ages. Parents should be guided by common sense. In general, children under 3 years of age do not need to be told anything. After the age of 3 years, children can usually understand if epilepsy is explained in simple language without the use of medical words. Parents need to keep it simple and be positive about the problem.

The book, *Lee, the Rabbit with Epilepsy*, is about a rabbit who has a seizure (see Appendix 4). This brightly illustrated book for young children describes how the rabbit visits the doctor, takes medication, and most importantly, continues to enjoy life. This book and other materials designed for children are available through the Epilepsy Foundation of America (EFA). Parents can show these materials to their children or study the materials themselves and use them as a model.

TELLING OTHERS WHO NEED TO KNOW

Anyone who is teaching, closely associated with, or caring for a child with epilepsy should know about the child's disorder. Lack of knowledge opens the door for potential problems.

Relatives

Relatives can be the most supportive and helpful people in the world or the most difficult. As a general rule, relatives should be told about a child's epilepsy. Who and how much to tell should depend on whether or not the relatives are likely to be alone with the child, and how they may react. Practically speaking, however, if one relative has been told, they have all been told! Just as it is important that one doctor manage a child's care, however, it is important that parents assume primary responsibility for their child's disorder. (As the child gets older, he or she should also help assume this responsibility.) One potential problem with relatives is that they love to give advice. Advice is fine and is often helpful, but the parents must do what they feel is best for the child.

School Nurses, Teachers, and Classmates

School is a major part of the child's day. For children with daytime seizures, school nurses and teachers should be told about the child's epilepsy. The school nurse is the advocate for the child in the school and a resource for teachers who need information about epilepsy. The school nurse is most likely to be called on if the child has a seizure or experiences adverse effects from medications. The nurse should have information about the child's seizures and the medications. The nurse should also have the parent's and doctor's telephone numbers. The school nurse is an important part of the child's health care team. Parents should make sure that the nurse is informed about changes in the child's medication or the type of seizures that the child has. In some cases, the school nurse may confer with the gym teacher or sports coach to discuss possible precautions during some activities.

The teacher should always know the type of seizures the child has, and what they look like. The teacher should also be asked to observe the child carefully for possible seizures or adverse effects of medication. If the teacher notices any unusual behavior, such as staring, lip smacking, repetitive hand movements, or involuntary movements, the parents and the doctor should be told. These behaviors may represent seizures. Further, certain problems such as tremor, lethargy, nausea, or double vision may occur only when the medication levels reach a peak during school hours. In this case, the teacher's observations will be critical in making dosage adjustments to relieve these symptoms. Thus, the teacher is an extension of the parents' and doctor's eyes and ears. The teacher must balance the careful observation of the child with the need to treat him or her just the same as the other children.

If seizures are frequent and occur during daytime hours, it is important to discuss the disorder with the other schoolchildren. A period of time can be set aside in class to discuss epilepsy and the classmate's seizures (see Chapter 31 for resources for in-class education on epilepsy). By discussing it openly, all of the children can be educated, and a sense of community is fostered.

The Child's Friends and Their Parents

> More than anything else, Pete just wants to be one of the kids. He has overcome a learning disability and is now in mainstream classes and doing well. He has a few good friends and loves intramural basketball. Although his seizures are now well controlled, he doesn't want anyone at school to know about his epilepsy. We have tried to convince him to tell his close friends, but he refuses.

Children with epilepsy should be encouraged to pursue friendships and social activities with their peers. Healthy socialization is essential for self-esteem and future success. The decision to tell a child's friends about epilepsy is often difficult. Children are immature and can be insensitive. In addition, the friends' parents, if uninformed about epilepsy, may unnecessarily fear for their children's safety or even potential "psychological trauma" if they were to witness a seizure.

Friends and their parents should be carefully told about the child's epilepsy; it should not just be casually mentioned. A discussion is warranted to explain the type of seizures, their frequency, how the seizures affect the child, and what to do in case a seizure occurs. Most important, they need to know that epilepsy is just another episodic medical problem, like asthma, that affects otherwise healthy, active children. Epilepsy is not something that a person can "catch." The child's friends and their parents should be asked if they have any questions.

The need to conform and to belong to a peer group makes many adolescents want to hide their epilepsy. Therefore, whether to tell their friends about epilepsy can be a difficult decision. *The adolescent must always be involved in the decision to reveal his or her disorder—whom to tell, how to tell, and how much to tell.* Because the maturity of children varies, some peers may be frightened by the disorder, whereas others may react with teasing and try to isolate the child. Although such negative reactions are becoming less frequent, ridicule remains a part of life for many high school children with epilepsy, especially in the earlier grades. When a child makes fun of another child with epilepsy, the most effective strategy is to pay little heed. It may be worthwhile to respond calmly that epilepsy is a medical disorder. Ask if they would make fun of their own mother or grandfather who had a heart condition, or an athlete who broke a bone? Most children are actually understanding and supportive. It may be a good idea for the young person to discuss it with his or her close friends and for the parent to discuss the disorder one-on-one with the close friends' parents. For adolescents whose seizures are not fully controlled, it is especially important that their friends know about the epilepsy and what to do in case a seizure occurs. However, the decision to confide should be the adolescent's, not the parents'. For adolescents with well-controlled seizures who have few or no adverse effects from medications, it is less important to tell other people about epilepsy.

Babysitters

Babysitters allow parents to have some independence from their children. Babysitters who are educated about the disorder can care for children with epilepsy. Although parents are right in thinking that no one will watch and care for their children the way they do, mature and responsible babysitters can do a very good job. It is also important for children's maturation for them to learn that their parents cannot be there for them every minute. This will pave the way toward successful separation from the parents when it comes time to go to school and camp.

Babysitters should be told that a child has epilepsy before they agree to watch the child. Because babysitters are left alone with the child, they should be knowledgeable about the epilepsy and basic first-aid measures. They should be reassured that dangerous situations and emergencies are extremely uncommon, but they must be prepared. Babysitters should know the type and frequency of seizures, medication dosage, where the medication is stored, and telephone numbers of those to call in an emergency, including the doctor's number. For children with seizures associated with incontinence, keeping a change of clothing on hand can be helpful.

The EFA has an educational pamphlet for babysitters. It gives basic information about children with epilepsy and describes basic first aid.

The Dentist

Although children with epilepsy rarely require special attention during dental procedures, dentists should be made aware of the child's seizure disorder. The dentist may want to speak briefly with the doctor about the child's condition. For children who have frequent tonic-clonic, myoclonic, or atonic seizures, a low dose of a benzodiazepine, such as lorazepam, may be helpful before dental procedures. Children with epilepsy who are taking medications that affect gum growth should receive regular dental care, in addition to conscientious brushing, and when the child is old enough, flossing.

Children with severe epilepsy, cerebral palsy, or associated neurological disorders may require general anesthesia for major dental work. Before such procedures, it may be helpful for the dentist and doctor to discuss the medications and precautions.

CHAPTER 19

Family Life, Social Life, and Physical Activities

The effects of epilepsy on children's behavioral, intellectual, and social development are extremely variable. The majority of children with epilepsy lead normal lives and have few or no restrictions on social or physical activities. Even if the seizures are well controlled, however, the diagnosis of epilepsy and the medical visits can be frightening to them. For some children, seizures and the effect of the antiepileptic drugs cause many difficulties. For other children, additional medical and neurological problems affect their lives. Regardless of the severity of the condition, children with epilepsy need special attention to ensure that their outlook and self-esteem are positive.

Children with epilepsy see the disorder through the window of their parents' eyes. How the epilepsy affects the child often depends on how the epilepsy affects the parents. On hearing the diagnosis of epilepsy, parents are likely to go through a series of responses: shock, bewilderment, disappointment, hopelessness, guilt, anger, and grief, but not necessarily in that order. The adjustment period is followed by the realization that life goes on, that the child and family can enjoy life and flourish. If the parents take a positive outlook, the child's outlook will be positive.

FAMILY AND SOCIAL LIFE

A child's illness complicates the existing challenges of family life. In the mildest cases, when a child has only minor seizures that are fully controlled, family life should not be unduly affected. When a child's seizures are more disabling, or the epilepsy is associated with physical or neurological disorders, family life is always affected. All relationships in the family are changed—the relationship of the parents with each other, the parents' relationship with the children, and the relationship of brothers and sisters to the child with epilepsy.

The changes that epilepsy in a child bring to a family deserve careful attention. The child with epilepsy has special needs, but so do the other children in the family. As their age and maturity permit, siblings should also be educated about epilepsy. They should not be neglected. Because the child with epilepsy will draw time and attention like a magnet, parents must make special time for their other children. This action will help prevent later resentment directed at both the parents and the child with epilepsy.

Just as it may be helpful for the child to join a group of children or have a buddy with epilepsy to share experiences with, it may be helpful for the parents to join a parents' group or to have other parents to talk with and share experiences occasionally. The parental "grapevine" for children with medical disorders is one of our most powerful communication networks. Parents share problems, frustrations, coping strategies, achievements, and joys, as well as information about doctors, hospitals, medications, and educational and recreational programs; parents also build strong bonds in the process. The local Epilepsy Foundation of America (EFA) affiliate may have parent groups. A pediatrician, neurologist, or comprehensive epilepsy center may be able to put parents in touch with other parents of children with epilepsy. A motivated parent can easily be the force to create a local group.

Getting on with Life

Initially, Jim and I were so consumed by Anthony's epilepsy that nothing else seemed to matter. Between the seizures, medications, doctor visits, tests, meetings with teachers, and our jobs, there was no time for anything else. It took us 6 months or so, but we have finally realized that life goes on for Anthony, for his older brother Paul, and for us. We do special things with Paul to let him know how much we love him. We also have our parents come every few months to spend the weekend with the kids so that we can just get away. Now we can give Anthony the attention he needs without resentment or guilt.

Once the child's epilepsy has been diagnosed, treatment begun, and some time has passed for understanding and accepting the disorder, it is time for the parents to get on with their lives. In the mildest cases, this is easy. In the cases of moderate severity, with intermittent seizures and some adverse medication effects, resuming normal life is a challenge. In the most serious cases, especially those with coexisting neurological disorders, assuming a normal life may seem impossible, but is is not. For families with children who have frequent and intense seizures and associated developmental problems, life can never be exactly the way it would have been if the child did not have these problems. However, this situation does not mean that the parents can never spend time alone together or enjoy their life. They can. They will have to work harder to get the time.

There are two steps toward resuming the life the parents want. The first is completely attitudinal. It is accepting the disorder and the associated disorders for what they are, and understanding the needs of the child with epilepsy and of the other children, as well as personal needs and the needs of a spouse. It means that parents must search for the best care for their child, decide how they want to live their lives, and most important, decide that they can do it. Some parents feel as if they are swept up in a current, and the current is pulling them. That is true for everyone at the beginning. They must not passively ride the current, however, or they will find themselves in a place they do not want to be; they must determine the direction.

The second step is acting on the commitment to a satisfying life. Parents must work toward a balance between their needs and the needs of their child with epilepsy and other family members. Their happiness and the integrity of their relationship with their spouse and other children will also positively affect the child with epilepsy. For some parents, it is a good idea to investigate family support, getting help around the house, community programs, respite programs, and the local EFA affiliate.

Counseling

I thought that Jake told us everything. We were positive and supportive about the epilepsy, and it seemed like he was doing great. We never suspected that things were bothering him—the epilepsy, feeling pressure to get good grades, and other kids in his school. It was building up inside for a while. When the school called to ask how he was doing, we realized that he had been missing classes for a while, telling the teachers he had seizures. It was all too much for him. The counselor has been a godsend. Jake needs us, but he also needs someone else.

Parents, brothers and sisters, grandparents, and teachers provide children with role models, advice, guidance, and support. In the vast majority of cases, none of these people has epilepsy. In most cases, family members and teachers provide a nurturing environment and a positive outlook. However, despite their best intentions and loving support, they often fail to ask, "How do you feel about having epilepsy?" "How do you think other kids react to you because you have epilepsy?" "Do you understand what the doctor said?" "What are your greatest fears?" If the diagnosis and treatment of epilepsy are confusing for the parents, they will certainly be bewildering to the child. In addition, the social impact of epilepsy, difficult for the parent, is often psychologically painful for the child.

Counseling can be an important support for children with epilepsy. The counselor provides the outside perspective that is often lacking. In the most well-meaning families, parental concern can be misdirected into telling the child how to feel and how to act. Although all parents feel that they know what is best for their children, it can be difficult to determine what is truly best. A dialogue is often much more helpful than a suggestion or an order. The successful counselor can help "open" the part of the child that epilepsy can hide. The essence of counseling is to provide understanding and help the person cope with the medical and social impact of the disorder. Counseling can be beneficial for the child or the entire family. The majority of children with epilepsy do not require formal counseling, but all of them require education about the disorder and help in learning to adjust to it.

Referral for Counseling

The recommendation for counseling can come from a doctor, social worker, teacher, or school guidance counselor. However, counseling is no benefit unless the child or family wants it.

Finding the right counselor is usually not difficult. The doctor, school guidance counselor or psychologist, social worker, or local EFA affiliate are potential sources of information and referral. The counselor must have some knowledge of epilepsy. In addition, there must be a good relationship and trust between the counselor and the child. If the "chemistry" between them is not good, it is not wise to pursue the relationship too long. It is better to find another counselor.

Benefits of Counseling

Counseling is helpful if there is a need for the child or family to gain a greater understanding of the disorder, accept the diagnosis and treatment, regain a sense of control over one's own life, or talk to someone about concerns. Counselors can help in a variety of ways. For some children and adolescents, understanding their epilepsy may be most important. They often have common fears and misunderstandings that go unasked and unanswered. Fear of dying or serious injury during a seizure is a fairly common hidden concern, but children often will not bring the subject up to parents or doctors, because they are too frightened, shy, protective of their parents, or do not know how to ask the question.

The relationship of stress to seizures is poorly understood, but seizures often are more common during or shortly after stressful times (see Chapter

6). The counselor can help to identify sources of stress, such as family or school problems. Simple techniques of stress management can be helpful, even for a child.

Poor self-esteem may be an obvious concern or an undiscovered problem. The parents and teachers of children with epilepsy may see them as "doing remarkably well," but deep inside, the children may remain insecure and have low self-esteem. To protect their parents and their own image, they may hide their feelings or overcompensate. Although this may be the exception rather than the rule, parents and others must look beyond what they want to see. Counselors can identify home and school situations and issues that have an impact on the emotional well-being of children with epilepsy.

Friendships

Children with epilepsy should be encouraged to socialize and enjoy friendships. Perhaps the most negative effect of epilepsy on children is the isolation and rejection that may accompany the disorder, often unnecessarily. Vigorous pursuit of regular social activities is the best protection against negative social effects and is important for normal intellectual and behavioral development (see Chapter 17). Children with epilepsy should be encouraged to pursue friendships and activities like other children.

A child must be given independence to pursue healthy friendships. Parents may face conflicting desires: they want the child to play with other children and they also want to protect the child from danger. Such conflicts are inherent in parenthood, but are exaggerated for parents of children with epilepsy. Physical injury can occur with seizures, and parents are often the best at recognizing a seizure and protecting their child. However, the emotional trauma of isolation is probably more painful and more long-lasting than the effects of seizures.

Many parents would like their child to be more active in friendships and social activities but find that the child is fearful of rejection or that the opportunities are limited. In some children, associated neurological and emotional disorders limit their social activities. In these cases, community programs and networking between parents can be helpful. It also can be beneficial for children to meet other children with epilepsy through camping or similar programs available through the local EFA affiliate.

Going to Camp

Camp can be enjoyed by all children with epilepsy. Well-controlled or occasional seizures should be no obstacle to attendance at a regular camp.

The range of activities and precautions must be individually specified, but children with epilepsy can usually enjoy a very full and active summer camp.

Children with frequent seizures, or children who have never met another child with epilepsy, may benefit from going to a camp with other children who have epilepsy. The EFA provides information about these camps, some of which include educational sessions on epilepsy for the children.

Some camps specialize in programs for children with severe epilepsy, cerebral palsy, or emotional disorders. They provide a wonderful social opportunity for the children and an important respite for parents.

SPORTS AND OTHER PHYSICAL ACTIVITIES

The balance between a child's safety and the ability to enjoy a full range of activities is tested when it comes to recommendations regarding sports. Because epilepsy affects each person differently, the approach to sports and epilepsy must be considered on a patient-by-patient basis. The seizure type and frequency of the seizures, the type of medication and its adverse effects, the child's ability to follow instructions and act responsibly, and the nature and supervision of the activity must all be considered.

Common sense should be the guiding force in making these decisions. The goals should be both safety and a lifestyle that is as normal as possible. No activity is completely safe. Making safety the exclusive concern will force unnecessary limitations on the child's activities. Restriction and isolation foster low self-esteem and emphasize the disability. Nevertheless, for some children with epilepsy, certain activities and sports can be dangerous, and safety concerns mandate that these activities be forbidden or carefully supervised. In the past, doctors and parents tended to put strict limits on physical activities. The current trend is to allow children with epilepsy to be children and to pursue as full a range of activity as reasonable.

The type of seizures and their frequency are critical in determining what activities are safe. Children whose motor control or consciousness is impaired during seizures are at higher risk for sports-related injuries. Children who have uncontrolled, frequent seizures should know that certain activities are restricted. For example, they should not swim alone (in fact, *no* child should swim alone), or play on high bars or climb ropes without a proper mat and supervision. Other activities, such as riding a bicycle or moped amidst traffic, should be forbidden. However, such activities may be considered in safer settings with special precautions (helmets, close supervision, limiting speed). For children whose seizures are more common at certain times, for example, within 2 hours of awakening, activities can be scheduled for the times when seizures are less likely to occur.

Seizures are only rarely provoked by exercise, but when this pattern is identified, physical exertion should be limited. However, it may be possible to devise a satisfactory program of exercise in which the level of exertion is gradually increased.

Children with epilepsy should be encouraged to participate in group and competitive sports, such as Little League baseball, community sports, and varsity sports. These activities are usually well supervised and require appropriate safety gear, and most children with epilepsy can safely participate without special accommodations. Most important, group activities are part of childhood and foster high self-esteem and independence. These benefits are extremely valuable, and the risks of participation must be serious to warrant prohibiting a child from joining group activities. Most potential hazards can be overcome. There are major league players with epilepsy in baseball, ice hockey, and other professional sports.

Serious injuries in children with epilepsy are uncommon and rarely occur during participation in sports. Believe it or not, bathrooms are much more dangerous than playing soccer or ice skating.

Stair Climbing

Our world is filled with stairs. For the vast majority of children with epilepsy, stairs should not be barriers to getting around. However, seizures that impair motor control or consciousness can cause serious injuries if they occur while the child is on a staircase. If a child has an aura, or warning, before a seizure, he or she may be able to sit down until the seizure is over. For a child who has frequent seizures that cause falling, it is not unreasonable to have him or her use elevators, not stairs. In school, however, this restriction can cause the child to be late for classes or to stand out from his or her peers. In these unusual cases, a "buddy" who is aware of the epilepsy may be able to accompany the child from one class to the next.

Swimming and Water Sports

Swimming is a pleasure all children should be encouraged to enjoy. Nonetheless, the water poses dangers for all children, and special dangers for children with epilepsy. Epilepsy, however, is not an insurmountable barrier to swimming. The issue of epilepsy and water safety is really a question of how much supervision is necessary. No matter how severe or frequent the epilepsy, a child can enjoy the water. A parent can hold a child in a shallow pool with little risk. In cases in which seizures are well controlled, swimming should be encouraged, although it is necessary to make sure that the child does not swim alone, and at least one person who knows the child has epilepsy, and who knows basic lifesaving, should be nearby. This person can be an older child.

The most difficult decisions about swimming arise when children have occasional seizures that impair motor control of consciousness. These children should be allowed to swim, but they must be closely supervised. There should be both a lifeguard who is responsible and aware of the child's disorder and another child in the pool who is the buddy. Unfortunately, lifeguards are often immature adolescents who may be more interested in observing the opposite sex than in watching children in the pool. It is important that the lifeguards know they *must* keep their eyes on the pool while the child is swimming. The buddy system, used by many camps for young children who swim (and by adult scuba divers), is another precaution to ensure a child's safety. The buddy should be responsible, understand the need for keeping an eye on the child, and should never go far away in the pool.

If a child with epilepsy wants to swim competitively, he or she should be encouraged. Competitive swimming practices and matches are usually well supervised. The coach should be aware that the child has epilepsy, however, and everyone involved, including the child, should recognize that there is some additional risk to this activity and make an informed decision about whether it is worth it.

Children with well-controlled seizures can snorkel and scuba dive. Children with uncontrolled seizures that impair consciousness or motor control should not scuba dive and should only snorkel in relatively calm water, in very close proximity to someone who has lifesaving skills.

Bicycling

Bicycles are a part of childhood. Yet a bicycle, if ridden on or near the street, presents a serious potential danger for a child with epilepsy. Even if a parent rides just behind the child on the sidewalk, during a complex partial seizure he or she may suddenly veer off the street, out of the parent's reach and protection.

Despite the dangers, children with epilepsy can learn to ride and enjoy bicycles. Because most serious bicycle injuries involve the head, everyone who rides a bicycle should wear a helmet. If the seizures are under control or do not impair motor control of consciousness, bicycle riding should be unrestricted. When the seizures pose a danger, bicycles can be ridden in a park or other place where there are no motor vehicles.

Stationary bicycles for exercise pose no serious danger for children with epilepsy. Ideally, the floor should be carpeted or padded. Low-seated bicycles are the safest.

Horseback Riding

Children with epilepsy, even small children with frequent seizures, can ride horses. Someone may need to walk alongside the horse. For children whose seizures are well controlled or always preceded by an adequate warning, horseback riding can be safe and fun. Children who have seizures that could cause them to fall off the horse must be closely supervised if they do ride. The risks and benefits of horseback riding must be carefully weighed for these children.

Competitive horseback riding often involves galloping and jumping and should only be considered for children with mild or well-controlled epilepsy.

Contact Sports

Contact sports such as football, rugby, basketball, soccer, and ice hockey are generally safe for children with epilepsy. The principal concern with contact sports is the chance of head or bodily injury. However, children with epilepsy who play contact sports are not necessarily more likely to be hurt than other children. If an absence or complex partial seizure were to occur during a game, there is a small chance of injury if someone were to tackle the child during the spell. Tackle football, rugby, and ice hockey have a higher incidence of injuries than most other sports; participation in these competitive sports should probably be limited to children with well-controlled seizures. There is nothing wrong, however, with a child who has occasional or even frequent seizures playing touch football in the backyard. The risks must be weighed against the benefits of the sport. The chances of serious injury are small compared with the positive effects of team participation.

It would be hard to recommend boxing for any child, and even less for a child with epilepsy. The goal of boxing is to inflict a head injury. Since a momentary lapse can mean taking a hard hit directly to the head, children with absence seizures or complex partial seizures are at particular risk of injury from boxing. Head injuries also can aggravate a seizure disorder. Children with epilepsy should avoid boxing, as well as fights with their peers.

Wrestling may be safe for children with well-controlled seizures or seizures that do not impair consciousness or motor control. It can be dangerous for other children with epilepsy.

High diving and some forms of gymnastics pose clear dangers for children with epilepsy. Only children with well-controlled seizures should consider high diving, or performing on the high bar or rings in gymnastics. Other gymnastic events, such as floor routines and the pommel horse, pose little risk. The parallel bars of intermediate risk; the risk reflects the specific exercises being done. Climbing a rope higher than 5 feet is also dangerous if seizures are not well controlled.

CHAPTER 20

Education of Children with Epilepsy

Children with epilepsy usually are of normal intelligence, but some do not do well academically. When this happens, it is important to find out why. Neurological impairment, frequent seizures, or adverse effects of anti-epileptic drugs can affect school performance. If a child is doing well in school, there is no reason to worry about the effects of epilepsy on learning. If the teacher reports problems or parents become aware that their child's performance is slipping, it may be worthwhile to consider interventions. First, the problem must be identified. It may be an attention deficit with easy distractibility, excessive tiredness from medications or poor sleep, or a specific learning disability, which may or may not be related to the epilepsy (see Chapter 17). Obtaining an educational assessment is the first step after talking with the child's teachers. Parents have the right to request an assessment of their child's problems and needs.

Public Law 94-142, discussed later, provides legal guarantees for educating children with handicaps. The child has the right to be taught in a regular classroom environment whenever possible and for as much of the school day as possible. The child has the right to be included in social and other activities provided by the school. Parents have the right to be directly involved in the process of planning the child's education.

In larger urban and suburban areas, parent advocacy groups are often active, and school systems recognize the special needs of children with handicaps. In these settings, parents may need to be assertive, a behavior that is not foreign to the urban environment. In contrast, in small rural communities, where there is often only one school system and one education "czar," children with handicaps and their parents face the greatest challenge. Parents are often extremely reluctant to challenge the school personnel and system. In this setting, suggestions from parents about their child's special needs or their desire to have their child attend regular (mainstream) classes can be met with indignation and ridicule. Knowing the child's rights under the law and some cautious assertiveness can go a long way toward ensuring the child receives the best possible education.

ATTENDING REGULAR CLASSES

Most children with epilepsy attend regular classes, even though in some cases they need special aides to work with them. Regular classes offer the opportunity for children with epilepsy and other disorders to enjoy their education and be in the social environment of other children, most of whom do not have disabilities. In regular classes, the children are stimulated by other bright children and have the chance to achieve their full potential. Further, by attending mainstream classes, children with epilepsy are more likely to consider themselves as regular children, not children with a disability, and to have social role models in the other children. That is not to deny the existence of the epilepsy. Rather, it emphasizes that most children with epilepsy have the potential to learn and accomplish all the things that other children can.

Regular classes do present potential problems for children with epilepsy. Children can be cruel. They may pick on or tease the child who has epilepsy. Other parents may forbid their children to play with a child who has epilepsy. If teasing or cruelty becomes a problem, it may be worth asking the school to conduct an educational program so that the children can better understand epilepsy. The "Kids on the Block" puppet show, sponsored by the Epilepsy Foundation of America (EFA) affiliates and other groups, is an entertaining and effective means of educating children about epilepsy. These and other programs help the child with epilepsy to be accepted by his or her classmates and help the other children to understand the human and medical sides of a health problem, and through that process, to mature.

SPECIAL EDUCATION

Special education programs are designed to meet the special needs of children with disabilities by supplementing or adapting the regular curriculum. These classes and programs recognize that some students are educable but have mental or physical impairments that make it essential to tailor their education to their special needs. The variety of special education programs reflects the types and severity of the disabilities, the educational emphasis, the student-to-teacher ratio, the funding for quality teachers and equipment, and other factors.

Special education includes instruction in regular classrooms or separate facilities for part of the day, as well as physical education, occupational and physical rehabilitation, musical education programs, home instruction, and instruction in hospitals and other institutions.

The vast majority of children with epilepsy are best served by mainstream classes. In addition, special education services can be delivered partly or entirely in the regular classroom. For children with frequent and severe seizures who also have orthopedic and emotional problems, the need for a specialized program is obvious. However, many children fall between these two extremes. If a child is not doing well in mainstream classes, it is often helpful to meet with the teachers to learn if the cause of the problems can be identified, through special testing if necessary. In addition, consultation with the child's doctor may provide insights. For example, attention deficit disorder may be causing the school problems.

Just because special education is recommended, it does not mean that it is necessary. In most cases, the recommendation is valid and should be followed, but if parents disagree with the school's placement, they can appeal or seek an outside assessment by a psychologist or neuropsychologist.

Emotional issues often arise when children are assigned to special education programs that require separate classrooms away from the mainstream. Sometimes the children are placed with other children who have severe emotional or behavioral problems and thus provide poor behavioral models. Schools are required to deliver services in "the least restrictive environment," meaning the regular classroom for as much of the day as possible. For some parents, the recommendation that their child attend special classes signals that the epilepsy or associated problems are severe and that their child is "not normal."

Although the goal should be to keep the child in regular classes as much as possible, some children require many special classes or a special school. Children who attend special education programs are aware that they are not in the mainstream, particularly if they were formerly enrolled in regular classes and had problems keeping up with the other children. The word "special" is key. Parents and teachers should emphasize that the child is special, not handicapped, disabled, or less bright. They should not deny or avoid discussing the disability or the epilepsy but should emphasize the positive. Depending on the child, parents may wish to discuss why he or she goes to a certain school while brothers and sisters or other children on the block attend another school. They can highlight some of the advantages of the special school, such as more teachers, more enjoyable activities, and more children who are like him or her.

PUBLIC LAW 94-142

The Education of All Handicapped Children Act (Public Law 94-142) was passed by the Congress in 1975 and ensures that all handicapped children receive appropriate education at no cost in the least restrictive environment. (In 1990, the law was renamed the Individuals with Disabilities Education Act.) All states that receive federal funds under this act must follow the rules for identifying, evaluating, and providing services to eligible children between 3 and 21 years of age. Federal funds are also provided to the states to develop early intervention services for infants and toddlers who have physical or mental conditions that are likely to cause developmental delay.

This act recognized the special needs of children with disabilities. This group includes children with mental retardation, hearing and visual impairments (including but not limited to deafness and blindness), serious emotional disorders, orthopedic impairments, autism, traumatic brain injury, learning disabilities, and other impairments that require special education and related services. Epilepsy is specifically included under the federal regulations defining the group of "children with disabilities." Children qualify who have epilepsy only, or they may have epilepsy and another disabling condition such as mental retardation. However, to qualify for service, the presence of a potentially disabling condition is not sufficient. The impairment must adversely affect the child's educational capacity to the degree that special education or related services are required.

In some children, although their epilepsy is not disabling and their intelligence is normal, other problems may require special attention. These include impairments of attention, reading, arithmetic learning, motor skills, memory, and behavior. They are often identified at a young age, permitting early intervention and treatment.

Public Law 94-142 requires, to the maximum extent appropriate, that children with disabilities be educated with children who are not disabled. Therefore, children with epilepsy and other disabilities should not be removed from the regular educational environment unless their disability makes it extremely difficult or impossible to educate them or other children in this setting. In most cases, children with epilepsy and other disabilities can be educated in the regular classroom with the use of supplemental aides and services. For example, a child with a disability may attend homeroom and four regular classes but also attend a special tutorial for a reading disorder and physical therapy instead of gym. In this case, the child enjoys the benefits of the mainstream environment and the benefits of special education.

Public Law 94-142 states that each handicapped child must have a written individualized educational plan (IEP) constructed jointly by the parents and school personnel. Parents are also provided with channels for exercising their appeal (due process) rights if they do not agree with their child's plan. The IEP is a written report describing the child's present level of development, the short-term and annual goals of the special education program, the specific educational services the child will receive, the date services will start and their expected duration, standards for determining whether the goals of the educational program are being met, and the extent to which the child will be able to participate in regular educational programs.

The IEP is usually developed during a series of meetings among the parents, teachers, and representatives of the school district. Because a child with epilepsy has special needs, it is essential that the IEP be written with care to meet those needs. Unless the parents request specific services such as physical therapy, speech therapy, or a barrier-free school, these needs may be overlooked.

Before or during the IEP process, parents should explore available educational programs, including public, private, federal, state, county, and municipal programs. They should observe classes and see for themselves which program is best suited for their child. Parents may bring a spouse, doctor, teacher, advocate, and others for support if they do not wish to attend the IEP meeting alone. They should be aware of the actions of everyone involved in their child's case. They must be assertive and persuasive advocates for their child during the IEP process. This does not mean that all school officials are adversaries, but it does mean that parents are a child's most important advocates; they know their child best. Parents are entitled to a copy of the IEP, and should request it if it is not offered.

Public Law 94-142 requires that schools provide all the additional services needed to help children with disabilities benefit from special education. These related services include transportation, audiology and speech therapy, psychological evaluation and treatment, physical and occupational therapy, recreation, therapeutic recreation, social work services, counseling, rehabilitation counseling, early identification and assessment of disabling conditions, and medical evaluations.

For children with epilepsy, related services include education for teachers and school nurses about epilepsy, how to administer medications, and first aid for seizures. Ideally, this education will be extended to include classmates, because social acceptance may be one of the greatest challenges for children with epilepsy.

THE REHABILITATION ACT, SECTION 504

Section 504 of The Rehabilitation Act of 1973 provides education rights for children and adults with disabilities. Although provisions of Section 504 and Public Law 94-142 overlap somewhat, Section 504 is primarily an anti-discrimination law, which says that it is illegal for any program or activity receiving federal funding to exclude or discriminate against qualified people with handicaps. It also requires that reasonable accommodations be made by educational institutions.

Section 504 covers "qualified" people with handicaps, that is, those who are of school age, or at any age during which state law requires that such services be provided to people with handicaps. In many cases, this includes not only elementary and secondary education but also adult educational services. This may include college, graduate, and technical schools. For schools of higher education, Section 504 prohibits them from making a preadmission inquiry as to whether an applicant has a disability. However, if academic or other accommodations are necessary, the student must request and justify them. Examples of such accommodations include adjustments in the class schedule to allow for rest and recuperation after medical treatment, modified test arrangements such as oral tests for those with certain learning disabilities, and transportation services for persons with impaired mobility.

CHAPTER 21

Epilepsy, Mental Retardation, and Cerebral Palsy

Children with epilepsy and mental retardation or cerebral palsy present a wider range of problems than children who have uncomplicated epilepsy. Children who are mentally retarded have below-normal intellectual ability and are often impaired in their ability to understand, communicate, solve problems, and function in social settings. Children with cerebral palsy have muscle spasms, difficulty standing or walking, or postural problems, and their intelligence may range from normal to subnormal. Mental retardation and cerebral palsy can also be associated with vision, hearing, and speech problems and possibly some physical deformity or emotional disturbance. Management of children with epilepsy and mental retardation or cerebral palsy requires the combined effort of doctors, therapists, and parents.

ACCEPTANCE AND ADJUSTMENT

When a handicapped child is born, the parents' distress is severe. The feelings of guilt, shame, despair, and self-pity can be overwhelming, and the agony of longing for a way out can be excruciating. Torturing questions tend to flood the parents' minds: What did I do wrong? Why did this happen to me? The turmoil may give way to sadness, a feeling of desolation and isolation, and a longing for the lost, normal baby.

The way in which the parents adjust to the situation is crucial for the future welfare of not only the handicapped child but also the whole family. A handicapped child needs to be loved and accepted as a normal child would be. When mutually enjoyable relationships develop between the child and the family, the child's personality is allowed to develop in the most favorable environment. Whether a child is normal or handicapped at birth, he or she will most easily achieve happiness and a satisfying adult social role if brought up in a loving, contented, and united family.

Adjusting to the shock of being told about the child's handicap is difficult, but families can receive assistance, support, and education from United Cerebral Palsy, Inc., or the Association for Retarded Citizens. As the distress lessens, the family must take stock of itself in relation to the task of doing its best for the new handicapped child. The child with mental retardation or cerebral palsy and epilepsy has the same emotional needs as other children. He or she needs love but not smothering, care but not over-indulgence, and above all, opportunities for achievement, self-control, and social growth toward an independent place in adult society.

The parents of a handicapped child are faced with the question of what to tell relatives, friends, and neighbors. The best answer is the truth. Friends and neighbors are bound to visit when the baby comes home from the hospital, and failure to tell them at once of the child's disability will only make it more difficult later. Parents should tell all inquirers, including their other children, as naturally as they can, that the doctors think the baby has weak arms and legs, or is severely mentally and physically handicapped, or has seizures, and treatment has begun. Few people will fail to be helpful and sympathetic. If the child's disorder only becomes apparent and definitively diagnosed months or even years after birth, it is still wise to tell the truth.

MENTAL RETARDATION

"Mental retardation" is a term loaded with fear for parents. In the past, it usually implied mental incompetence, and was often a ticket to institutionalization. Mental retardation means slowed or delayed mental development. Children with mental retardation and epilepsy are not incapable of learning; they just do not learn as rapidly as other children.

Until recently, about two thirds of children with cerebral palsy were thought to have mental retardation. Epilepsy was also frequently associated with retardation. But now, thanks to early intervention and advanced technology, many children with serious movement and communication problems are better able to demonstrate their true potential. As a result, experts believe the rate of mental retardation among children with cerebral palsy may be as low as 25%. (It is 2% among children in the general population.) Among children with epilepsy, mental retardation occurs in 9%. Factors associated with an increased risk of mental retardation in children with epilepsy include early age when seizures begin (especially before age 2 years), prolonged duration of epilepsy, multiple seizure types, and use of several antiepileptic drugs in high dosages.

Parents need to keep in mind that the intelligence quotient (IQ) is based on a standardized way of measuring cognition (intellect) and intellectual achievement (fund of knowledge). Many children with cerebral palsy are penalized on IQ tests because their movement impairments can interfere with test-taking performance. Children with epilepsy may be slowed by medication or by seizures that are not obvious to others. Therefore, intelligence testing may not provide an accurate indication of a child's true potential.

If a child with epilepsy scores in the mentally retarded range, his or her development will probably be slower than that of other children of the same age. However, as in children without physical or mental handicaps, children with mental retardation have a wide range of abilities. The IQ score is only one measure of intelligence. Psychologists can also measure a child's adaptive level, or ability to manage common daily activities such as feeding, dressing, toileting, and social interaction. Because of movement problems, mentally retarded children with cerebral palsy and epilepsy may be delayed in these areas. The accuracy of these tests depends on the expertise and experience of the test administrators. An assessment by professionals from different disciplines is essential for an accurate picture of a child's potential. By integrating the different observations and test results, these professionals can reach a depth of understanding that could not be provided by one person.

What mental retardation means for a child depends on the nature and severity of the problem. Just as there is a wide range of intelligence among children without intellectual handicaps, there is also a wide range among children with mental retardation. Mental retardation is classified as mild (IQ of 69 to 55), moderate (IQ of 54 to 40), severe (IQ of 39 to 25), and profound (IQ of less than 25).

Although a child's IQ may place some restrictions on what he or she learns and the rate at which he or she learns it, early intervention and special education programs can reduce the impact of mental retardation on cognitive development. Programs for children with epilepsy and mental retardation tailor their curriculum so that children can learn at a rate that gives them confidence in their emerging new abilities. Therefore, parents must recognize their child's developmental strengths and weaknesses so that they can help plan an educational program that will help achieve their child's potential. When the curriculum is appropriate, a child is less likely to experience stress and more apt to appreciate his or her own achievements (see Chapter 20). Skill development, not high scores on intelligence tests, should always be the goal. It is true that a handicapped child's pace of learning may be somewhat slower than other children's, but that does not make the achievements any less meaningful.

Parents of children with epilepsy who also have mental retardation must remember that they learn new skills more slowly than other children and find it harder to acquire advanced skills such as reading, math, and complex problem solving. They also may not be as motivated as other children to learn new skills, but it does not mean that they cannot learn. Given a good educational program and support from family and friends, almost all children can make important, steady progress in intellectual abilities.

CEREBRAL PALSY

About 25% to 35% of all children with cerebral palsy have epilepsy. Epilepsy and cerebral palsy are separate disorders, but both can result from the same abnormality of the brain. Epilepsy does not cause cerebral palsy. Cerebral palsy does not cause epilepsy. The two conditions simply coexist.

Cerebral palsy is not a specific medical diagnosis but rather a descriptive name given to a group of disorders that affect control of movement resulting from a central nervous system abnormality. The neurological disorder is referred to as "stable" or "static" because the condition does not worsen over time. The neurological injury may occur while the fetus is in the womb, during or shortly after childbirth, or during the first year of life. Even when the injury occurs in the womb or at birth, not all children born with cerebral palsy show any clear signs of the disorder immediately after birth, and the symptoms vary in severity depending on the type and degree of abnormality involved.

Usually, the child's intellectual functioning is not diminished by the disorder. However, mental retardation occurs in approximately one third of children with cerebral palsy, and some children with epilepsy and cerebral palsy are also mentally retarded. The major problems for children with cerebral palsy are poor muscle control such as difficulty in sucking, holding up the head, delay in rolling over, delay in walking or inability to walk, incoordination, muscle tightness, and muscle spasms.

Cerebral palsy is classified according to six principal abnormal movements, all of which are not under a person's voluntary control; that is, they are involuntary movements. Many children with cerebral palsy have a combination of the movements, and their symptoms may vary from time to time. The abnormal movements are:

- *Spasticity.* Tense, stiff, contracted muscles.
- *Ataxia.* Poor sense of balance and impaired coordination; for example, when walking, the child may sway or lose balance; when reaching

for an object, the child's hand may stop before, then move past the target, and then finally reach the desired object.

- *Rigidity.* Tense, stiff, contracted muscles that resist movement. The difference between the spastic and the rigid forms of excessive muscle tightness is based mainly on other neurological findings (athetosis and dystonia [see below] with the rigid form, and weakness and increased reflexes with the spastic form).
- *Athetosis.* Uncoordinated, writhing, or wormlike movements of the head, limbs, and eyes that occur without deliberate effort.
- *Dystonia.* Unnatural and sustained postures of a body part, such as the hand, leg, or neck.
- *Tremor.* Trembling or shaking.

There are two main types of cerebral palsy: pyramidal and extrapyramidal. The pyramidal and extrapyramidal systems are the two principal motor systems of the central nervous system, which is composed of the brain and spinal cord. The pyramidal system is primarily concerned with strength and control of fine movements of the arms and legs, especially the hands and feet. The extrapyramidal system is primarily concerned with more basic aspects of movement and exerts greater control over muscles of the trunk, body, shoulders, and hips, although it also controls muscles in the arms and legs. Many children with cerebral palsy and epilepsy have overlapping features of these two types. Children with either type of cerebral palsy may have ataxia, tremor, or other neurological impairments such as mental retardation.

Pyramidal Cerebral Palsy

More than 80% of children with cerebral palsy have the spastic form, a pyramidal type of cerebral palsy that occurs either alone or in combination with the extrapyramidal type. These children usually have weakness, increased muscle tone (spasticity), and increased reflexes as, for example, when the doctor taps the knee and the leg jumps forward. The injury in this disorder is either to the brain cells in the frontal lobe area that control voluntary movement or to the nerve fibers that pass from this area in the depths of the brain into the spinal cord. The patterns of damage give rise to different types of impairment.

Spastic Hemiparesis

Hemiparesis refers to weakness on one side of the body. This is the most common form of spastic cerebral palsy, and most often results from an injury of the opposite side of the brain. The damage may affect either the motor area, or the nerve fibers, or both. Stroke from blockage of a blood vessel or bleeding in the brain is the most common cause of hemiparesis; other causes include trauma or an abnormality in brain development. In most children, the arm is weaker than the leg, with the hand often being severely impaired. (The hand and fingers have a large representation in the motor area of the brain [see Fig. 4].) Depending on how severely the leg is affected, children with spastic hemiparesis can usually walk with a limp. An operation to release tight tendons, or braces for the ankle, can improve the child's ability to walk. Because the injury is relatively restricted to one area of the brain, most children with spastic hemiparesis are not retarded.

Because the cerebral cortex of the brain is often damaged, children with spastic hemiparesis often have epilepsy. The seizures are partial seizures and are treated with medications for partial epilepsy. In most cases, the seizures can be controlled with antiepileptic drugs, but if not, surgery can be considered.

Diplegia

In children with diplegia, both legs are weak and stiff. The arms are usually quite functional and may be entirely normal. This disorder most often occurs in children who are born prematurely, and usually results from injury to the nerve fibers in the deep parts of the brain. Because the cerebral cortex is usually not affected, neither seizures nor mental retardation are common.

The main problem for children with diplegia is walking. Physical therapy, braces, orthopedic surgery, or the use of a wheelchair can improve function and the quality of life.

Spastic Quadriparesis

Quadriparesis refers to weakness of all four limbs. In this severe form of cerebral palsy, the injury often affects multiple and widely distributed areas of the brain. The weakness is often severe and affects not only the limbs but also the muscles of the trunk, neck, mouth, and face. In addition to a severe movement disorder, the children have epilepsy and mental retardation, which often are also severe.

The seizures in children with the spastic quadriparetic form of cerebral palsy usually begin early (during the newborn period or in the first year of life) and are difficult to control with medications. The first seizures are often infantile spasms, followed later by the Lennox-Gastaut syndrome, with multiple types of seizures that are only partially controlled with high dosages of medications.

Extrapyramidal Cerebral Palsy

The extrapyramidal type of cerebral palsy is characterized by abnormal involuntary movements, which include dystonia (sustained postures, such as the fingers curled up), athetosis (wormlike, writhing movements), chorea (irregular, spasmodic, dancelike movements), and tremor. The extrapyramidal motor system is deep within the brain. Because it is so far removed from the cerebral cortex, mental retardation and seizures are uncommon in children with this type of cerebral palsy. However, they commonly have impaired balance and coordination.

This type of cerebral palsy has become less common, as babies born with different blood types than their mother's (Rh incompatibility) are now successfully managed. Babies with this problem often had severe metabolic changes that injured the extrapyramidal parts of the brain. Extrapyramidal types now comprise approximately 20% of children with cerebral palsy. (About half of these have only extrapyramidal problems, whereas the other half have both pyramidal and extrapyramidal types, called mixed cerebral palsy.)

Treatment of Cerebral Palsy

Comprehensive child development clinics (centers for neuromuscular and developmental disorders) can identify, assess, and diagnose children's general health conditions; identify emotional and learning problems; refer children with special problems to specialists; provide instruction and counseling for parents; serve as a source of referral to other programs; and provide physical, occupational, and speech therapy. Treatment of children with cerebral palsy and epilepsy varies according to their age, the severity of their symptoms, and the type of cerebral palsy. Common measures include corrective lenses, braces, and corrective surgery for affected limbs, drug therapy to reduce spastic tension in muscles, speech and physical therapy, psychological counseling to assist with adjustment issues, and referrals to appropriate resources.

Exercise is an essential part of the therapy for children with cerebral palsy. Babies who are developing normally are seldom still; their arms and legs are in almost continuous motion. As they reach for objects and manipulate them, roll, crawl, and get into and out of sitting positions, they are exercising without making a conscious effort. For babies with cerebral palsy, this kind of healthy, spontaneous exercise is more challenging. Because some may be capable of only a few movements, babies with cerebral palsy are often relatively inactive. Despite their limitations, exercise is crucial for children with cerebral palsy. Movement through all ranges of motion can prevent contractures or joint limitations, thereby helping a child's body maintain its potential. Weight-bearing exercises can prevent bone loss. The motor and sensory input that exercise provides is an important building block for the future development of motor and cognitive skills.

The parents of a child with epilepsy and cerebral palsy must make sure the child gets all the exercise he or she needs. Consequently, if the child is passive and content to lie back and watch the environment, the parents need to foster activity. For young children with cerebral palsy, one of the best ways to encourage movement is through the roughhouse play that other children instinctively make a part of their regular exercise. The touch and movement that are so much a part of this type of play are essential to the development of normal tactile (touch sensation) and vestibular (balance and sense of head and body position) systems. A child can enjoy roughhousing if the parents keep in mind the principles of good handling and pay attention to the child's body. For example, if rapid movements such as playfully raising and lowering make the child stiff, it is better to try a slower activity involving some trunk rotation and leg separation to reduce the child's stiffness or increased muscle tone (muscle tone refers to the firmness and consistency of muscles at rest and with movement). A good alternative might be the merry-go-round, in which the parent holds the child face-to-face with the child's legs straddling the parent's waist and twirls around. Children with low muscle tone (floppy or hypotonic) generally respond well to fast movements, and children with increased muscle tone (stiff or rigid muscles) respond better to a slower pace.

Ideally, the child's exercise should be a part of the daily routine; it can be incorporated into such activities as diapering, dressing, and feeding. The child's occupational and physical therapists can provide specific tips on how to do this, but here are two general guidelines: (1) place objects far enough away from the child that he or she needs to reach for them or crawl to them, and (2) encourage the child to do all the physical activities he or she is capable of, even if it sometimes seems easier for someone else to do them.

In addition to fitting exercise into their child's daily routine, some parents of children with epilepsy and cerebral palsy also enroll the child in formal physical fitness programs. Gym classes, movement experiences, and other programs for young children are blossoming, and many are quite receptive to children with special needs. It is not absolutely essential to find a program with a staff trained in dealing with children with special needs, although the instructor should be helpful and cooperative. Generally, it will be up to the parent to apply the correct principles of reducing or increasing muscle tone and to encourage normal movement. The physical or occupational therapist can tell parents whether the child might benefit from any program they are considering.

As the child grows older, it becomes increasingly important for his or her exercise routine to include outdoor activities. Walks in the stroller or in a backpack are good ways to provide opportunities for fresh air and learning about the world outside the house. Just spending time lying or sitting on the grass while parents do yard work can be a special event. Outdoor smells, sights, and sounds all stimulate the child's developing sensory system. With proper precautions, the child may also enjoy riding on the back of the parent's bicycle. Parents may have to be creative in thinking of outdoor play activities that are within the child's abilities, but because playing outdoors is the most enjoyable form of exercise for many children, the more activities parents can come up with, the better. For example, horseback riding can provide both good physical therapy and fun for children with cerebral palsy. As with many aspects of raising a child with cerebral palsy, much trial and error is involved in finding enjoyable exercises that are right for the child.

INDEPENDENCE FOR PERSONS WITH EPILEPSY AND CEREBRAL PALSY

Some children with epilepsy and cerebral palsy have normal or close-to-normal intelligence and mild to moderate physical problems. These children usually achieve independence during later adolescence and adulthood, but others are not so fortunate. Children who are also mentally retarded and whose physical problems limit their mobility or prevent the mastery of self-help skills will continue to depend on others to some extent for the rest of their lives. In these cases, parents should strive to have their children become as independent as possible. The needs of persons with epilepsy and cerebral palsy for special education or other services depend on how the disorders affect them. These services can be provided through the school system, employment programs, and residential or community-based programs.

Education and Outlook for Success in Life

The "education" of children with cerebral palsy and epilepsy may begin shortly after birth. With the proliferation of infant stimulation programs, many children begin receiving services soon after the diagnosis is made. The best infant stimulation programs almost always involve the parents as teachers of their own children. These programs stress stimulation of the child's visual, auditory, olfactory, and tactile senses and include activities that promote language, cognitive, social, and self-help development. Some programs include specialists such as physical or speech therapists, in addition to specially trained teachers. Most parents are very receptive to infant stimulation programs, because their involvement fulfills their need to "do something" to help their children.

Children with cerebral palsy and epilepsy are often educated in regular classes, but, if they need them, they are eligible under Public Law 94-142 for special education programs (see Chapter 20).

The outlook for children with epilepsy and cerebral palsy has never been brighter. Advanced therapeutic and surgical techniques are helping to minimize the effects of cerebral palsy and its complications, and new medications and treatment methods are helping to control seizures. In addition, special equipment is helping children with these disorders to unlock their potential as never before. For example, computers are giving voices to children who might not otherwise be able to speak, and orthotics and mobility devices made from lightweight plastics and metals are granting new freedom of movement to children with limited motor skills.

Increased opportunities in education are also helping these children make giant steps toward conquering the effects of their disabilities. Another bright spot for children with epilepsy and cerebral palsy is that their parents are taking increasingly larger roles in helping the children reach their potential. Therapists, for example, now routinely train parents to reinforce their child's movement and speech skills at home. Teachers usually confer with parents when deciding how and what children with cerebral palsy and epilepsy should learn in school. Most professionals recognize that parents are the experts on their child's special needs and are often able to help the child receive the most appropriate services. These parent-professional partnerships naturally foster greater progress.

Some children with epilepsy and cerebral palsy graduate from regular academic high school programs and go on to college. Others succeed in completing vocational high school programs. Still others spend their school years in programs designed to help them become as self-sufficient as possible. Likewise, some children with epilepsy and cerebral palsy grow up to hold jobs that enable them to support themselves, whereas others need varying amounts of financial help throughout their adult lives.

Today, all children with epilepsy and cerebral palsy have the potential to live rich, fulfilling lives and to enjoy good health, good friends, and good feelings about themselves and their accomplishments. The right therapeutic and educational programs will help get the children started on the road to a rewarding future; motivation and support will help to keep them on track.

Vocational Training Programs

In the past, persons with epilepsy whose cerebral palsy was severely disabling were excluded from receiving vocational training services, because they likely could not achieve the goals of competitive full-time or part-time employment. People with epilepsy only were often excluded for the same reason. Amendments to Public Law 94-142 (see Chapter 20) made services and training available to people with severe disabilities. They are eligible even if the most they will achieve is "supported employment," which means employment in a setting with a job coach, special training, or other services that allow an individual to perform work.

The department of vocational rehabilitation in each state, sometimes called "DVR," or "OVR," or "voc rehab," are charged with carrying out the law (see Chapter 26). Under these programs, adults with epilepsy and cerebral palsy can continue to receive vocational education after they reach age 21. The state vocational rehabilitation department, United Cerebral Palsy (UCP), or a local UCP affiliate can be contacted for specific information on available services.

Living and Working in the Community

New trends are emerging in efforts to enable people with epilepsy and other disabilities to live independently and productively. The focus of these efforts is to help people with disabling conditions to overcome the physical limitations that in the past too often meant lives spent in institutions.

Personal assistance services are available for people with disabilities who need help with daily care and mobility in order to live in the community. In some programs, a personal assistant can help with cooking meals, cleaning house, and grooming so that a person with cerebral palsy can live independently. The extent to which Medicaid will help fund these programs varies from state to state.

Another current trend is the movement away from caring for people with severe cerebral palsy and epilepsy in large public or private facilities, called intermediate care facilities. The trend is to provide funding and services for independent living within the community. Programs in the state for adults with epilepsy and cerebral palsy should provide a variety of community living and working arrangements.

Protecting the rights of people with epilepsy and cerebral palsy to employment and equal opportunity in the community is of utmost importance. In 1990, The Americans with Disabilities Act was passed to protect people with disabilities from discrimination in employment, public accommodations, transportation, telecommunications, and other areas (see Chapter 26). The Epilepsy Foundation of America (EFA) may be helpful in providing additional information.

Driving

Persons with cerebral palsy and epilepsy have the same right as everyone else to obtain a driver's license if their seizures are completely controlled by medication for a specific period of time (usually 3 months to a year). If they can pass the written test (given verbally if the person is unable to write) and the driving test, persons with these disorders can obtain a license to drive (see Chapter 23).

Income Maintenance and Medical Assistance

Two federally funded income maintenance programs can provide additional income to persons with cerebral palsy, mental retardation, or both: Supplemental Security Income (SSI), a public assistance program, and Social Security Disability Insurance (SSDI), a disability insurance program (see Chapter 30). Both provide a monthly income to qualified persons with disabilities. The Social Security Administration regulations prescribe a set of tests for making the determination of disability. The test of severity is somewhat different for children and adults. A child with epilepsy and cerebral palsy meets the test of severity if he or she meets these criteria: Severe motor dysfunction, *or* less severe motor dysfunction with an IQ of 69 or less, *or* a seizure disorder (with one major seizure in the year before application), significant interference with communication, *or* a significant emotional disorder.

The Medicare and Medicaid programs (see Chapter 30) are important to people with epilepsy and cerebral palsy, but each has its own eligibility requirements and rules for recipients. Both of these programs may be available to children with disabilities who are under 18 years of age. Medicaid provides medical assistance to people who are eligible for SSI and to other people with incomes that are insufficient to pay for medical care. Because eligibility is based on financial need, placing assets in the name of children with epilepsy and cerebral palsy or providing those children with income through a trust, can disqualify them. However, trust funds designed to supplement benefits may not be disqualifying if they are properly drawn up. Medicare is not based on financial need. Anyone entitled to receive Social Security benefits is also entitled to Medicare coverage after a 2-year waiting period.

CHAPTER 22

After the Parents are Gone

No one wants to think about the reality of growing old or dying. For parents of children with uncontrolled seizures and serious physical and neurological disabilities, planning for the future is critical. The more the child depends on the parent, the more that planning is needed.

All adults should have a will. If there is no will, the state's rules for this situation—called intestacy rules—will apply. The intestacy rules, rather than the individual's desires, will govern the distribution of assets as well as the ultimate guardianship of any minor children. A will can be drawn up inexpensively, and it is the only way that parents can guarantee that their children will be cared for as the parents desire and that their assets will be distributed in accordance with their wishes. A will is a necessity for parents of young children and adolescents with epilepsy and for parents of older children who are unable to fully care for themselves. A will allows parents to designate someone to take care of their children, to manage the money they leave behind for the children, and to supervise the proper distribution of their estate.

CHOOSING A GUARDIAN

Guardians have the legal responsibility for a child (or a legally incompetent person) if the child's natural parents die. Whether a guardian is required depends on the age of the child and the child's ability to manage his or her own affairs. Because of these awesome responsibilities, parents must choose a guardian carefully.

Choosing a guardian is one of the most difficult decisions any parent has to make. Parents should consider their values and how they would want their child to be brought up. The guardian should share the parents' values and principles about raising a child or overseeing the well-being of an adult with severe seizures and related disabilities. Parents should discuss their concerns and wishes with the potential guardians. Even after talking things over, it is a good idea for the parents to put their thoughts in writing.

Family members and close friends are usually considered possible guardians. The guardians should be responsible and mature, but they should also love, or at least have the capacity to love, the child. The guardians should have a stable family structure. If the guardians have children, parents should make sure that their child will not be an added burden and the source of resentment.

TRUSTS AND ESTATE PLANNING

After deciding on the guardian, parents must next decide on the trustees and executors of their will. The executor is the person who oversees the administration of the estate and the distribution of the assets. The trustees are the people who are responsible for administering the trust funds for the child. Attorneys who specialize in estate planning can be helpful in creating trusts with terms that parents find in their child's best interest.

The terms of the trust will vary depending on the amount of assets, the immediate and long-term needs of the child, the maturity and age of the child, and other factors. A trust instrument can be very flexible. It can provide that the trustee have the discretion to distribute money as required for the health, welfare, and maintenance of the child. In some cases, the child can be given the interest earned in addition to these discretionary distributions. In other cases, the child can receive the interest until a certain age and then, if the trustee feels the child can manage the money, the entire assets or a fraction of the assets can be given to the child.

When parents write their will, it is often a good time to consider estate planning. No one wants to pay the government more taxes than they need to legally. When there is a child with special needs, assets assume even greater importance. There are several things that parents can do to protect the amount of money their child receives from their estate. First, every year, each child can receive a maximum gift of $10,000 from each parent. This money, and the interest that it generates over time, can go into a carefully drawn trust fund designed to supplement the child's other benefits. This money will not be subject to estate taxes when the parent dies. The gift to the child's trust can be in the form of cash, investments, or insurance policies. For example, a parent can purchase a whole-life insurance policy that is owned by the child's trust. The cost of the premiums can be paid as part of the child's yearly gift. If structured correctly when the parent dies, the child receives the death benefit without its being subject to estate taxes.

Similarly, whole-life policies can be obtained that are payable to the trust only when both parents have passed away. These policies are often much less expensive than policies on a single parent, and the benefits from these policies can be used to pay estate taxes, leaving the assets to go to the children. A variety of other strategies may be worth considering. The laws regarding estate taxes and exemptions are complex, so parents should consult an attorney who is knowledgeable about estate taxes.

When an adult child needs assisted living arrangements and cannot be self-supporting, he or she will qualify for a range of services through state and federal agencies. However, eligibility for these programs can be lost if there is a transfer of funds when the parents pass away. Trusts must be set up to *supplement* the benefits, not to replace them. It is important that the proper legal steps are taken and that the whole family knows that bequests to the affected family member must go to the trust, not directly to the person.

PART FOUR

Epilepsy in Adults

CHAPTER 23

Living with Epilepsy

One of the biggest questions for adults with epilepsy concerns whether and how much to restrict their activities of daily living. There must be a balance between safety and the need to pursue employment, fulfill household responsibilities, and enjoy leisure activities. That balance can best be achieved by common sense. For persons with rare or fully controlled seizures, most activities can be safely pursued. For those who have frequent seizures with impairment of consciousness and a period of confusion afterward, certain activities must be restricted, with the hope the restrictions can be lifted when seizure control improves.

RISK-BENEFIT DECISIONS

Life for all of us is never free of risks. Making decisions about the risks and benefits associated with different activities is not unique to people with epilepsy. The high-risk activities of skydiving, hang gliding, bungee jumping, motorcycle riding, and scuba diving can potentially cause injury or death, yet millions of people participate in these activities every year. Those who do so feel that the benefits—enjoyment, economical transportation, employment—outweigh the risks. Many more of us engage in lower-risk activities such as driving a car or snorkeling. Our decisions ultimately reflect our personal philosophy of life and how we define the benefits and risks. The risk-benefit decisions of persons with epilepsy should be influenced by their seizure control. For persons whose seizures are well controlled, the situation is essentially no different from that of someone without epilepsy. For persons with frequent, uncontrolled seizures, precautions are needed for some activities such as swimming and bike riding, whereas other activities such as driving a car or flying a plane are simply unsafe. The most difficult situations and decisions arise for persons who have occasional seizures.

It is important that persons with epilepsy consider the impact not only on themselves but also on others of having a seizure during a specific activity. For example, cigarette smoking by persons with epilepsy can present dangers other than the well-known ones that affect all smokers. If someone is smoking and has a seizure, the fallen cigarette can start a fire, and the fire can be deadly to the one who started it, as well as to other, innocent victims.

PREVENTION OF SEIZURE-RELATED INJURIES

Most seizures do not cause physical injury. Unfortunately, however, serious injuries can occur during tonic-clonic and tonic or atonic seizures. During these attacks, patients usually fall and can bruise or cut themselves, fracture their bones, chip their teeth, dislocate their shoulders, or sprain their joints. Because of the dangers, persons with frequent, uncontrolled seizures that cause them to lose control of their muscles or to become unaware of their surroundings should take special precautions in the kitchen, and should not work in places where they could be injured by heat, electricity, or dangerous equipment (such as an electric saw), unless special safety features are in place or they always have a warning (aura) of an approaching seizure. *Prevention is the best strategy for avoiding seizure-related injuries.* When cooking, for example, persons with frequent seizures may be safer using a microwave oven or putting guards around an open flame, and, whenever possible, bringing individual dishes to the source of hot food rather than carrying kettles or saucepans. Other safeguards in the home include carpeting the bathroom, putting a temperature monitor on showerheads, lowering the temperature of the water heater, putting guards around radiators, using a laundry for clothes that have to be ironed, avoiding electric carving knives and slicing machines, and perhaps even living in a first-floor or elevator-served apartment or a single-story house to avoid falls on stairs.

QUALITY OF LIFE

A 40-year-old married man with two children was referred to an epileptologist after he asked his neurologist to recommend a doctor who could give a second opinion on his care. He had juvenile myoclonic epilepsy, had had seizures for more than 15 years, and was being treated with high doses of two antiepileptic drugs, which caused him to sleep 12 hours a night, yet feel constantly tired. He complained that he was "always a bit foggy, a little down and depressed; it's not me, I know it's the medications." Despite the therapy, he continued to have two or three tonic-clonic seizures a year. The epileptologist took the old drugs away and prescribed another antiepileptic drug. The man has been seizure-free for more than a year and has almost no adverse reactions to the new drug. He says, "I feel as if I have been reborn. I am another person. Everyone at work, at home can see the difference. I am awake, my spirits are great. I can think. I am so happy."

The concept of "quality of life" is relatively new in medicine. Quality of life is difficult to measure. Simply stated, it reflects the patient's, not the doctor's, perspectives on an illness and its effects on life. Although it would seem that the patient's and doctor's views on the quality of life would be similar, they can be quite different. In different fields of medicine, quality-of-life studies have provided new insights into the effect of disorders and treatments on patients and into ways of improving their lives.

There has been increasing recognition that the quality of life is often impaired in persons with epilepsy, but doctors may not be aware of it. Many doctors who care for people with epilepsy consider occasional seizures "acceptable" and minor adverse effects of medications "tolerable." Of course, in some cases, the seizures cannot be entirely controlled, and adverse effects invariably occur despite the doctor's best attempts to adjust the medications. Too often, however, the doctor does not aggressively try to control the seizures further or to reduce the adverse effects of the medication. The problem is often one of perception: The doctor does not see a problem worthy of attention, but the patient does. A person who has occasional seizures may have restrictions on driving, difficulties with getting a job or career advancement, and problems with finances, social and family life, and self-esteem. Fear of another seizure may be the person's greatest disability. The stigma of epilepsy, which unfortunately is still too often encountered, may have altered the person's view of society and affected his or her possibilities of employment. In some cases, however, the person's perception of the stigma may be greater than any actual discrimination. Others may find that tolerating an occasional seizure offers a better quality of life than the adverse effects that accompany more aggressive treatment.

Achieving the best possible quality of life for persons with epilepsy is a challenge. On one hand, doctors must pay greater attention to patients' expectations and their actual experiences of living with epilepsy. On the other hand, patients must help doctors to understand how epilepsy, and its treatment, affect their lives.

MOTOR VEHICLE DRIVING

A driver's license is a passport to adulthood. In both rural and suburban areas of the United States, access to a motor vehicle is often essential for independence and employment. Even in many urban areas, driving is required for a variety of jobs or to reach certain locations for work or pleasure.

Driving is a privilege, and the applicant must meet the criteria set forth by their state to qualify for a driver's license. In all states, to obtain a driver's license, the applicant must be older than a minimum age (usually 16 or 17 years), must not have a medical disorder that would make driving dangerous, and must pass a written test, a vision test, and a driving test.

Licensure of Persons with Epilepsy

The laws determining which medical conditions disqualify someone from obtaining a driver's license vary from state to state. In many states, the laws have become more liberal over the past decade, resulting in fewer restrictions for people with epilepsy. The laws are written to protect public safety and to grant the privilege of driving to people who are the most unlikely to have an accident. Compared with those of most European nations, however, our state driving restrictions are quite liberal. In some European countries, for example, a single tonic-clonic seizure in adulthood prohibits holding a license for the rest of the person's life.

Many people do not recognize that, in addition to tonic-clonic seizures, absence and complex partial seizures while driving are dangerous and can be deadly. Furthermore, the risk of injury or death is not restricted to the driver and passengers but applies to pedestrians and people in other vehicles. Studies have shown that motor vehicle accidents are more common in people with epilepsy, but nowhere near the rate for those who drink and drive. In some cases, accidents involving epilepsy are caused by people, especially men, who are driving without a license or who fail to report their epilepsy when applying for a license.

In most states, for a person with epilepsy to obtain a driver's license, he or she must be free of potentially dangerous seizures for a certain period of time and must submit a doctor's statement of opinion of the person's ability to drive safely. The seizure-free period varies from state to state. During the past decade, there has been a trend away from an "absolute period" of being seizure-free toward a shorter interval of freedom from seizures. Although some states still require a period of at least 1 year during which the person with epilepsy is seizure-free, most consider exceptions that would permit someone to drive after a shorter seizure-free interval. In most states, the doctor who cares for the person with epilepsy must fill out a form stating that it is safe for the person to drive and recommending licensure. This recommendation is used as one of several factors in making a decision. In states that do not require a specific seizure-free period, the doctor's recommendation often carries much weight.

The Review and Decision Process

In most states, the medical information submitted by the applicant and the doctor is reviewed by personnel in the state's department of motor vehicles (or equivalent department). In complex cases, or those in which the decision is uncertain, the information is usually forwarded to a consulting doctor or the state's medical advisory board. This board is active in most states and also hears appeals concerning decisions to deny or revoke drivers' licenses.

Decisions made by the motor vehicle department can be appealed by requesting an administrative hearing before the medical advisory board, or other designated body, within a specified period. If the administrative decision is not favorable, the applicant can request a judicial review. Such requests must be made within a specified period.

Someone with persistent seizures may be allowed to drive if the seizures do not impair consciousness or control of movement, occur only during sleep, are consistently preceded by an aura, are restricted to a certain time of the day (such as within an hour after awakening), or occur only when the antiepileptic medications are reduced or stopped on the advice of a doctor. A letter from the doctor confirming the presence and consistency of these features is often required by the state motor vehicle agency. Evidence that the person takes the prescribed medications is often required, and the level of the antiepileptic drug in the blood is usually provided as confirmation of compliance.

Restricted and Commercial Driver's Licenses

In many states, persons who do not meet the requirements for a regular driver's license may be granted a restricted license. This license may grant a person with epilepsy or other disabilities the privilege to drive under certain conditions, such as during daytime only, to and from work within a certain distance from the home, or only during an emergency.

The US Department of Transportation (DOT) regulations prohibit anyone with a history of epilepsy from driving a truck between states. These regulations are currently under review, however. For advice about the current rules, a person with epilepsy should contact the DOT. The blanket denial of a commercial driver's license to any person with a history of epilepsy is unfair for several reasons. Some childhood epilepsies, such as benign rolandic epilepsy, are associated with a high remission rate; the seizures in some persons may have been fully controlled for years; and some types of seizures are not dangerous if they occur while driving.

Regulations for driving a truck or bus within a state vary from state to state. Some states have restrictive policies that prohibit such driving by any person with a history of epilepsy, and others take the more reasonable approach and review each case individually.

Maintaining a Driver's License

Most states that grant driver's licenses to people with epilepsy require periodic medical reports. These reports document that seizure control has not deteriorated and that the person is taking or does not need to take medications. If the seizures have stopped or have been controlled for more than 3 to 5 years, most states will no longer require periodic medical reports.

Regardless of the reporting requirements, if the seizures recur and impair consciousness or control of movement, it is imperative to stop driving and consult the doctor, who may be able to suggest alterations in lifestyle (such as more sleep) or adjustments in medications that may restore seizure control. If a driver's license is revoked because of a breakthrough seizure surrounded by extenuating circumstances (reduction of medication on a doctor's advice or unusual stress such as the death of a loved one) the driver may appeal the decision, as described earlier.

Potential Liability and Physician Reporting

A person with epilepsy may face civil or criminal charges because of a motor vehicle accident caused by seizures. Liability may occur when someone drives against medical advice, without a valid license, without notifying the state department of motor vehicles of the medical condition, or with the knowledge that driving is prohibited because of a particular reason.

In 1994, six states, California, Delaware, Nevada, New Jersey, Oregon, and Pennsylvania, had laws mandating that doctors report people with epilepsy and other disorders that may make driving hazardous. These laws generally require that the doctor notify the department of motor vehicles of the person's name, age, and address. The specifics of when a doctor must report someone can be vague. In New Jersey, for example, the law states that the doctor will report any person 16 years of age or older for recurrent convulsive seizures or for recurrent periods of unconsciousness or for impairment or loss of motor coordination due to conditions such as, but not limited to, epilepsy in any of its forms when such conditions persist or recur despite medical treatments. However, it remains unclear what constitutes "medical treatments." The plural usage indicates that more than one treatment has failed to control the seizures but does not specify how many dosage adjustments or medications must have been tried.

Mandatory reporting laws should be repealed, as was done by Connecticut in 1990. However, if a physician in Connecticut cares for a person whose seizures are so poorly controlled that driving would present a serious risk to public safety, and there is evidence that the person continues to drive, the doctor can report the person with immunity. Such cases are rare. Connecticut's approach to mandatory reporting is a reasonable middle ground, as it strikes a balance between the rights of the individual and the public's safety.

The chief problem with mandatory reporting is that it can destroy the doctor-patient relationship. In many cases, a person who must drive is forced to lie to the doctor about his or her condition in order to avoid mandatory reporting and potential loss of the driver's license. This is the worst of two worlds: the person is not receiving the best medical care and is driving. If the doctor and patient can work together, the seizures are more likely to be better controlled, and the person can drive more safely, thus ensuring both the driver's own and the public's safety.

In states with mandatory reporting, doctors may be liable for negligence if they fail to report a person with epilepsy who is later involved in a motor vehicle accident. The most common penalty for failure to report is a fine, usually ranging from $5 to $50. In states that require mandatory reporting, the rates of reporting vary widely between different doctors.

Doctors who state that it is safe for a person with epilepsy to drive and recommend licensure could also face some liability in case of an accident, although it appears to be minimal. Very few cases have been brought against a doctor by a third party who was injured in a motor vehicle accident allegedly caused by a person with epilepsy. Doctors should not be liable for recommendations made to the department of motor vehicles if their opinions are reasonable and consistent with the standard of care. Some states grant immunity from liability to doctors who make recommendations about driving privileges.

SPORTS AND OTHER PHYSICAL ACTIVITIES

Common sense must reign in making decisions about sports and other potentially dangerous physical activities. The discussion in Chapter 19 concerning sports and other physical activities for children and adolescents is relevant to adults. There must be a balance between an active, full life and safety. For most persons, the balance is easily achieved, because most sports can be safely pursued by adults with epilepsy. Persons with well-controlled seizures, seizures occurring only during sleep, or seizures that are always preceded by a warning should have few or no restrictions on sports or other physical activities. For persons who continue to have complex partial or tonic-clonic seizures, even if they are preceded by warnings, safety mandates the application of some restrictions. For example, in skydiving, the person may be able to pull the ripcord if the seizure occurs after jumping but would have no control over the descent, increasing the risk of landing in trees or power lines; without control, even hitting the ground could be deadly. Similar restrictions apply to scuba diving, unless the dive depth is under 10 feet and, of course, as with any scuba dive, the person is accompanied by a buddy.

Most sporting activities can be pursued by persons whose seizures are not fully controlled. These activities include water skiing, sailing, windsurfing, snorkeling, bicycling, gymnastics, soccer, football, baseball, handball, squash, tennis, basketball, volleyball, archery, skiing, sledding, hiking, and many others. When a person is engaged in any of these activities, certain precautions can be taken to minimize the risk of injury. For example, when water skiing, sailing, windsurfing, or participating in other water sports, wearing a life vest reduces the risk of drowning if the person ends up in the water; its use is required of water skiers in many states. None of these activities should be pursued by a person with epilepsy unless someone is nearby who is familiar with the condition and with basic lifesaving skills. Snorkeling can also be enjoyed by persons with seizures, but they must use caution about where they snorkel. In some areas, the rocks, corals, and sea urchin spines form a maze close to the water's surface. If the water stirs, even an experienced snorkeler can get cut or injured. Such areas should be avoided by persons whose seizures are not fully controlled, because their ability to navigate through the sharp objects in the maze could be impaired. Although diving from the edge of a pool, dock, or low diving board is generally safe, diving off a high diving board is dangerous. For all of these activities, persons with epilepsy must weigh the benefits and risks.

Although hiking can be safely pursued by persons with recurrent seizures, mountain climbing can be dangerous. Whether a person uses ropes or climbs along difficult paths, the activity can be dangerous even for the most alert and agile climber. Even a brief lapse of concentration or a small problem with control of movement could be deadly. Nature is not forgiving. Climbers should carefully consider the specific trail or mountain before starting and remember that there is no glory in proceeding when they reach an unexpected and dangerous obstacle.

Hunting can be safely pursued by persons with epilepsy. When hunting, a person whose seizures are not fully controlled should be accompanied by someone else who maintains a close position. If the person with epilepsy has a warning of a seizure, he or she should lay the gun down immediately. If a warning does not always occur before the seizure, it may be best only to load the rifle shortly before shooting, and if no shot is taken, to unload the weapon.

Persons with frequent, uncontrolled seizures can also vigorously pursue sporting activities, although the safety issues assume even greater importance. They must use greater precautions and more carefully consider the risks.

SMOKING

The toll of tobacco on our society is enormous. Smoking contributes to the death of approximately 500,000 people each year from heart disease, stroke, and cancer. Smoking tobacco is not known to have any definite effects on seizure control. Persons with epilepsy not only are susceptible to all the usual lethal effects of smoking but also are at increased risk of injury or death from another effect of smoking: fires.

Consider what happened to one of my patients and her daughter. The patient, a 35-year-old woman with absence and tonic-clonic seizures, and her 5-year-old daughter rented an apartment in New York City. One evening, while smoking, the woman had a tonic-clonic seizure. When she awoke in the hospital, she had first-degree burns on a large part of her arms and body. Her daughter suffered severe smoke inhalation and brain damage. The girl, now 13 years old, is severely retarded, uses a wheelchair, and is in an institution. The woman, who has gone through a long emotional process of dealing with what happened, finally appears to have won another battle— she has stopped smoking for 3 years.

The risk of smoking, unlike the risks of many other activities for persons with epilepsy, can severely injure or kill others. Therefore, any person with epilepsy who has episodes of impaired consciousness should make a special effort to stop smoking. There are a variety of programs and methods that can help a smoker to stop smoking. The use of nicotine patches is safe for people with epilepsy. For those who find it impossible or unacceptable to stop smoking, the risk of a dangerous fire can be substantially reduced by smoking with someone else nearby. Of course, all places where people smoke should be equipped with working smoke detectors.

ROMANTIC RELATIONSHIPS AND MARRIAGE

Persons with well-controlled or infrequent seizures should have no serious problems dating or developing and maintaining a stable, intimate relationship. For persons with uncontrolled seizures, dating and romantic relationships can be more difficult. Nevertheless, some people with frequent seizures have adjusted well to their condition and are successful in pursuing an active romantic life. All persons with epilepsy sooner or later face some important questions: "Do I tell this person that I have epilepsy?" "When should I tell him or her?" "How much should I tell?"

There is no reason to rush the disclosure of epilepsy. Unless the seizures are so frequent that one might occur on the first date, it is best to wait until the ice is broken and trust and openness have developed in the relationship. These positive developments may happen on the first date or the tenth date, or they may never happen. If the two persons are obviously incompatible, there is no reason to discuss the disorder. If the relationship is developing slowly, but is promising, it is reasonable to discuss the epilepsy earlier rather than later. It is best to tell someone in person, not over the telephone or by letter.

The way in which the disorder is presented is often how the other person will see it. The person with epilepsy should be honest and tell the other person the truth about the disorder and how he or she has been affected by it. The other person should be allowed to react to what he or she has heard. The person with epilepsy has had time to adjust to the disorder, but the friend needs time to ask questions and to reflect on the disclosure. Epilepsy should not be made the focus of the conversation. The two people should discuss it and then move on to other subjects. A person with epilepsy, like everyone else, is defined by many traits and attributes, likes and dislikes; the disorder should not be allowed to be the defining feature.

Anyone who dates and gets involved in romantic relationships is likely to experience rejection at some time or another. Someone may say no to the first date, others may say no to the second date, and others may break up the relationship after an extended period of dating. Rejection is, unfortunately, part of dating and relationships for everyone; it is not unique to persons with epilepsy. People are rejected for a variety of physical characteristics, personality traits, social beliefs, and other reasons. We all have numerous observations and feelings about other people, and as they merge in the subconscious parts of our minds, we end up attracted to some people and not to others. Although epilepsy may contribute to the reasons for rejection by some people, it may be "attractive" to others who have a need to nurture or care for someone. However, a healthy and long-term relationship is more likely to develop when the other person is attracted to someone's personal qualities and is able to put epilepsy in its rightful place as a medical problem.

Sex Life

Persons with epilepsy can enjoy all the sexual feelings and pleasures others enjoy. Epilepsy is not generally associated with restrictions on sexual activities. Most persons with epilepsy have normal sex lives. There is no convincing evidence that seizures are more likely to occur during sexual activities. Very rarely, seizures may be more likely to occur during physical exertion. In this case, some modifications may be needed for the enjoyment of an active sex life.

Sexual dysfunction, a common problem in the general population, refers to an inability to experience sexual feelings or perform sexual activities. For example, the failure of a man to achieve an erection (impotence) or the inability of a man or woman to achieve an orgasm (anorgasmia) are forms of sexual dysfunction. In the general population of people without epilepsy, many women do not routinely achieve orgasm, and intermittent impotence is a problem for young men and even more of a problem for older men. Impotence is more common in men with epilepsy than in men in the general population. Antiepileptic drugs, mainly the barbiturates (phenobarbital and primidone), can cause or aggravate the impotence. In some cases, the epilepsy itself, and not antiepileptic drugs, contributes to sexual dysfunction, especially if the seizures are poorly controlled. If depression is present, its treatment may lead to resumption of normal sexual functioning.

Studies suggest that some persons with epilepsy have a reduced libido, or a lower level of interest in sexual activity, compared with people in the general population. Only a minority of persons with epilepsy have such a problem, and they are not usually concerned about it. More often, a spouse feels that the partner's interest in sex is less than he or she would expect. If sexual dysfunction is a problem, a person should not hesitate to discuss it with the doctor.

Fertility

The majority of men and women with epilepsy have normal sex lives, are fertile, and are able to have perfectly healthy children. Nevertheless, epilepsy, its treatment, and associated disorders may affect fertility and reproduction. Men with epilepsy may have slightly reduced fertility. Hormonal changes associated with the seizures may contribute to the problem. In addition, sperm production may be reduced in men who take antiepileptic drugs. Women with epilepsy also have somewhat higher rates of infertility than women in the general population. Antiepileptic drugs and irregular menstrual cycles probably contribute to this infertility.

Infertile couples in which one member, or both, have epilepsy should consult with an infertility specialist. Common causes of infertility, such as endometriosis (abnormal location of the lining of the womb) in women or a varicocele (abnormal collection of veins in the scrotal sac) in men, should be investigated and treated. Infertility should never be dismissed as simply a problem of the epilepsy or the antiepileptic drugs used to treat it.

CHAPTER 24

Pregnancy in Women with Epilepsy

Planning a family and expecting a child should be joyous activities. The fears that accompany pregnancy and parenthood are compounded for persons with epilepsy, especially for women with epilepsy. Our society has taught us that taking medications during pregnancy is unsafe. Yet, most women with epilepsy are unable to safely stop their antiepileptic drugs during pregnancy.

Defining the potential dangers and ways of reducing these risks is a starting point for family planning. The risks associated with pregnancy for women with epilepsy are fairly well defined. Many of the steps to reduce the problems for both the mother and the child must be taken before the pregnancy. There should be good communication among the couple, the neurologist, and the obstetrician to ensure that the need for seizure control and the desire for a healthy baby are met to the highest degree possible and are well balanced. Potential parents should know that more than 90% of women with epilepsy have perfectly healthy babies.

BEFORE PREGNANCY

During the past decade, much greater attention has been focused on the subject of epilepsy in women of childbearing age. Perhaps the most important realization is that planning for pregnancy is essential, but which persons with epilepsy should plan for pregnancy? Most people answer this question incorrectly, saying that women with epilepsy who want a family should make plans. The correct answer is that all women of childbearing age who have epilepsy should learn about pregnancy. Many babies are born each year to women with epilepsy who were not planning on becoming pregnant. Men with epilepsy who are potential fathers also need to know about family planning. Men often ask: "What is the risk of epilepsy in the baby?" "Are the antiepileptic drugs I take dangerous for the baby?" "Can I care for the baby?"

Risk of Epilepsy in the Baby

Children whose parents have epilepsy have a slightly higher risk of developing epilepsy. The lifetime risk of developing epilepsy in the general population is approximately 3%. If the father has epilepsy and the mother does not, the risk to the children is only slightly higher than 3%. If the mother has epilepsy and the father does not, the risk is somewhat higher but still under 5%. If both parents have epilepsy, the risk is a bit higher than if only one parent has the condition.

A couple in which one or even both partners have epilepsy should not decide to forgo having children because of fear that the children will have epilepsy. The risk of epilepsy is low, many children outgrow epilepsy, and in the vast majority of persons with epilepsy, the seizures are well controlled by a single drug.

Birth Defects and Antiepileptic Drugs

The healthiest women have a 2.5% chance of having a baby with a major birth defect. The chance increases to approximately 6% in women with epilepsy. The reasons for the increased risk in women with epilepsy are not fully understood. We know that the risk is increased by the use of antiepileptic drugs but not by seizures before or during pregnancy. Genetic factors definitely contribute to an increased risk of birth defects in the general population. It remains uncertain, however, if women or men with epilepsy are at increased risk of having children with birth defects because of genetic factors. If there is a family history of birth defects, then the parents should seek genetic counseling.

Antiepileptic drugs taken by the mother shortly before conception and during the first 3 months of pregnancy clearly present the greatest danger to the developing baby. The danger of antiepileptic drugs taken by the father is less clear. Some studies show a slight increase in birth defects among babies whose fathers took antiepileptic drugs, and others show no increase.

Women with epilepsy are faced with a difficult decision. The use of antiepileptic drugs during pregnancy has risks for the baby, but most women need to continue taking the drugs. It is an understandable but misguided and dangerous practice to reduce or stop the medication without a doctor's recommendation. Seizures can be dangerous to both the woman and the baby.

The first trimester (first 3 months) is the critical period for development of the baby's major organ systems, and the second and third trimesters (last

6 months) are critical for its growth and maturation. In a relatively small number of cases, exposure to antiepileptic drugs during the first trimester can cause major congenital malformations (birth defects) such as cleft lip and cleft palate (a gap in the middle of the lip or palate) and structural defects of the heart. Other major malformations affect the central nervous system, the gastrointestinal system, the genitourinary system, and the skeletal system. These defects are serious but often compatible with normal development after surgical correction or other forms of treatment. Minor malformations result from exposure to antiepileptic drugs during the last 6 months and include widely spaced eyes, a small and upturned nose, and short fingers and toes. Minor defects are actually not rare in the general population, and may "disappear" after the first year of life.

The three new antiepileptic drugs (felbamate, gabapentin, and lamotrigine) have not been associated with major congenital birth defects in animal studies, in contrast to all of the currently available first-line antiepileptic drugs. However, the safety of these new drugs in women during pregnancy has not been established. We are anxiously awaiting this additional and vital safety information.

Treatment with one antiepileptic drug in the lowest dosage that will control the seizures presents the least risk for the baby's development. Any woman of childbearing age who is taking two or more antiepileptic drugs, and who would consider having a baby if she became pregnant, should ask her doctor if she could be treated with one medication. In some cases, because of the difficult nature of the seizure disorder, more than one drug may be necessary. However, many women can be safely treated with one drug, and some can remain seizure-free with lower dosages than usually taken. Women who are thinking of discontinuing their antiepileptic drugs may find no better time to try it, under a doctor's supervision, than before pregnancy.

Knowing the approximate risks is not always reassuring. Some couples are relieved to learn that the risk of major birth defects is only slightly greater than if the woman did not have epilepsy. Others focus on the relative percentages, noting that the risk of birth defects is approximately double that of the general population. It is important to discuss pregnancy ahead of time and to feel comfortable with family-planning decisions. Most experts recommend that women and men with epilepsy should feel free to pursue parenthood.

DURING PREGNANCY

Regular medical care is essential for all pregnant women. The doctor can identify common problems of pregnancy before they become serious.

Because of the increased risk of problems during pregnancy and the potential for problems with seizure control, regular visits to both the obstetrician and the neurologist are critical for women with epilepsy.

Vaginal bleeding during and after pregnancy is the most common obstetrical problem in women with epilepsy. Other common problems include abnormalities of the placenta (the organ that nourishes the baby) and complications around the time of birth, such as high blood pressure (preeclampsia) and premature delivery.

Taking Vitamins

Taking vitamins before and during pregnancy can help reduce the risks of malformations in the baby. Folate (folic acid) appears to be the most important vitamin, but the best dose remains unknown. The recommended daily minimum in the general adult population is 0.4 milligram, the amount of folate found in most high-potency vitamins. For women taking antiepileptic drugs, a supplemental dose of 0.4 to 2 milligrams per day is reasonable. For women taking antiepileptic drugs who have a family or personal history of birth defects, a dose of 1 to 4 milligrams per day is reasonable. In addition to folate, women with epilepsy who may become pregnant should probably take a high-potency multivitamin pill. During pregnancy, women with epilepsy may have an additional need for vitamins, which can be discussed with the obstetrician.

Effects of Pregnancy on Seizure Control

Pregnancy brings about dramatic changes in the body. It affects metabolism, fluid balance, hormone levels, and other physical functions and has a psychological and emotional impact. The net result of all of these changes is complex and makes seizure control unpredictable. Among women with epilepsy who become pregnant, one fifth have an increase in seizure frequency, one fifth have a reduction, and more than half have no change. Seizures are more likely to increase in the last 3 months of the pregnancy. Good seizure control during one pregnancy does not necessarily predict that seizures will not increase during subsequent pregnancies. Women can help keep their seizures well controlled during pregnancy by taking their medications as prescribed. If nausea and vomiting become a problem, the doctor should be informed immediately, because the absorption of antiepileptic drugs can be seriously affected.

Doctors and pregnant women face difficult decisions about adjusting drug dosages during pregnancy. Monitoring blood levels of the drugs may be helpful, but the patient's condition should be the principal guide for maintaining or changing therapy. If the seizures have been well controlled before pregnancy, most doctors do not increase the dosage of antiepileptic drugs during the first 3 months, even if the blood levels of the drugs decline. If the frequency of the seizures increases, however, a higher dosage may be needed.

The decline in blood levels of antiepileptic drugs during the course of pregnancy is associated with the amount of "total" and "free" drug in the bloodstream. The total amount of drug consists of two parts: drug that is bound, or attached, to proteins in the blood, and drug that is unbound, or floating freely, in the blood. Only the unbound, or free, drug crosses from the blood to the brain and helps to control seizures. When a blood drug level is monitored, the results are usually reported as the total drug level and not the free level. Although the total blood levels of all antiepileptic drugs are moderately reduced during pregnancy, the free levels of most drugs (phenobarbital is the major exception) are usually reduced only slightly. A doctor who considered only the total blood drug level might predict that seizure control would worsen, but if he or she considered the more meaningful free level, the prediction for a change in seizure control would be more realistic.

Effects of a Woman's Seizures on the Baby

Absence seizures, simple partial seizures, or complex partial seizures during pregnancy pose no danger to the baby unless the woman injures herself during the seizure, which is rare. Convulsive (tonic-clonic) seizures in the woman, however, can be dangerous for the developing baby. Most women who have one or two tonic-clonic seizures during pregnancy have healthy babies, but during a convulsion, there is a risk of trauma to the abdomen, potentially injuring the baby. The temporary interruption of breathing that accompanies tonic-clonic seizures, which is rarely of any significance for the woman, can lead to oxygen deprivation in the baby. The baby's heart rate slows for as much as 30 minutes after a tonic-clonic seizure. The greatest dangers are prolonged or repetitive tonic-clonic seizures, which can impair the supply of oxygen to the baby's brain and other organs.

Women who are pregnant should avoid the stressors that are known to provoke seizures (see Chapter 6), as well as alcohol, illegal drugs, caffeine, and smoking.

LABOR AND DELIVERY

Women with epilepsy have cesarean deliveries much more often than women without epilepsy. The reasons for this difference are poorly understood. Women with epilepsy who are taking high dosages of antiepileptic drugs may have slightly weaker contractions of the womb (uterus) during delivery. The high rate of cesarean sections in women with epilepsy may have more to do with the perceived risks of complications in a vaginal delivery than with the actual risks.

The use of agents to induce labor is approximately three times more common among women with epilepsy than among women in the general population, although the reasons for this are not fully defined. The vast majority of women with epilepsy do not need drugs for the induction of labor. Epilepsy itself is not a reason to induce labor, as most women with epilepsy are able to have normal, spontaneous labor and deliveries. In selected situations, however, it may be prudent to induce labor in women with epilepsy. The potential benefits of an induced labor must be weighed against the risks, which include prolonged labor as well as uterine and physical exhaustion, and can lead to the need for a cesarean section.

For women who have only simple or complex partial seizures, myoclonic seizures, or absence seizures, there should be no problems with a natural vaginal delivery. Similarly, well-controlled or infrequent tonic-clonic seizures present no reason not to try a natural vaginal delivery. However, for women who have uncontrolled tonic-clonic seizures during pregnancy or those with tonic-clonic seizures during labor and delivery (approximately 1%–2% of women with epilepsy), cesarean section may be indicated.

The increased frequency of seizures during labor and delivery and the first 2 days after delivery (an additional 1%–2% of women may have tonic-clonic seizures during this period) may be due to the failure or inability to take antiepileptic medication, sleep deprivation, hyperventilation, stress, and physical pain. It may not be possible to eliminate these factors completely, but some can be partially prevented. Women should prepare for labor with a reminder to take medications as scheduled, and they should tell the doctor if unable to do so because of nausea or pain. Fortunately, despite many of these problems, the large majority of women do not have tonic-clonic seizures around the time of delivery.

Spinal anesthesia is safe for women with epilepsy. If general anesthesia is required, it also can be given safely. The anesthesiologist should be informed about the woman's history of epilepsy and the antiepileptic drugs she is taking (as well as about other medical disorders and medications).

CHAPTER 25

Parenting by People with Epilepsy

Few if any joys equal those of parenthood, and epilepsy should not be viewed as a restriction on becoming a parent. Although laws against marriage and parenthood existed during this century in many states, all these prohibitions have been repealed. There are no legal barriers between epilepsy and parenthood, except for those associated with custody suits. Chapter 29 addresses legal rights related to child adoption by persons with epilepsy.

Parenthood, however, is not for every person or couple. Becoming a parent is a major commitment of time and resources. The responsibility of caring for a child is difficult to understand before the child is born. A baby is completely dependent on its parents or caregivers for food, clothing, diaper changing, and protection. Caring for a child can be as frustrating as it is joyful.

CARING FOR INFANTS AND CHILDREN

Caring for a baby or child means loss of freedom and personal time, as well as a new sense of responsibility. The maternal and paternal instincts are strong. After having made it through the potential hazards of a pregnancy with epilepsy, the parents may sigh with relief, feeling that the dangers of epilepsy have passed. Persons with well-controlled epilepsy have no restrictions on child care, but women or men with episodes of impaired consciousness or control of movement must take special precautions when caring for a baby or a young child. The precautions will depend on the child's age, its nature, and other circumstances.

If at all possible, a parent with uncontrolled seizures should not bathe the baby alone. The baby should be placed in a safely designed baby bath and transferred to and from the bath relatively close to the floor, and the drain should be open if the baby bath is placed inside a larger tub. The bathroom should be carpeted if possible. The parent should always heed an aura, or warning, of a seizure while bathing the baby.

A parent with uncontrolled seizures should be extremely careful when carrying the baby. That is not to say that persons with epilepsy should not carry a baby, but care must be exercised in many cases. Some persons get enough warning of a seizure that they have time to place the baby in a safe place. Others have no warning of an impending seizure, and must be especially careful when caring for a baby. Breast feeding and diaper changing by women who are at risk of having a seizure are best done on the floor or on a low and soft surface where the baby would be safe from falling.

The baby or young child of a parent who has epilepsy is better off sleeping in its own crib or bed. There is a chance the child could be injured if the parent had a seizure, especially a tonic-clonic seizure, while sleeping.

As the baby becomes a toddler, other potential dangers confront a parent whose seizures are not fully controlled. For example, walking on a busy street with an impulsive, active 2-year-old could be potentially dangerous if the parent had a complex partial seizure. During the minute or two of the parent's impaired consciousness, the child's ball could bounce into the street, and the child might run after it. Although instances such as this are rare, it is worthwhile considering ways of reducing the risk. In this case, the child might be given another toy that is less likely to bounce into the street, or the child's hand and the parent's hand might be linked by a colorful plastic coil that will keep them close together.

If a parent's seizures are not fully controlled, the disorder should be discussed with older children. Children understand more than adults give them credit for, and they may be aware of the seizures and frightened by them. Explaining to the children what a seizure is, why the parent takes medication, and why they should not worry is comforting to children. As the children get older, they should be told more about epilepsy and what to do if first aid is needed.

Missed medications, sleep deprivation, and stress can aggravate seizures. For new parents, sleep deprivation and stress are unavoidable, but not unmanageable, and dramatic changes in the daily schedule can easily lead to missed medications. It is important to recognize these potential problems and plan to reduce their impact. A mother with epilepsy who chooses to breast feed might want to use a formula supplement so that her husband or another person can feed the baby once during the night. Caring for a baby is stressful and exhausting, and enlisting family or other help is a good idea.

BREAST FEEDING

Breast feeding is recommended for most women with epilepsy, because breast milk confers a variety of benefits to the baby, including protection against infection. However, the benefits of breast feeding must be weighed against the risks when the mother takes antiepileptic drugs.

The percentage of the mother's blood drug level found in breast milk ranges from a low of 10% for valproate to a high of 90% for ethosuximide. Other drugs have intermediate percentages: phenytoin 30%, carbamazepine 50%, phenobarbital 60%, and primidone 75%.

Phenobarbital and primidone, both barbiturates, cause the most problems with breast feeding. Although the percentage of these drugs excreted in the breast milk is only slightly higher than that of other drugs, the baby's digestive system is particularly good at absorbing these drugs, and they linger for an unusually long time in the baby's blood. A single dose of phenobarbital may last more than 15 days. Because of the high amount of ethosuximide found in breast milk, it can also cause problems. The antiepileptic drugs in babies who are breast fed cause fussy feeding habits, sedation, and irritability. Some irritability and gas pains are normal, however, and should not be interpreted as medication effects. The mother can contact the pediatrician if she has any doubts.

When a woman breast feeds and takes two antiepileptic drugs, or takes barbiturates or ethosuximide, the baby should be watched closely for signs of adverse reactions to the drugs. The baby of a woman who breast feeds and then stops taking a barbiturate should be observed for signs of drug withdrawal.

CHAPTER 26

Employment and Military Service for People with Epilepsy

People with epilepsy face severe discrimination in the job market. Employers have discriminated against them because of the stigma associated with epilepsy, misconceptions about the medical and social aspects of epilepsy, unfounded fears of legal and medical liabilities, and the misconception that people with epilepsy are not as productive as other people. These biases have led to discrimination and considerable hardship for those who have epilepsy, but new laws have begun to change the American landscape of employment opportunities for people with epilepsy and other disabilities.

PROTECTION AGAINST JOB DISCRIMINATION

Public Law 101-336, the Americans with Disabilities Act (ADA), makes discrimination based on disability illegal in employment, activities of state and local governments, public and private transportation, public accommodations, and telecommunications. In the 1980 census, 20% of Americans were found to be disabled. Epilepsy, because it is a disorder of the nervous system that can substantially limit major life activities, is considered a disability. Title I of the ADA provides that people with disabilities cannot be excluded from employment unless they are unable to perform the essential requirements of the job. An employer may *not* discriminate in:

- Recruitment, advertising, and job application procedures
- Hiring, upgrading, promotion, demotion, tenure, transfer, layoff, termination, return from layoff, and rehiring
- Rates of pay or other compensation and changes in compensation
- Job assignment, job classification, position descriptions, lines of progression, structures, and seniority lists

- Leaves of absence, sick leave, or other leave
- Fringe benefits, whether or not administered by the covered entity
- Selection and financial support for training, including apprenticeships, professional meetings, conferences and other related activities, and selection for leaves of absence to pursue training
- Activities sponsored by a covered entity, including social and recreational programs
- Any other term, condition, or privilege of employment

The ADA applies to all employers, employment agencies, labor organizations, and joint labor-management committees in which at least 15 (after July 26, 1994) employees work for each working day in each of 20 or more calendar weeks. The ADA excludes the federal government or entities that receive a certain level of federal support (because of similar protections offered by Sections 501 and 504 of the Vocational Rehabilitation Act), Indian tribes, or private-membership clubs that are exempt from taxation.

In the following sections, the use of the term "employers" refers only to employers covered by the ADA. However, state and local laws against employment discrimination can actually provide protection equal to or better than the ADA and cover a wider range of employers.

Criteria for Employment

Persons with epilepsy or other disabilities must be both qualified and able to perform the *essential* job functions. The ADA does not require employers to alter the fundamental duties of jobs to meet the needs of individuals with disabilities. The Equal Employment Opportunity Commission (EEOC) holds that removing an essential function would fundamentally alter the position. The word "essential" is often critical in determining whether or not there is discrimination. For example, if a job description for a department store stock person requires that the person work in high places, but no one in this position has actually had to work in high places during the past several years, this function is not essential.

Driving privileges are often restricted for people with epilepsy. Because driving is essential for jobs such as a pizza delivery service, traveling salesperson, or a bus or taxi driver, driving privileges are essential for these jobs. Some positions may require an applicant to have a driver's license, but further examination of the position may show that driving is not an essential part of the job. Some jobs have driving requirements that are marginal and can be accommodated through job sharing.

Stereotypes, Myths, and Segregation

Employers are not allowed to discriminate against people with disabilities because they have fears about the stereotypes and myths that surround certain disorders. Epilepsy, which historically has carried a stigma, has often produced discrimination against job applicants. Discrimination includes limiting, segregating, or classifying an applicant or employee in a negative way based on his or her disability. Determining what constitutes discrimination requires an individual approach. Each case must be viewed separately. This is especially important for people with epilepsy, because the type and frequency of seizures vary from person to person.

Employment decisions must be based on facts, not on presumptions and rumors about people with a certain disability. For example, a department store could not categorically deny the position of salesclerk to a person with epilepsy because "we are afraid that seizures will frighten off the customers." Employees must not be segregated on the basis of their disability. For example, it would be illegal for a company to sponsor the annual office party on a boat and not invite an employee who has epilepsy because it fears the liability if the person were to have a seizure on the boat and be hurt. Similarly, it would be illegal for a company to deny facilities such as an employees' exercise room to an employee with epilepsy. However, it may be reasonable for the company to obtain medical clearance from the employee's doctor.

Contractual Arrangements

It is illegal for employers to use an employment agency and ask the agency to screen out applicants with epilepsy or other disabilities. It is also illegal for an employer to have a contractual arrangement with another entity that discriminates against a person with epilepsy. For example, if a company provides that all of its employees can use a health club, but the health club excludes people with epilepsy, the employer is violating the ADA's provision requiring equal benefits and privileges to all employees. Furthermore, the health club is unfairly discriminating against people with epilepsy under the ADA's public accommodations provisions.

Reasonable Accommodations

The ADA requires that covered employers make reasonable accommodations for people with disabilities. Therefore, it is illegal for an employer to hire an individual who does not have a disability over a disabled individual who is equally qualified for the same job simply because the employer will have to make a reasonable accommodation for the disabled person.

Reasonable accommodation is defined as "any change in the work environment or in the way things are customarily done that enables an individual with a disability to enjoy equal employment opportunities." There are three categories of reasonable accommodations; these provide accommodations for (1) equal opportunity in the application process, (2) performing essential functions of the position held or desired, and (3) enjoying equal benefits and privileges of employment as are enjoyed by employees without disabilities.

A broad range of reasonable accommodations could apply to people with epilepsy. The following are some examples:

- Providing extended time to take an entrance examination
- Job restructuring; that is, redistributing *nonessential* or marginal job functions, such as driving, to other employees
- Temporary changes in job responsibilities or time required to perform certain tasks while someone is adjusting to new medications or to changes in an existing regimen
- Replacing a flickering light or loud banging noise if it could provoke a seizure
- Installing a safety shield around a piece of equipment
- Installing carpet on a concrete floor
- Asking a supervisor for written, as opposed to oral, instructions for someone with memory loss caused by antiepileptic medications
- Allowing an employee who experiences fatigue as an adverse effect of medications to take more frequent breaks
- Allowing an employee to take an extended break after a seizure

Determining what accommodation is reasonable can be difficult. The applicant or employee should notify the employer of his or her need for accommodation. The employer may require that the need for the accommodation be documented by a letter from the doctor. The EEOC recommends that, in making the determination of what accommodation is reasonable, the employer and qualified person with a disability undertake a "flexible, interactive process." Because epilepsy affects each person differently, the input of both the employer and the employee is essential to provide the most helpful and efficient accommodations. When there are questions about what types of accommodations are best, employers may obtain useful information from the EEOC, an Epilepsy Foundation of America (EFA) affiliate job placement program, their state vocational rehabilitation agency, or the Job Accommodation Network (800-526-7234 Voice/TDD; for calls within West Virginia, 800-526-4698).

Health Insurance, Life Insurance, and Disability Benefits

The ADA requires that employers offer equal benefits to employees with disabilities. The ADA does not require an employer to offer health or other forms of insurance. However, if the employer does offer benefits to its other employees, it may not exclude people with disabilities. Employers may not refuse to hire people with disabilities because of a feared or actual increase in insurance costs. Similarly, employers cannot refuse to hire the parent of a child with a disability because of perceived or actual increases in insurance benefits for employee dependents.

The ADA does not affect the preexisting condition clauses included in many insurance policies. Therefore, employers may continue to subscribe to health insurance plans that do not cover preexisting conditions. This exclusion may be permanent (that is, they never cover preexisting conditions) or temporary (for example, preexisting conditions are only covered after 1 year of employment).

Bringing a Claim of Discrimination

The ADA requires that for a claim of discrimination to be valid, the individual with a disability must establish that (1) the disability is covered under the act, (2) the employer in question is a covered entity required to comply with the law, (3) the individual is qualified for the essential functions of the job in question, and (4) the employer violated one or more of the prohibitions of the act.

The employer has the burden of proof to show a valid defense to the employee's claim of discrimination. Several defenses can be used by the employer, including direct threat and undue hardship. The direct threat provision states that there is "a significant risk of substantial harm to the health or safety of the individual or others that cannot be eliminated or reduced by reasonable accommodation." It must be demonstrated that the applicant or employee with a disability presents a significant risk, not merely a slightly increased risk. The undue hardship provision is a limitation on the employer's obligation to provide a reasonable accommodation to an applicant or employee with a disability. The employer must prove that the accommodation would be "unduly costly, extensive, substantial or disruptive, or would fundamentally alter the nature or operation of the business."

THE APPLICATION PROCESS

The ADA makes it illegal for an employer to use any job application that requires individuals to disclose their disability. Applications cannot list medical, neurological, or psychiatric disorders such as diabetes, epilepsy, or depression, and ask people to check off those that apply to them. Further, a question such as, "Do you have a health condition that would affect your ability to do the job?" is also prohibited by the ADA because it is overly broad. Similarly, application forms cannot ask if someone has previously filed a workers' compensation claim. However, an application can ask questions about the applicant's ability to perform essential job duties and request that the applicant list any type of reasonable accommodation that may be necessary during the application process. For example, someone may need more time to complete a written examination.

If the disorder is under control, an applicant may elect not to disclose the epilepsy. When seizures impair consciousness or control of movement, however, they present potential dangers if the person drives, works on ladders or high places, works as an electrician, works as a plumber with very hot water, or works in a position where he or she is responsible for the safety of others, as in, for example, a job as a ski lift operator or lifeguard. That is not to say that someone with epilepsy cannot work in these jobs. Rather, special consideration must be given to the person's specific seizure condition and the essential duties of the specific job for which he or she is applying. The doctor is often asked to write a letter regarding the safety of the person with epilepsy in a specific situation. Unfortunately, no one can guarantee safety for anyone. Depending on the specific case and job, the doctor's letter can state that the person is able to work at the job and that the epilepsy does not represent a significant risk for injury.

Some employers still discriminate against people with epilepsy, even though it is illegal under the ADA. Therefore, before applying for a job, it may be helpful for a person with epilepsy to speak with a local affiliate of the EFA regarding discrimination laws and restrictions on employers asking questions about a prospective employee's health, or with the protection and advocacy staff of the state human rights commission, the EEOC, or a social worker who specializes in employment issues.

The Job Interview

As on the application form, the ADA prohibits employers from asking any interview question that would require individuals to reveal their disability. The employer may ask about the applicant's ability to perform both essential and marginal job-related functions, but these questions cannot be phrased in terms of disability. For example, a flower shop owner who needs a delivery person can ask whether the applicant has a driver's license, which is essential for the job. If the response is no, the employer cannot ask if the applicant has epilepsy or a visual impairment. Although the employer can ask about the applicant's ability to perform marginal or nonessential job functions, the employer cannot refuse to hire someone with a disability because he or she is unable to perform these functions.

During the interview, the employer may ask if an accommodation is needed during the application process. If the applicant informs the employer that he or she has epilepsy and that the medications affect the ability to respond quickly to written questions, then the employer may ask how much extra time is needed during an examination. However, the employer cannot probe and ask, "How long have you had epilepsy?" "How many medications do you take?" "What caused your epilepsy?" or other such questions.

If a disability is known or disclosed during the course of the interview, then the employer is limited in questions that can be asked about how the applicant's disability would interfere with performance of essential job functions. However, the employer may ask how the applicant would perform an essential function, with or without a reasonable accommodation.

If it becomes necessary to discuss one's epilepsy during the interview, the applicant should be honest and direct and should not argue or become defensive. If questioned as to how the epilepsy might have an impact on the job, the applicant should pause to collect his or her thoughts and answer the question in a calm but assured manner. Applicants should be familiar with the ADA, as such questions before a job offer may be illegal, and they may not have to respond. The individual should know his or her type of seizures, how often they occur, if there are certain times when seizures are especially likely to occur, if there is a consistent warning (aura) that allows him or her to go to a safe place, the types of supportive measures that may be needed, and how long it takes to recover after a seizure. It might be helpful to mention one's own "seizure safety" history; that is, during past jobs or schooling, did seizures ever cause physical injury or require special treatment? It is worth emphasizing that epilepsy is a common disorder (approximately 1%–3% of the population will have epilepsy and 5%–10% a single seizure), that people with epilepsy continue to be effective in all segments of society and workplaces (ranging from the Congress of the United States to professional sports), that epilepsy does not affect the intellect or everyday behavior of most people who have it, and that injuries at work related to epilepsy are rare. Indeed, most persons with epilepsy have no increased risk of work-related injuries.

Medical Examinations

Before offering a job, employers are not allowed to conduct any type of medical examination unless the position has established criteria that require medical examination. Examples of these positions include airplane pilots and cabin attendants, air traffic controllers, train conductors, and certain construction positions.

After a conditional offer of employment has been given (that is, once it has been determined that the applicant is qualified for the job), the ADA allows employers to require medical examinations of its employees with disabilities *if* there is a need to determine whether the employee can perform essential job functions. Employers may require medical examinations of job applicants with epilepsy if such examinations are required of *all* applicants. If a disability such as epilepsy is disclosed during the medical interviews and examination, then the employer cannot use the disability to refuse to hire the applicant if essential job functions can be performed, with or without reasonable accommodation.

The ADA requires that all information obtained during a medical examination remain confidential and only be disclosed to supervisors and managers, if necessary, regarding necessary restrictions on the work or duties of the employee and necessary accommodations, as well as to first aid and safety personnel, and to government officials investigating compliance with the ADA.

Testing for Illegal Drugs

Employers are allowed to test for use of illegal drugs during any stage of the application process or during employment. The ADA does not consider drug testing a medical examination. However, the employer cannot use the results of a drug test to discriminate against a person with a disability. The EEOC's regulation emphasizes that if the results of a drug test "reveal information about an individual's medical condition beyond whether the individual is currently engaging in the illegal use of drugs, the additional information is to be treated as a confidential medical record."

Tests for illegal drugs may be required before a conditional offer is made, but the employer cannot use information regarding drugs taken for medical conditions, such as epilepsy, to refuse to hire an individual. Positive drug tests should be repeated, as laboratory errors do occur. In addition, the applicant should be aware that antiepileptic drugs can show up in standard drug testing, depending on the specific test.

EXPLAINING SEIZURES TO COWORKERS

A person with epilepsy whose seizures are not well controlled should prepare for the possibility of a seizure occurring at work. The preparation will vary depending on the type and frequency of seizures. The first, and most important, step is to discuss the seizures with the supervisor and coworkers. They will be the first ones to see the seizure and to administer first aid. Although there may be one person with whom the new employee is particularly close at work, he or she should never rely on one person, especially if the seizures are frequent or intense. That person may be on vacation or out of the office when the seizure occurs. Depending on the work environment, the people, the employee's relationship with various people, and the nature of the epilepsy, a person with epilepsy may choose to tell only a few people or all of his or her coworkers. People can be told individually or in a group. It is often a good idea to review first aid measures in a group setting.

The coworkers need to know what happens during a seizure. It is normal for them to be frightened when first watching a seizure. They must be reassured that the risk of serious injury is small, and that the seizure does not cause pain. The employees should know the type of seizures their coworker has and what they should and should not do if one occurs. They should know not to stick something in the person's mouth, because the belief about swallowing the tongue is a myth. They should know when to call for medical personnel or an ambulance, but it should be emphasized that this is rarely necessary for a person with epilepsy who has a single seizure. The local EFA affiliate may be able to provide in-service education for the coworkers. First aid cards, a videotape, and other educational materials are available from the EFA.

Complex partial seizures may cause some work-related problems. Although the pattern of activity (for example, staring, rubbing the hands, or mumbling a phrase) stays fairly constant from one seizure to the next, marked changes in behavior can occur during a seizure. The coworkers need to know that complex partial seizures usually last 1 to 2 minutes and that automatic acts are common. These automatisms can be misinterpreted. For example, someone having a complex partial seizure might crumple a sheet of paper or bang on a desk without being aware of it.

The period after the seizure should be discussed. Many well-intentioned people try to restrain a person who has had a seizure. Restraint, even gentle restraint such as holding a hand, can occasionally provoke agitation. Coworkers should know that a person may be confused after a seizure but should be left alone if he or she is in a safe place and seems to be all right. They should not hold or restrain the person unless it is absolutely necessary for safety.

It is always helpful for the person with epilepsy to have a clear description of what happens during a seizure. A coworker may be willing to write a brief description of the event. There may also be some question as to whether consciousness is impaired during a seizure. A coworker might also be asked to test the person's responsiveness ("show me your left thumb") and memory (remember a word) during the seizure.

When the person has fully recovered from the seizure and returned to work, he or she should acknowledge what happened, thank the people who were helpful, and ask if they have any questions.

VOCATIONAL REHABILITATION

People with epilepsy may have problems with employment as the result of recurrent seizures and their aftereffects, adverse effects of antiepileptic drugs, associated neurological or medical disorders, and the negative feeling that some people still have about epilepsy. Vocational rehabilitation provides specialized training for people with disabilities to develop skills that will enhance their chances for employment.

The Rehabilitation Act of 1973, a landmark law, provides employment rights for people with disabilities. This act changed the face of federal and state vocational rehabilitation programs, making services to people with disabilities a national priority.

An extensive number of vocational rehabilitation services are available. These services include, but are not limited to, diagnosis and evaluation for determining eligibility and appropriate vocational training; counseling and psychological therapy; physical therapy; occupational training; books, instructional tape recordings, and other goods; transportation; and job-placement services, including supported employment, independent-living services, personal assistance, and transition services.

Eligibility for Vocational Rehabilitation

Vocational rehabilitation programs are administered at the state level, although the federal Rehabilitation Act authorizes federal funds to the states for these programs. To be eligible, one must meet two criteria: (1) there must be a substantial impediment to employment and (2) the person can benefit in terms of an employment outcome. The first criterion requires that there be a mental or physical disability that impairs occupational performance. A "substantial handicap" is not precisely defined and must be determined on an individual basis. However, the law mandates that those with severe disabilities be given the highest priority for services. There is now a presumption that an individual can benefit from services despite the severity of the disorder.

If vocational rehabilitation is denied, or if the range of services provided is believed to be inadequate, there is an appeal process. The initial appeal is conducted by a state agency's supervisory staff, and is known as the informal or administrative appeal. If the decision is not favorable, one can request a hearing with an impartial hearing officer. Finally, if this decision is not favorable, a final appeal can be made to the director of the state vocational rehabilitation agency. The Client Assistance Program is present in every state and is available to inform and assist all clients and applicants regarding their benefits and protections under the law.

Individualized Written Rehabilitation Plan

The person with a disability and the vocational rehabilitation counselor must jointly develop an individualized written rehabilitation plan. If appropriate, the disabled person may be joined by a parent, guardian, or someone else who can assist in developing the plan. The plan must identify the goals, services, and goods that are needed to obtain and continue with employment and must include a statement that the client has been told that he or she can challenge any agency decision.

The Vocational Rehabilitation Dilemma

People with epilepsy may fall through the cracks in the current system. They may unfairly be in a "Catch 22" situation, in which the alternatives actually cancel each other out, leaving no means of escape from a dilemma. If seizure control is the only factor used to establish the relative severity of a person's disability, the counselor has an incomplete view of why it presents a barrier to employment. As a result, people may be deemed ineligible for vocational rehabilitation services because their disability is not considered to be severe. Other difficulties—like memory loss and adverse effects of medication—should be included so that the picture is clearer. If seizures persist despite treatment, the reviewer may consider the person with epilepsy to be unemployable, although recent changes in the law may make this less possible. To ensure that people with epilepsy are given fair consideration, it is critical that all the details of the individual case be clearly presented.

Although the seizures may be fully or partially controlled, the stigma associated with epilepsy and the effects of medications can be significant barriers to employment. Nevertheless, many people with seizures can be successfully employed in a wide range of positions, and it is important that the vocational rehabilitation counselor understand the full context of the person's condition in order to establish the severity of the disability and the potential for benefits through the vocational rehabilitation system.

The EFA sponsors the Training Applicants for Placement Success (TAPS) national program (see Chapter 31). This program has effectively helped to train and employ more than 12,000 people with epilepsy. TAPS offers a variety of vocational rehabilitation services, including the establishment of employment goals, counseling about possible jobs based on preferences and skills, help to improve interviewing and other skills needed to get a job, identification of available positions, peer support during the job search, and help with problems that may arise once the person is working. Because epilepsy remains poorly understood by most employers, TAPS staff provide educational training to employers and fellow employees about epilepsy. They also communicate with other community service providers to coordinate a variety of services to support people as they move to independence through employment. Information can go a long way in dispelling false beliefs.

WORKERS' COMPENSATION

Every state has laws that guarantee compensation for job-related injuries. These laws protect both employees and employers. For employees, an injury that results from performing their job, whether or not their negligence contributes, will be covered and compensated. Employers, therefore, must either be self-insured or insured through the state workers' compensation program. For employers, these laws serve to limit liability and costs. Employees are legally prohibited from receiving anything more than workers' compensation. The rates set by workers' compensation for medical care are often low, and many doctors and surgeons do not accept the reimbursements paid by workers' compensation.

Work-related injuries are only covered if the injury occurred during work (not while getting ready to go to work or traveling from home to work) and was clearly a result of the employment. Therefore, if someone with epilepsy falls at work and is injured, the accident could be viewed as independent of the employment, and dependent only on the person's medical disorder. In the past, claims for falls due to seizures were denied. However, there has been a trend toward liberalization of workers' compensation coverage to include falls, even if the conditions at work had little or nothing to do with the fall.

Work-related factors could cause or contribute to seizure-related injuries. For example, excessive overtime and stress can lead to sleep deprivation or exhaustion, which can make seizures more likely to occur. In such a case, the seizures could be viewed as "arising from the employment."

Some states and territories allow employers to demand that an employee waive his or her right to workers' compensation. In 1994, these are Massachusetts, Maryland, Iowa, Virginia, Tennessee, and the Virgin Islands. Other states permit employees to waive benefits "voluntarily." Laws demanding employees to waive their compensation rights should be abolished.

These laws discriminate against people with disabilities by incorrectly assuming that their disability would be the cause of any injuries at work.

Premium Rates for People with Epilepsy

People with epilepsy do not have higher rates of accidents or absenteeism. Further, overall work performance does not differ between people with epilepsy and other employees. Employers often fear that if they hire a person with epilepsy, their premiums for workers' compensation will go up. There is little evidence to support this fear. Premiums for workers' compensation do not increase because of a new employee's medical history and are rarely affected by a seizure-related work injury. For the majority of employers, especially large companies, workers' compensation premiums are based on the class of employees in a specific industry, not on the work or medical histories of individual employees.

Second-Injury Funds

Second-injury funds guarantee employers that hiring a person with a disability will not increase their workers' compensation premiums. Second-injury funds cover the difference in costs between the workers' compensation insurance and the total costs of the injury. For example, if a person with epilepsy falls and is injured at work, and the injury is found to result from a preexisting condition and not from the conditions of employment, the second-injury fund would compensate the employee for the fall. These funds have been adopted in many states and encourage employers to hire people with disabilities. Applications, criteria for coverage, and types and amounts of coverage vary from state to state.

Second-injury funds in most states provide coverage for employees with a "permanent preexisting impairment" that could interfere with obtaining employment. Epilepsy may or may not be included in this category, depending on the state. In many states, for the second-injury fund to provide coverage, the employer must be informed of the epilepsy at the time of hiring, or proof must be provided that the employee was retained after the employer learned of his or her epilepsy.

MILITARY SERVICE

The United States armed services (military services, Coast Guard, and State National Guard) requires that its members be available for duty 24 hours a day and have no condition that could impair their performance under adverse conditions. Because sleep deprivation and lack of medication are considered adverse conditions and can cause seizures in people with epilepsy, there are relatively strict regulations regarding the enlistment of people with epilepsy.

Prior to 1982, the armed services excluded any person with a history of seizures after age 5 years. The current regulation requires that the individual be seizure-free without medications for at least 5 years. Cases are reviewed on an individual basis, and an appeal can be made for persons who are seizure-free for less than 5 years, depending on the medical history, prognosis, and the specific position for which the person is applying. For example, an appeal could be made for a young woman with benign rolandic epilepsy who applies to the military at age 18. Her last seizure was a nocturnal simple partial motor seizure at age 14 years, and she had stopped all antiepileptic drugs at age 13 years. She has had normal electroencephalograms (EEGs) during the past 3 years. Her prognosis for remaining seizure-free is excellent, and she should be able to serve successfully in a variety of positions.

Persons with paroxysmal disorders of any kind are excluded from flight training. The only exception is for individuals who had febrile seizures before age 5 years and who have a normal EEG.

When seizures or epilepsy develops in a member of the armed services, he or she may be discharged because of the disorder. The military retains a limited number of people with disabilities who cannot actively serve in various parts of the world or under adverse conditions. However, the number of such positions is restricted, and members of the armed services have no legal or constitutional right to be retained in the service. Furthermore, the armed services have no obligation to accommodate an individual's disability by changing the work environment or position.

Because behavior during and after some seizures may be mistaken for intentional actions, persons with epilepsy in the armed services may, on occasion, be less than honorably discharged. The military has review boards to which the discharge status may be appealed. It is the applicant's burden to prove that the discharge was unfair or improper.

ACKNOWLEDGMENT

This chapter is based largely on *The Legal Rights of Persons with Epilepsy* (see Appendix 4).

CHAPTER 27

Mental Health of Adults with Epilepsy

People with epilepsy are often subject to depression, anxiety, irritability, and even psychosis. The psychological and psychiatric disturbances may be unrelated to epilepsy or may be related to their emotional reactions to the disorder, the effect of the medications, the cause of the disorder, or the disorder itself. Although people with epilepsy are often said to display more aggressive behavior than other people, there is little evidence to support such a claim, except in unusual cases such as when people are restrained after a seizure. Experiencing unusual and bizarre episodes is a problem for some people with epilepsy, but the spells are often simple partial seizures preceding other seizures.

DEPRESSION

Depression is a common experience of both people in the general population and people with epilepsy, but it occurs more often in those who have epilepsy. All people feel sad at some time in their life, and the depth of sadness varies. The borderline between sadness and depression is imprecise, but, at some point, when sadness is prolonged and impairs a person's ability to enjoy life and to work, there is a problem.

Depression causes feelings of sadness, helplessness, hopelessness, and guilt and an inability to experience happiness. Other problems include difficulty with sleeping (insomnia or sleeping excessively), decreased libido (sexual desire), and appetite disturbances (loss of appetite or overeating).

In persons with epilepsy, depression can result from a psychological reaction to having the disorder or being treated differently because of it; from medication effects; from the cause of the epilepsy, such as head trauma or stroke; or from the epilepsy itself. Controversy persists regarding the relative contribution of the different factors. In some cases, the depression is related to loss of a job or a loved one or to a flurry of seizures. The depression related to the psychological effects of living with epilepsy and other problems of life can be effectively treated in most cases by therapy and counseling. Discussion of troublesome feelings with a therapist—a psychiatrist, psychologist, or counselor—can be extremely helpful.

Antiepileptic drugs, especially barbiturates, can cause depression. The depression associated with the barbiturates (phenobarbital and primidone) is often dose-related; that is, the higher the dose, the greater the risk of depression. Taking one or more other antiepileptic drugs in combination with a barbiturate can also increase the risk of depression. It is rare that only a barbiturate can control epilepsy. Therefore, if a person is feeling depressed and taking a barbiturate, he or she should explore a medication change with the doctor.

Injury to the brain, whether from a stroke, oxygen deprivation, head trauma, or infection, can cause depression. Because the brain controls our emotions and moods, it is not surprising that disruption of normal brain functions can cause depression. Studies suggest that people with injury to the left side of their brain, especially in the front portions (frontal and temporal lobes), are more prone to depression. Depression can also occur with injuries to other parts of the brain, but the majority of people with brain injuries do not become depressed.

The role that epilepsy itself plays in directly causing depression remains controversial. As more information accumulates, however, it appears that epilepsy does contribute to the problem in some cases. Often, several factors contribute to the depression. When possible, the cause should be treated. Serious depression requires antidepressant medication. Some psychiatrists and neurologists fear that antidepressants can aggravate the seizure disorder. Although some evidence supports this fear, the majority of people with epilepsy who are treated with antidepressant medications do not experience an increase in their seizure frequency.

The most serious complication of depression is suicide. Just as the rate of depression is increased in people with epilepsy, there is also an increased rate of suicide in people with epilepsy compared with people in the general population. Patients, family members, and doctors often fail to recognize the presence or severity of depression. If there is any question, seek help. Anyone who expresses thoughts about hurting himself or herself should be taken extremely seriously. Finally, if someone who is depressed discusses a specific plan to hurt himself or herself or gives away treasured items, psychiatric consultation should be obtained as soon as possible. Depression can be treated with counseling and medications and in very severe cases, with electroconvulsive shock therapy.

ANXIETY

Anxiety disorders are quite common in the general population and appear to be even more common among people with epilepsy. We all experience feelings of anxiety and nervousness. It becomes a disorder when these feelings are frequent or intense, occur spontaneously or follow a trivial provocation, and interfere with our functioning. As with depression, several factors, including psychological stress related to the epilepsy, medication effects, associated neurological or psychiatric disorders, and the epilepsy itself, can contribute to the cause of anxiety disorders. Anxiety disorders can be effectively treated with counseling, therapy, and medications.

IRRITABILITY

We all get irritable. People in the general population vary considerably with regard to how often they get irritable and what triggers it. People with epilepsy are also subject to irritability. Only a few studies have compared irritability in people with and without epilepsy. Some of them suggest that people with epilepsy may be more prone toward irritability. Irritability in people with epilepsy usually has the same causes as in people without epilepsy but may also be related to medications, especially the barbiturates (phenobarbital and primidone), to brain abnormalities in areas that regulate emotions, and possibly to the epilepsy itself.

In some people, a change in medications or improved control of the seizures is associated with a reduction in anxiety and irritability. For the few people with epilepsy in whom irritability is a serious problem, it would be worthwhile consulting with the doctor. A new medication, a change in dosage of an existing regimen, treatment of an underlying depression or sleep disorder, or some form of counseling or therapy may be beneficial.

PSYCHOSIS

Psychosis is a serious mental disorder characterized by disturbances in the content and form of thought (disorganized, incoherent, delusions), perception (hallucinations and distortions of sensation), emotional functions (lack of emotions or inappropriate emotions), sense of self, volition (decreased drive and motivation), interpersonal behavior (social withdrawal and detachment), and physical activity (hyperactive, immobile). Psychosis can occur as a pure psychiatric disorder, as in schizophrenia, or can result from brain injuries such as viral encephalitis or from certain medications such as amphetamines (stimulants).

There appears to be a slightly increased rate of interictal psychosis ("in between" seizures—not occurring only around the time of seizures) among people with epilepsy. This issue remains controversial, however. Overall, the chances that someone with epilepsy will develop an interictal psychosis are very small.

The best-documented form of psychosis in epilepsy occurs after seizures, usually after a cluster of complex partial or tonic-clonic seizures. In this setting, the person often appears well for a few hours or days and then expresses disordered thoughts and delusional ideas (for example, paranoid thoughts that someone is going to hurt him or her). Such psychoses are usually relatively brief and can be effectively treated with medications (antipsychotic and tranquilizing drugs). Prompt recognition and treatment of this disorder are most important. Because antipsychotic drugs can occasionally cause seizures, if the drugs are needed by someone with epilepsy, they should be used at the lowest effective dosage.

AGGRESSION

The false association between epilepsy and aggressive behavior is one of the most damaging stigmas cast on people with epilepsy. As a group, there is no clear evidence that people with epilepsy are more likely than other people to commit violent crimes or to be involved in other types of criminal activity. Unfortunately, however, the stigma still lingers in social and medical communities.

There is some evidence that in a few children and adults with epilepsy, aggressive behaviors can occur and may be related to antiepileptic drugs, underlying brain abnormalities, or the confused (postictal) state after certain seizures. Children are less able to control their impulses than adults and translate thoughts into actions more readily. The brain continues to develop and mature over the course of childhood and, therefore, control over social behavior and aggressive impulses is acquired relatively late in childhood. Some children with epilepsy, and with other neurological disorders such as mental retardation, are reported to have higher rates of aggressive behaviors than other children. In part, this results from injury to brain areas that are important in developing social skills and learning to control impulses. Similar aggressive behaviors may develop in adults who have brain injuries after motor vehicle accidents, even if they never have a seizure.

Certain medications can make aggressive behavior more likely to occur, especially in persons with a preexisting injury in areas that regulate aggressive behavior. The barbiturates (phenobarbital and primidone) are most likely to cause aggressive behaviors. In susceptible individuals, however, other antiepileptic drugs and some stimulants, such as methylphenidate or dextroamphetamine, can trigger aggressive behaviors. Elderly persons can be paradoxically agitated with barbiturate therapy.

During a complex partial seizure, directed aggressive behavior is exceedingly rare. After a tonic-clonic seizure, during the period of confusion, aggressive behavior can occur, usually because someone tries to restrain the person. If such a reaction is provoked, the best response is to remove the restraint.

UNUSUAL SEIZURES

Some persons with epilepsy, especially those with partial seizures, may experience unusual and bizarre phenomena during seizures. The experiences can be fascinating, frightening, or both. Very often, people are reluctant to discuss strange symptoms or experiences for fear of being considered bizarre or crazy. However, symptoms that begin suddenly and last for a brief time can be a seizure, no matter how strange they seem.

The following are descriptions of unusual seizures. These descriptions were often provided only after specific questions were asked:

- I had a feeling of extreme embarrassment, as though I had made a very foolish remark.

- I feel that someone else is in the room behind me, that I am not alone.

- Looking into the mirror, I noticed that the right side of my face was missing.

- On the left half of space there were colored balls of light. As I looked at them, they changed to multiple figures of small men. On later occasions, I recognized these as myself—tiny replicas that would approach and then recede.

- I have a flood of thoughts; I don't know where they come from; I can't shut them off.

- Scenes appear in my mind's eye. I have never lived them, they must be imaginary, not real memories, but they appear real. During this time I sort of know what is going on around me, but I am also a bit tuned out.

- My seizures start with a warning of fear, and then I feel as if I am a character in the PacMan video game and the monster is going to eat me. I am actually in the machine, running away from the PacMan.

- It is the most frightening feeling, as if I know the worst thing in the world is about to happen, I don't know what, just that something horrible is imminent.

There is a forced recollection of childhood memories that flash in front of me like a slide show in fast motion. They are all real memories, things that happened that I haven't thought about for decades. It's like what people describe before they die.

The next thing I knew I was floating just below the ceiling. I could see myself lying there. I wasn't scared; it was too interesting. I saw myself jerking and overheard my boss telling someone to "punch the timecard out" and that she was going with me to the hospital. Next thing, I was in space and could see Earth. Next thing, I woke up in the emergency room.

These experiences are not typical seizure symptoms. However, the spectrum of seizure symptoms is so broad that almost any emotion or experience is possible. Although most seizure symptoms are brief (last less than 3 minutes), on rare occasions they are prolonged (last more than 10–15 minutes). The important feature is the sudden onset, although obviously many symptoms and experiences unrelated to epilepsy also begin suddenly.

Patients who experience phenomena such as the ones described should mention them to their doctor. If the symptoms precede definite complex partial or tonic-clonic seizures, then they are almost certainly part of the seizure (a simple partial seizure).

CHAPTER 28

Epilepsy in the Elderly

Epilepsy spares no age group. Although epilepsy is often considered a disorder of childhood, it can begin at any age, and in some people persists from childhood to old age. There is actually an increased rate of newly diagnosed epilepsy in the elderly as compared with middle-aged adults. As in younger people, the cause of epilepsy often cannot be determined when it begins in the elderly. In approximately half of the cases, the cause is stroke (often a small one that did not cause other symptoms), head injury, or tumor (either benign or malignant).

EFFECTS OF SEIZURES ON OLDER PEOPLE

There are special concerns about the effects of seizures on older people. The body becomes less resilient with age. The effects of tonic-clonic seizures can be more severe. They cause stress on the heart and potential problems for people with heart disease. Similarly, breathing is affected during a tonic-clonic seizure, which poses potential problems for people who have pulmonary (lung) disorders. Bones are more fragile in elderly people; the risk of neck or back pain, or even a fracture, during a tonic-clonic seizure is increased. Despite these and other potential problems, most older people who suffer tonic-clonic seizures have no serious aftereffects.

EFFECTS OF ANTIEPILEPTIC DRUGS AND OTHER MEDICATIONS ON THE ELDERLY

A 74-year-old woman began to experience twitching movements on the right side of her face. A computed tomography (CT) scan showed a benign tumor—a meningioma, growing from the membrane that covers the brain—on the surface of the left frontal lobe. She was treated with phenytoin, and the seizures stopped. An operation was performed to remove the tumor. She had no seizures for 6 months after the operation, but then the twitching movements recurred. She took phenytoin (400 milligrams) in the morning. Most of the twitching movements occurred in the late evening or would awaken her from sleep at night. She complained of tiredness and unsteadiness around lunchtime, which she attributed to the drug. Because of the seizures, her doctor increased the dose to 500 milligrams a day, but the adverse effects became worse. Two months later, her internist prescribed sucralfate for a stomach problem, and she had a brief tonic-clonic seizure during sleep several weeks later. The next day, the neurologist measured the blood phenytoin level early in the morning, before she took her five phenytoin pills, and found it was low. The blood phenytoin level was measured again, around lunchtime, when the adverse effects were most severe. The blood level was at the top of the therapeutic range. The phenytoin was divided into two doses and eventually adjusted to 200 milligrams in the morning and 230 milligrams at night. Sucralfate, which can lower the blood phenytoin level, was discontinued, and another medication that did not interact with phenytoin was prescribed. The patient's blood phenytoin level became much steadier, the adverse effects almost completely disappeared, and the seizures were fully controlled.

This case report illustrates several important aspects of therapy for epilepsy in older patients. People become more sensitive to the effects of medications as they grow older. The adverse effects that occurred when the blood phenytoin level was in the therapeutic range are common for older people using all types of antiepileptic drugs and other medications, and drug interactions can occur (see Tables 6 through 9). It is important that the doctors treating an older person know of all the medications he or she is taking. Finally, older people (and sometimes younger ones) may need to go on a twice-a-day regimen of phenytoin or other antiepileptic drugs to "smooth out" their blood levels of the drugs, thereby reducing the chances of both seizures and adverse effects.

Some medications that are often used in the elderly may, in certain cases, provoke seizures. These include the drugs used to treat behavioral and psychiatric problems, asthma, heart disorders, and infections. Therefore, all persons with epilepsy or with a history of epilepsy should make it known to their doctors, because a medication prescribed for an unrelated problem could make seizures more likely.

PART FIVE

Legal and Financial Issues in Epilepsy

CHAPTER 29

Legal Rights of People with Epilepsy

Unfortunately, discrimination against people with disabilities, and especially epilepsy, continues in public accommodations and housing. A variety of state and federal laws have been enacted to protect people with disabilities against discrimination. The Americans with Disabilities Act (ADA), a federal law passed in 1990, protects the rights of people with disabilities. Most states also have laws prohibiting discrimination in public places, housing and real estate, and credit transactions.

People with epilepsy or other disabilities also may face unjust accusation of antisocial or criminal behavior after a seizure in public, denial of adequate medical care in correctional facilities, and problems in child adoption or child custody cases. In many of these areas, the rights of disabled people are secured by federal or state laws prohibiting discrimination. In others, such as false arrest, persons with epilepsy can take precautions to avoid mistreatment or unfair judgments.

MEDICAL CARE

In the United States, no one has a legal right to medical care. However, most hospital emergency departments do not refuse medical care to someone who has a serious medical problem. The greatest problem for many people is availability of insurance to cover office visits to the doctor, outpatient tests, and nonemergency hospitalizations.

PUBLIC SERVICES

Some state laws protecting the rights of people with disabilities are extensions to their civil rights laws, whereas others are part of a comprehensive handicap discrimination law. In some states, protection against discrimination for people with disabilities extends to services rendered directly by the state or those that are regulated or funded by the state. Thus, state laws may also provide protection in areas such as education, insurance, licensing, and access to transportation.

PUBLIC ACCOMMODATIONS

Persons with epilepsy are sometimes unfairly prohibited from entering public places such as hotels, doctor's offices, and restaurants. Although such instances are rare, seizures may recur when a person has previously had a seizure in that place. Although there are legal avenues of redress, it may be easiest to inform the supervisor or manager of the place about your disorder and describe the type and frequency of your seizures and any first aid measures that may be helpful. It is also worth reminding them that they must comply with the ADA.

The ADA prohibits places of public accommodation (excluding religious organizations and private clubs) from discriminating against individuals with disabilities. Such persons are entitled to full and equal enjoyment of goods, services, facilities, privileges, advantages, or accommodations. To enforce the ADA, individuals may bring a private lawsuit or file a complaint with the US Attorney General through the Department of Justice.

HOUSING

The Fair Housing Amendments Act (FHAA) of 1988 prohibits discrimination in the sale, rental, or financing of housing because of a disability. The FHAA mandates that housing providers make "reasonable accommodations" in rules, policies, and services to allow people with disabilities an equal opportunity to use and enjoy housing. Multifamily housing built after March 13, 1991, must meet minimum standards allowing access so that the housing can be used by people with disabilities.

Complaints of housing discrimination can be filed with the US Department of Housing and Urban Development or in federal district court.

AIRLINE TRAVEL

People with epilepsy can be passengers on airplanes, because there is no evidence that seizures are more likely to occur during or shortly after airplane flights than at other times. For those who have uncontrolled seizures, it may be worthwhile considering special precautions. If the person is traveling alone, it may be helpful to inform flight attendants about the disorder. Then, if a seizure occurs during the flight, they will be much less likely to overreact. When a tonic-clonic seizure occurs in someone without a known history of epilepsy, the airline may divert a coast-to-coast flight to have the person treated in a city en route.

FALSE ARREST

After complex partial or tonic-clonic seizures, some persons will appear to be confused or under the influence of alcohol or illegal drugs. In this setting, persons with epilepsy may be unfairly arrested and charged with being drunk and disorderly or creating a public disturbance. During complex partial seizures, some persons may perform automatic acts that are misinterpreted as willful and criminal. For example, they may undress in public or pick up something in a store and break it or place it in a pocket. In these cases, a careful description of the act; the person's behavior before, during, and after the aberrant behavior; and a statement from family members or friends of the person's behavior during previous seizures can be extremely helpful. Unfortunately, a person's first seizure may be the one for which he or she is unjustly accused of criminal behavior. A doctor can usually determine whether the behavior occurred during or after a seizure, and a doctor's report can lead to dismissal of the charges.

Restraint after seizures should be avoided, as even relatively mild restraint can lead to violent reactions. During and after a seizure that impairs consciousness, the person is in a confused state, may interpret physical contact as an aggressive act, and may respond in an aggressive manner. The person with epilepsy can then be charged with assault or resisting arrest or be injured or more aggressively restrained by law enforcement officers or others, further stimulating more aggressive behavior. In the worst case, because some police officers and other public employees are unfamiliar with epilepsy, seizures and their aftereffects are mistaken for criminal behavior, and the person with epilepsy is jailed, denied medication, and suffers additional seizures.

Persons with epilepsy can do several things to help avoid mistreatment and possible unjust arrest. They should wear a bracelet or necklace identifying them as having a seizure disorder, and it should include the telephone numbers of their doctor, pharmacist, and the person to call in case of an emergency. In addition, people with epilepsy should carry their medications in the bottle from the pharmacy or carry a copy of the prescription or a doctor's note. If stopped by police or security personnel (for example, at an airport during the search of carry-on bags), problems may arise if prescription drugs are not in their original containers.

RIGHTS OF INMATES OF CORRECTIONAL FACILITIES

Epilepsy is more common among prisoners than in the general population. This is largely the product of sociological factors, including a higher rate of epilepsy in impoverished groups, the people who are more likely to become incarcerated. Prisoners also have an increased incidence of head trauma, alcoholism, and drug abuse, problems that can cause seizures and epilepsy.

Prisoners have grave health care problems. Although their need for better medical care is well recognized, the delivery of that care is still lacking. Although the health care in many federal and state prisons has improved, it is still deficient in many aspects. The greatest problems remain in local jails, where persons with epilepsy may be denied medication or are given medication in unreasonable ways and may, thereby, be forced unnecessarily to suffer additional seizures.

For inmates who believe they have been denied adequate medical care, the simplest solution may be to have the doctor who cared for them before incarceration contact the prison doctor or nurse. If this is either impossible or unsuccessful, the attorney who represented the person in the criminal trial or an attorney recommended by the local Legal Aid office or the American Civil Liberties Union, may be helpful in obtaining better health care.

CHILD ADOPTION

Persons with epilepsy can adopt children. Laws concerning adoption are written with safeguards to ensure the child's best interests. The fitness of a potential adoptive parent may be questioned because he or she has seizures. Although no state law specifically mentions epilepsy, many states have adoption laws that require consideration of the mental and physical health of prospective parents. If seizures are fully or partially controlled, there should be no restrictions on the ability of a person to be a parent.

California has a law that allows adoptive parents to annul the adoption if, within 5 years of adoption, the child shows evidence of a developmental disability due to a condition that existed before the adoption. This law unfairly stigmatizes children with disabilities and can have a devastating effect on their emotional development.

CHILD CUSTODY

Persons with epilepsy can obtain custody of their children. Courts deciding custody matters primarily consider the best interests of the child. A parent's epilepsy should not affect most custody decisions.

For a parent whose seizures are completely or partially controlled, the custody decision should not be based on the epilepsy. Unfortunately, negative attitudes toward epilepsy still persist, and some courts may unfairly deny custody on the basis of perceptions, not facts.

The parent with epilepsy should be ready to provide detailed information about the type, duration, and frequency of seizures and about medications taken. If the seizures impair consciousness or control of movement, it may be helpful to discuss specific safeguards that will be taken to protect the child. If the other spouse claims that the child was injured during a seizure, the event should be carefully investigated and the direct relevance of the seizure examined.

If epilepsy has been a factor in making a custody decision, and the disorder later comes under better control, the parent should present a doctor's statement of the improvement and request a change in the custody decision.

The claim may be made that even if the seizures cause no physical harm to the children, they will be psychologically harmful. There is no evidence to support this claim. No study has found that children of parents with epilepsy have higher rates of psychological problems than children in the general population.

ACKNOWLEDGMENT

This chapter is based largely on *The Legal Rights of Persons with Epilepsy* (see Appendix 4).

CHAPTER 30

Insurance and Benefits for People with Epilepsy

People with epilepsy, like most people in our society, have to be concerned not only with health insurance to cover the cost of medical care but also with the many other kinds of insurance, such as life insurance, mortgage insurance, and disability insurance, that are available to provide security for themselves and their families. In addition to the financial protection afforded by private insurance, two income maintenance programs, administered by the Social Security Administration, are sponsored by the federal government.

HEALTH INSURANCE

Lack of affordable health care is one of our nation's gravest problems. More than 30 million Americans have no health insurance, and another 20 million have inadequate health care. Despite a concerted effort by state and national regulatory agencies, insurance companies, and hospitals, health care costs are increasing. As the costs increase, private health insurance moves further from the reach of individuals, families, and businesses.

Health insurance policies are expensive, especially for people with preexisting conditions such as epilepsy. Although people with epilepsy have always had trouble obtaining affordable health care, the problem is growing more acute. One cost-cutting tactic employed by many health insurance providers is to exclude coverage for preexisting conditions such as epilepsy. A 1989 Epilepsy Foundation of America (EFA) study found that most companies base their underwriting decisions on outdated statistical information contained in the Medical Impairment Study prepared by the Society of Actuaries. These underwriting guidelines do not reflect important advances in the diagnosis and treatment of epilepsy.

People with epilepsy who are fortunate enough to have health insurance may find that certain diagnostic procedures and treatments are not covered. For example, some plans do not cover expensive outpatient tests such as ambulatory electroencephalograms (EEGs) and magnetic resonance images (MRIs). Other policies deny coverage for specialized inpatient services such as video-EEG monitoring. In some cases, the persistence of both the patient and the doctor in documenting the need for specialized services will overcome the resistance of insurance carriers. However, the process of getting approval for these specialized services is often unduly prolonged and, in some cases, coverage is ultimately denied.

There are different categories of health insurance. Commercial or private indemnity insurance policies are the most expensive, but they provide the most comprehensive coverage of hospital, doctor, and outpatient services. They allow the patient to choose the doctor and hospital. These plans typically pay all or a large portion of the hospital and doctor bills. Some plans pay a large percentage of outpatient charges as well.

Health maintenance organizations (HMOs) and Preferred Provider Organizations (PPOs) are alternative health care delivery systems formed by groups of doctors and hospitals. Medical care is usually rendered only by the individuals and institutions within the system. Usually little or no fee is charged for medical services, but patients have to select a doctor or hospital from a specified list. Further, to help reduce costs, these organizations can limit the number of diagnostic procedures. If the HMO or PPO does not have an epileptologist, a neurologist with expertise in treating epilepsy, or a facility that performs studies such as video-EEG monitoring, the organization may approve consultation with one. However, there are strong financial incentives for the HMO or PPO to restrict the number of patients receiving health care outside its system. Nevertheless, if seizures remain poorly controlled, medication adverse effects are intolerable, or the epilepsy has a significant impact on the quality of life, a consultation with an epileptologist should be considered.

Managed health care plans are also becoming more common. These plans use a group of doctors, laboratories, and hospitals. A single doctor often acts as a "gatekeeper." He or she must approve all tests and referrals to doctors within or outside the system.

Medicare

Medicare, administered by the federal Health Care Financing Administration, is health insurance for all members of our society age 65 or over and for people who receive Social Security Disability Insurance (SSDI) benefits for at least 2 years. Medicare benefits are divided into two parts: Part A and Part B. After a deductible payment by the patient, Part A covers hospital services, skilled nursing services, and home health services. Part B covers doctor services, home health services, and nondisposable equipment.

Medicaid

Medicaid, a federal-state program administered by the states, provides financial assistance and health insurance to families with children, older Americans, and people who are blind or have disabilities. Eligibility and benefits vary from state to state. Most states provide coverage for hospital and doctor services; inpatient and outpatient services and prescription drugs are usually included. In many states, a person who is eligible for Supplemental Security Income (SSI) is automatically eligible for Medicaid.

Although Medicaid covers doctor services, the majority of private practice ("fee-for-service") doctors do not accept Medicaid. The reimbursement from Medicaid often does not cover the doctor's expenses for maintaining the office (rent, utilities, staff, malpractice insurance). However, many private practice doctors are willing to see a limited number of patients who have Medicaid. Further, a patient who consults a doctor who does not accept Medicaid may pay the fee (or work out a payment schedule) and use Medicaid to help with inpatient hospital costs, outpatient tests, and medications.

LIFE INSURANCE

There are few things as complicated as life insurance. The buyer faces aggressive salespeople, a smorgasbord of policy types and amounts, and a variety of companies offering slight variations on the same themes. Before buying a life insurance policy, buyers need to define their goals in obtaining life insurance, determine the type of policy and the amount of insurance they need, and do comparative shopping.

Most people begin their quest for life insurance with the goal of providing financial security for their family when they die, so it is most important to insure family members who provide significant income. After they have met with one or two insurance salespeople, however, their initial goal becomes clouded with terms like "investment," "cash value," and "retirement planning." Buyers must never lose sight of their goals. All forms of life insurance get more expensive as the insured gets older, so it is worth considering now rather than later. However, it pays to be careful. It is too easy to buy life insurance that is not needed. As a medical student, I was approached by aggressive salespeople who pushed a whole-life policy. They came in with impressive graphs and used a language that was foreign to me. I made the correct decision—not to buy then. Had I not resisted the sales pitch, I would have owned a policy that was a financial burden at the time and would have become meaningless for my current needs.

The two main types of life insurance are term and whole-life. A third type, universal (flexible) life, has become popular in the past decade. Term insurance is cheaper; it is pure insurance, and has no growth potential as an investment. Whole-life insurance is more expensive, but accumulates value; the insured can withdraw money after a period of time depending on the specific policy. With term insurance, a certain premium is paid each year. A rate can be locked in for a certain number of years, and so can an option to buy more term insurance at a certain rate. Term policies can be structured so that the cost increases on a yearly basis, or the cost can be averaged over a period of years so that the yearly payment remains constant. It is important to find out if the insured can renew the term insurance policy without taking another physical examination.

Whole-life insurance has the advantage of building a nest egg that can be used during the insured person's life or to increase the death benefit to survivors. Whole-life policies have a yearly premium that continues as long as the insured person is living. Most policies are structured so that the insured pays extra for the first 10 or 15 years. Then, based on current rates of investment return, the interest income will cover the yearly premium, and no additional money is paid out. The differences in the cost of whole-life policies largely reflect the projected income of the company. It may be dangerous to choose a company because it offers the cheapest rates. For example, one company, heavily invested in junk bonds, offered policies at less than half the rate of the major AAA-rated insurance companies. When the junk bond market crashed, the cost of the yearly premiums skyrocketed. Remember, whole-life insurance is an investment. If an insurance company's investments do poorly, the premiums can go up significantly.

There are several types of universal-life policies. In some, the policy owner can direct how the cash value of the policy is invested. This transfers the risk of how well things go from the insurance company's investment team to the insured. The policy owner may elect relatively conservative and low-yield investments; aggressive, speculative, and high-yield investments; or a mixture of the two. In other universal-life policies, the investments are controlled by the insurance carrier, but the yearly premium varies more depending on the prevailing interest rates and other economic factors.

Epilepsy can influence a person's eligibility for life insurance, as well as the life insurance rates. Insurance companies rely on statistics regarding lifestyle habits and life span in different diseases and disorders when deciding on whether to offer, and how much to charge for, life insurance. People who smoke or have a history of heart disease pay higher rates. Because epilepsy is not a disorder with a uniform course among different people, it is unfair for insurance companies to lump together everyone with a history of epilepsy. Most insurance companies are aware of this, and ask for a medical history, usually from the doctor. Lying about a history of epilepsy on a life insurance application can backfire badly. If the insurance company investigates at the insured's death and finds that the disorder had been concealed, it may be able to deny any benefits, even if death was in no way related to epilepsy.

Finally, a word on life insurance salespeople. It is often better to buy a policy from an independent agent, who represents a variety of companies, rather than an agent who sells only a single company's policies. Always obtain quotes from at least two salespeople, and compare both the details of the policies and the rating of the companies. Insurance agents are adept at telling potential buyers why the other agent's policy is not as good as theirs.

MORTGAGE INSURANCE

Mortgage insurance is a kind of life insurance. In case of the insured's death, it will pay off the remainder of the mortgage. It provides another form of security for the family and is worth considering. As with life insurance, mortgage insurance can be more difficult to obtain and more expensive for people with epilepsy. However, providing accurate medical information will help the buyer to obtain a policy at a good rate.

DISABILITY INSURANCE

For people younger than 45 years old, chances are greater that they will be disabled in the near future than that they will die. People whose income is critical for their own or their family's support should consider disability insurance. Unfortunately, it is expensive even though it resembles term insurance. That is, you pay as you go and build no savings in the process. Furthermore, disability insurance gets more expensive as a person gets older.

People with epilepsy may find disability insurance more difficult to obtain and more expensive than it is for people without epilepsy because some of them have a greater chance of becoming disabled.

Disability insurance policies vary considerably. Some of the most important questions a buyer should ask are: "How long do I have to be disabled before benefits begin?" "Can I renew the disability insurance without another physical examination at the end of the 'term' period?" "Do I have to be completely disabled or only unable to work at my current job to obtain benefits?" "What amount of benefits will I receive?" "Are the benefits lifelong or only until a certain age?" "Is the cost of the insurance stable for the duration of my coverage, or does it increase?" It is also important to make sure that the insurance company is well rated; AAA is the highest rating. Most reputable insurance agents do not sell insurance that is not rated.

SUPPLEMENTAL SUPPORT AND INCOME

Social Security Disability Benefits

The federal government's Social Security Administration (SSA) sponsors two programs that provide monthly income payments to individuals whose disabilities are expected to prevent them from working for at least 12 months. For these programs, disability is defined by the inability of the person "to engage in any substantial gainful activity by reason of any medically determinable physical or mental impairment which can be expected to result in death or which has lasted or can be expected to last for a continuous period of not less than 12 months."

The first program, SSDI, pays benefits to eligible workers under age 65 (and their dependents or survivors) who have worked for a minimum period and have paid Social Security taxes. There is a 5-month waiting time between the determination that one is disabled and the initial payment.

The second program, SSI, is based on need and does not require prior payment of Social Security taxes. To qualify (these criteria are subject to change; the SSA should be contacted for current criteria), the applicant must have no more than $2000 in assets, which includes cash or other property that could be converted to cash and used to help support that individual. Disabled children under age 18 who live at home are considered to have their parents' income and assets, and are therefore usually not eligible. Special rules may apply to some children, however. SSI payments begin as soon as the person is determined to be eligible and are retroactive to the first month in which the application was filed.

Establishing eligibility for Social Security disability benefits can be a difficult process. Criteria are strictly enforced, and many deserving applicants are initially denied benefits but later approved on appeal. Persons who believe that their benefits were wrongfully denied can contact an attorney who can help file an appeal. If the appeal is successful, payments are retroactive to the date of the initial application.

Applying for Benefits

An application should be filed, in person if possible, at the local SSA office. The applicant should be prepared for lots of questions about his or her disability, medical history, work history, and financial status. When applying, the applicant should bring the following information:

- A list of all doctors, clinics, and hospitals where the applicant has been treated.
- A detailed letter from the patient's doctor on the nature of the disability and how it prevents the patient from working; if there is more than one physical or mental disability, the doctor should describe all of them.
- A list of activities of daily living (cooking, cleaning, grocery shopping, and so on) that the applicant cannot do.
- A list of past jobs that the applicant can no longer perform; if possible, a letter from a previous employer concerning inability to continue at the previous job.
- Names, addresses, and telephone numbers of all social workers and counselors the applicant has been to see.

Social Security Administration Criteria for Eligibility

The SSA considers epileptic seizures in two broad groups: *major motor* (tonic-clonic [grand mal]) and *minor motor* (absence [petit mal], complex partial [psychomotor], and focal motor). Major motor seizures must occur at least once a month despite at least 3 months of treatment. There must be either daytime seizures with loss of consciousness or convulsive seizures, or nocturnal seizures with residual effects that interfere significantly with daytime function. Minor motor seizures must occur more often than once a week despite at least 3 months of treatment. There must be "alteration of awareness or loss of consciousness and transient postictal manifestations of unconventional behavior or significant interference with activity during the day." (The SSA regulations regarding epilepsy are subject to review; the SSA should be contacted for current regulations and requirements.)

If epilepsy is the cause of the disability, the SSA requires documentation of the disorder with an EEG and a detailed description of a typical seizure. Although the SSA requires an EEG, they recognize that a normal EEG does not preclude the diagnosis of epilepsy. In cases of a normal EEG, however, it may be helpful to have the neurologist write a note confirming that normal EEGs occur in people with epilepsy and also to submit a statement from a textbook confirming that fact. Detailed documentation of a typical seizure is essential. The description should include whether or not there is an aura (and the features of the aura, if present), tongue biting, loss of bladder or bowel control, injuries caused by the seizure, and postseizure symptoms such as confusion or sleepiness. The doctor who provides the seizure description should state the source of the information and whether corroboration was obtained from more than one person. If a health professional has witnessed a seizure, the observations should be included and the source noted. Although the patient's doctor will provide information about the seizures and the patient's examination, SSA has the right to request that the applicant see an agency-paid doctor.

Several other issues may be relevant to the determination of disability benefits on the basis of epilepsy. First, although the actual seizure count for the last 2 months may not fulfill the SSA criteria, the average seizure frequency over the past 6 to 12 months can be used, because seizures often occur in clusters. This point must be emphasized, as a cluster of three seizures in 2 days can be extremely disabling. Although this criterion is not yet recognized, it could be argued that this seizure frequency is equivalent to the one currently used and has a similar meaning for determining the presence of a disability. Second, if seizures can only be controlled with very high dosages of medications, then the disabling effects of these drugs must also be considered. Third, blood levels of the antiepileptic drug are requested and help to confirm that the person is taking the prescribed medications. If the levels are in the subtherapeutic range despite compliance with the regimen, then the person's doctor should note that the subtherapeutic levels are not the result of noncompliance but may be due to problems with absorption or rapid metabolism.

Review and Termination of Benefits

After Social Security disability benefits have been approved, the SSA conducts periodic reviews to determine if the condition has improved and the person is now able to be gainfully employed. The SSA may request documentation from both the person and the doctor regarding the current status of the disability. Benefits may be terminated if the SSA finds that the impairment is gone, did not exist, or is no longer disabling.

If a person believes that his or her benefits have been terminated unfairly, he or she should immediately file a request to have the decision reconsidered. The person may also want to make a separate request, which must be done within 10 days of receiving the notification of termination, to have benefits continue while the appeal is pending. A disability hearing must be requested within 10 days of receiving notification of benefits termination. This hearing is available only if the termination is based on medical factors. If the termination is based on new information regarding income or assets, reconsideration is made only by review of the file. If a disability hearing is not requested, or if it is determined that the person is no longer disabled, the person still can request a full hearing before an administrative law judge. He or she must request such a hearing within 60 days of the disability hearing decision or notification of disability benefits termination. The request that benefits be continued pending the decision of the administrative law judge must also be renewed.

Work Incentive Programs

Social Security disability benefits may continue when a person enters a work incentive program. These programs encourage disabled people to work, with the hope that they can become self-supporting. Individuals receiving either SSDI or SSI may participate in a vocational rehabilitation program. These programs are designed for persons who improve medically and are no longer considered disabled by the SSA. The SSA determines whether the benefits will continue, based on the likelihood that the individual's participation in the program will allow gainful employment on a long-term basis. Benefits can continue until the vocational rehabilitation program ends.

SSDI and SSI have different rules regarding the amount of participation and income that are allowed while benefits continue. Information regarding these rules can be obtained from the local SSA office.

ACKNOWLEDGMENT

The section on supplemental support and income is based largely on *The Legal Rights of Persons with Epilepsy* (see Appendix 4).

PART SIX

Resources for People with Epilepsy

CHAPTER 31

The Epilepsy Foundation of America

The Epilepsy Foundation of America (EFA) is the only national voluntary health organization devoted to helping people with epilepsy. The EFA is committed to the prevention and cure of seizure disorders, the alleviation of their effects, and the promotion of independence and optimal quality of life for people with these disorders. The EFA is a voice for people with epilepsy at national and local levels to promote legal rights and provide information and assistance in a variety of areas. The EFA's growth in size and scope during the past quarter century has been dramatic. The EFA seeks to accomplish its mission through support of research, education, advocacy, and service.

ADVOCACY FOR PEOPLE WITH EPILEPSY: FORMATION OF THE EFA

People with epilepsy have faced severe stigma, isolation, and discrimination since ancient times (see Chapter 1). The misunderstandings and misconceptions that formed the image of epilepsy in earlier times have been thoroughly discredited, but the damage of these false views still persists. Members of older generations may still hold that epilepsy is a curse and a shame, a disorder that should be shrouded in secrecy and never revealed to the outside world. Some of these false views survive in old medical textbooks, as well as in folklore. The misrepresentation of epilepsy has exacted a bitter price from people with epilepsy in the form of job bias, discrimination, and restrictive legislation directed against them. During the first half of this century, laws passed in several states forbade people with epilepsy from marrying, permitted sterilization, and barred children from attending regular schools.

At the end of World War II it became clear that a lot of wounded veterans had developed epilepsy as a result of serious head injury, and there was renewed interest in rehabilitation and fairer treatment. The late 1940s

297

and the 1950s saw the emergence of a movement to help people with epilepsy. Public education campaigns to demystify epilepsy and remove the stigma and discrimination began. Local groups were created to provide information, medical referrals, and emotional support. Some of them established clinics. They raised funds for vital equipment, such as electroencephalogram (EEG) machines, and provided medications for people in need. Individual and group efforts combined to repeal many of the laws that restricted and discriminated against people with epilepsy, and efforts were made to improve their acceptance in the schools.

The EFA was established in 1968, formed by a series of mergers of local and regional epilepsy advocacy groups. The initial task of the EFA was to obtain greater recognition for the problems faced by people with epilepsy, to help direct public opinion away from misinformation and misunderstanding to a more realistic and open view of epilepsy, and to stimulate increased federal funding for research and other programs. As the epilepsy advocacy groups grew in strength and number during the 1950s and 1960s, so did federal interest in epilepsy and other neurological disorders. A special institute was formed to fund research in these areas. Today, the National Institute of Neurological Disorders and Stroke (NINDS), a part of the National Institutes of Health, supports research on epilepsy at its own clinics and laboratories and at universities across the nation. With the active encouragement of the EFA, the NINDS has played a critical role in the establishment of comprehensive epilepsy centers and the development of new antiepileptic drugs.

In 1975, Congress responded to pressure from the EFA and passed a bill calling for the establishment of a commission to study the treatment of epilepsy in the United States. The Commission for the Control of Epilepsy and Its Consequences concluded that (1) epilepsy was widely misunderstood throughout society, (2) there was a chronic lack of information about it, (3) people with epilepsy wanted to be more involved in their own care, and (4) people with epilepsy wanted to become as independent as possible.

The commission's findings were based on many hours of testimony by people with epilepsy and their families, dozens of papers by leading experts in the field, and the active participation of the EFA. Its report helped prepare the ground for the funding of many important federal initiatives, including the increased growth of epilepsy centers to evaluate the whole patient while providing state-of-the-art medical care. These came to be known as comprehensive epilepsy centers. The commission also made important recommendations to the executive branch of the federal government, urging that people with epilepsy be included in key programs and services such as those provided through the Education of All Handicapped Children Act (Public Law 94-142) and by the Rehabilitation Service Administration.

The commission's recommendations provided a blueprint for action, and the EFA responded enthusiastically. It pushed successfully for Food and Drug Administration approval of a new drug that the commission believed should be available in the United States, and it strengthened its own programs to provide information about epilepsy to individuals and families and to stimulate research in key areas of inquiry, especially some of the social problems associated with epilepsy.

In 1982, the EFA fulfilled a commission recommendation when it established the National Epilepsy Library at its Landover, Maryland, offices. Since then the EFA has built its library into the largest single source of information on the social and medical aspects of epilepsy in the world.

The EFA has worked tirelessly to remove barriers that prevent the entry of people with epilepsy into the mainstream of American life. Its representatives have testified in legislatures across the country; it has filed friend-of-the-court briefs in lawsuits that test legal issues of importance to people with epilepsy; and it was a major force in the campaign to craft and subsequently secure passage of the 1990 Americans with Disabilities Act, which opened new doors of opportunity for people with epilepsy in many areas of life.

Studies have shown that 25 years of public education, sponsored by the EFA and its affiliates, have begun to pay off. Its annual campaigns on television and radio to change the negative image so long associated with the condition are beginning to have an effect. Public opinion about epilepsy has changed. There is greater acceptance of people with epilepsy and greater recognition that it can be effectively treated in many cases.

Today, the EFA wants to build on that understanding by helping the public to see that there is a spectrum of disability and that, although some people can now do very well, the disorder is by no means conquered. For those with severe seizures or associated disabilities, or those who have to take so much medication that their lives are severely limited, epilepsy is still a major barrier to a normal life.

EFA PROGRAMS AND ACTIVITIES

The EFA supports programs at the national and local levels to improve the lives of people with epilepsy and their families. The EFA works closely with international and national organizations, including the American Epilepsy Society, the professional association of doctors and other health care workers. The EFA also maintains contacts and works with government agencies and organizations at the federal, state, and local levels. The national EFA has affiliates in most states. The affiliates are independently organized state and local groups that are bound to the national organization by an affiliation agreement.

The national office of the EFA helps to coordinate the activities of the more than 85 affiliates, and it runs the educational, research, legislative, and other national programs. The national EFA leadership includes an all-volunteer board of directors and a professional advisory board of leaders in the scientific community, who provide expertise, guidance, and oversight for the EFA's programs and services. The national office also produces a range of materials for use by the EFA affiliates and provides technical assistance to them as they conduct programs on the local level. The number of programs offered by the affiliates varies depending on the local needs and the level of support from the surrounding community.

Information and Referral Services

The national EFA office receives more than 30,000 calls and letters each year requesting information about epilepsy. Since a toll-free number (see Appendix 3) was installed in 1986, the number of requests has increased dramatically. The calls come from people with epilepsy, their family members, doctors, and other people in search of information. People who call or write the EFA for information receive a personal letter in response. Callers and writers are given current information on a wide range of epilepsy-related topics and are provided with information on resources in their local areas.

One of the most important services provided by the local EFA affiliates is the distribution of basic information about epilepsy and local services. Although the EFA pamphlets often contain answers to most of the basic questions, a personal explanation is often more gratifying. Local medical, psychological, social, and other service referrals can be provided.

National Epilepsy Library

Requests for technical information are referred to the National Epilepsy Library. The library provides doctors, research scientists, nurses, people with epilepsy and their family members, and others with the most up-to-date information on medical and other aspects of epilepsy. Literature searches on the latest developments in research and clinical aspects of epilepsy for doctors and other health care professionals are provided free of charge. A quarterly update lists recently acquired documents and is available to health care professionals on request. The National Epilepsy Library has its own database of more than 6000 entries and is linked with major research collections. It is available to the medical community through the BRS Colleague System.

The National Epilepsy Library responds to thousands of requests for information each year. For information, call the National Epilepsy Library's toll-free number (see Appendix 3).

Information and Education

The EFA produces and distributes a variety of educational materials about epilepsy to individuals and groups. These materials include pamphlets, video tapes, posters, and books. More than 750,000 pamphlets are distributed annually by the national office. People can choose from more than 30 pamphlets, covering topics such as basic information, medicines, legal rights and issues, employment, first aid for seizures, information for babysitters of children with epilepsy, parenting children with epilepsy, and epilepsy and learning disabilities. Pamphlets and posters specially designed for the African-American and Spanish-speaking communities are also available.

The EFA actively promotes epilepsy education and spreading of information through the information media. Public services messages are sent to magazines, radio, and television stations nationwide.

Through its educational campaigns, the EFA seeks to improve the public's understanding of epilepsy and people with epilepsy while correcting outdated and incorrect views; to provide people with epilepsy and those around them with information on medical, social, and other aspects of epilepsy; and to bring the interests of people with epilepsy to public attention.

Advocacy Programs

The national EFA advocacy program helps fight discrimination; promotes access to health care, education, and employment; and supports independent living. Through position papers, congressional testimony, and legal briefs, the EFA attacks the inequities and barriers that people with epilepsy face. As already noted, in 1990, the EFA worked with other national health agencies to support passage of the Americans with Disabilities Act, landmark legislation that prohibits discrimination on the basis of disability in private sector employment and many other areas and that will help to open the doors of the American workplace to people with epilepsy.

Each year EFA representatives testify in support of essential government programs related to the needs of people with epilepsy. These include medical research, improved quality of medical care, better access to insurance, financial assistance for the disabled and ill, and employment and rehabilitation programs.

Legal advocacy is another important EFA program. Staff attorneys provide general information about epilepsy-related legal issues. Staff lawyers work with local attorneys and, in some cases, file friend-of-the-court briefs in cases that have far-reaching significance for people with epilepsy. Such cases are ones in which a precedent or point of law may be established that can advance the well-being of others with epilepsy.

Advocacy programs of the local affiliates are designed to support the interests of people with epilepsy, by speaking up on their behalf and getting the message out to those in a position to affect their lives. The advocacy can be on a personal level to solve a dispute or misunderstanding. In one instance, a woman with absence seizures was accused of being on drugs because she was "so spacy." An explanation to her supervisor from the doctor on the local affiliate's professional advisory board not only resolved her employment problem, but, for the first time, made the doctor aware that her absence seizures were frequent. With adjustments of her medications, she has better seizure control, and a more secure job.

Advocacy can also help people with epilepsy pass through the maze of bureaucracy and red tape that pervades society. The "Catch 22s" of life—problems in which the solutions create new problems or make the original one worse—can often be resolved through advocacy efforts. In some cases, advocacy programs provide experts to write a letter to legislators or agencies or to testify in support of better services or a needed facility, such as additional disability benefits or a living unit for young adults learning independence for the first time.

In some instances, advocacy simply provides recognition for people with epilepsy. One local affiliate recently secured a letter of recognition from New York's governor to a boy who was graduating from high school. Despite uncontrolled epilepsy, cerebral palsy, and serious learning disabilities, he persisted and graduated from his public high school. When his name was called, he received a standing ovation. When the letter from the governor was presented, the crowd could not stop applauding.

Employment Programs

The EFA's employment service programs help more than 1500 people with epilepsy find work each year. Since 1976, EFA has sponsored a Training Applicants for Placement Success (TAPS) program in 13 cities in cooperation with its affiliates. The program is funded by the Department of Labor and helps adults and young people with seizures through job-search training, job counseling, and placement assistance. Many EFA affiliates offer similar programs in their own communities. EFA affiliates work with local job clubs and business people to help find employment opportunities. Support groups for adults with epilepsy may be available and help to identify barriers to employment and means to successful employment. In some instances, education of employers about epilepsy and follow-up services after employment are also available.

Research Support

Advancing knowledge about the prevention, diagnosis, and treatment of epilepsy through research is one of the EFA's primary goals. Research can provide new insights into the causes of epilepsy, help discover new drugs to stop seizures, and promote a better understanding of the medical and social disorders that occur in people with epilepsy. Every year the EFA funds research projects by both young and established investigators. This support helps to uncover new information and to stimulate the careers of young scientists and doctors interested in epilepsy research.

Epilepsy Advances is a quarterly newsletter for the medical and scientific community. This newsletter provides summaries on what is new in the basic sciences (for example, laboratory studies on brain cells) and clinical research.

Professional Education

The EFA sponsors educational programs and produces a variety of materials about epilepsy for health care and other professionals. It produces videotapes and booklets for primary care doctors, doctors in training, nurses, and other health care professionals on how to diagnose and treat seizures. It also sponsors training courses and seminars at professional meetings and funds training and fellowships for students and doctors.

Local affiliates, together with local medical centers, coordinate educational programs to bring up-to-date information about epilepsy to health care and other professionals in the community. These programs include full-day courses for doctors, seminars for nurses, lectures to police officers and fire fighters about recognition of and first aid for seizures, and in-service presentations for personnel directors. These educational services help to keep health care professionals knowledgeable about epilepsy and help other professionals do a better job in serving people with epilepsy.

Membership Services

Anyone can join the EFA. Members' benefits include a subscription to *Epilepsy USA*, the EFA newspaper, which carries regular features on living with epilepsy and covers stories on medical and research breakthroughs, national developments, activities of the local affiliates, useful information on legal rights and social problems confronted by those with the condition, and other topics relevant to people with epilepsy. EFA members of any age are able to purchase medications through the prescription pharmacy program of the American Association of Retired Persons. Members are also informed about new pamphlets and educational materials produced by the EFA and others and are provided with advance programs of the EFA national conference.

For information about membership, call or write to the EFA (see Appendix 3).

National Conference

The annual conference of the EFA brings together representatives of its local affiliates, the national EFA staff, health care professionals, people with epilepsy, and their families. Depending on its theme, each conference includes lectures and workshops on specific aspects of epilepsy. Experts in different fields present information about new developments in treatment, medications, surgery, quality-of-life concerns, and the occurrence of epilepsy in select populations.

Winning Kids Program

The Winning Kids program was designed to change the negative stereotypes that children with epilepsy had to face, but it has evolved to celebrate the ability of children to overcome adversity and enjoy success in life. The program promotes self-esteem and rewards achievements large and small in these children. Every year, local EFA affiliates enter children as their Winning Kids. Although only one of them is chosen to represent the others as the national Winning Kid, in the EFA's view, they are all winners.

Parent and Family Networks

Outreach to families struggling with the challenges of epilepsy is very much a part of the EFA's mission. It is currently establishing a series of parent teams to contact and work with other parents in a cooperative effort to solve common problems. In some communities, these Parent and Family Networks are being operated with the assistance of the local EFA affiliate, but they are operating in other areas without an affiliate.

Counseling Programs

Professionally staffed or peer-group support programs involving people with epilepsy or their parents are offered by many of the affiliates. Counseling sessions may cover such issues as adjusting to and living with epilepsy and parenting a child with epilepsy.

Self-Help Groups

Self-help groups are designed to allow people to gain strength from shared experiences and the recognition that their feelings, frustrations, and joys are not unique. Depending on local resources, support groups may be provided for adults, teenagers, parents, or even children. If one is not available, anyone can work to generate the interest and get one started.

School Alert Program

The School Alert program is a locally conducted, national educational program to improve the school environment for children with epilepsy. Information about epilepsy is made available to teachers, school nurses, students, and other school personnel through videotapes, manuals, pamphlets, and in-person presentations. For young children, the "Kids on the Block" puppet show is offered by many affiliates; the shows have been warmly received and present the information in a way the children can understand. With this understanding, their classmate with epilepsy can be more easily accepted and be seen as "just another kid."

Speakers' Bureau

The Speakers' Bureau is an educational service through which EFA affiliates provide trained speakers to talk to groups and clubs about epilepsy.

Epilepsy Month

November is Epilepsy Month, a month devoted to providing the public with information about epilepsy. The intensive education campaign includes press and publicity materials, radio and television messages and stories, and fund-raising efforts; it is conducted on both the national and the local level.

Independent-Living Centers

Some EFA affiliates operate residence programs for adults with epilepsy who need assistance with activities of daily living but who are not so disabled that they need more care. Many other affiliates are in contact with agencies that operate independent-living centers and can be helpful in getting places in such facilities. These centers range from large houses in which residents have individual bedrooms, to individual apartments, to day-care centers.

Camping and Recreational Programs

A growing number of EFA affiliates are offering camping experiences, often combined with epilepsy education, for children with epilepsy. Parents whose children go to these camps frequently find they are more independent and self-confident afterward. Other recreational programs include day camps and weekend retreats for the whole family.

Respite Care

When a child has severe seizures or associated disabilities, parents need an occasional time out. Some EFA affiliates are offering respite care in the form of trained people to relieve parents and other family members for predetermined periods of time.

GETTING INVOLVED WITH THE EFA

The EFA was created and has grown through the efforts of people with epilepsy and their families and others devoted to seeing people with epilepsy achieve greater success and an optimal quality of life.

Anyone who has epilepsy or who is the parent or other family member of someone with epilepsy, should consider joining the EFA and becoming active at the local level. Members can be helpful in various volunteer efforts, speaking at school gatherings, fund-raising, and organizing and participating in support groups.

THE EFA TODAY AND IN THE FUTURE

The EFA continues to grow and serve people with epilepsy and their families in new and innovative ways. The positive changes in public perception about epilepsy need to be reinforced. We must make sure that people with epilepsy reap the benefits obtained through the passage and implementation of the Americans with Disabilities Act. Most of all, we must work together to prevent seizure disorders, to find a cure for them, and to pursue activities that will improve opportunities for people with epilepsy to be independent, employed, and enjoy their lives. This is the EFA's mission for the future.

CHAPTER 32

Other Resources for People with Epilepsy

Although the Epilepsy Foundation of America (EFA) is the national organization for people with epilepsy, other resources may also be helpful for some people. People with epilepsy often face specific individual challenges. No matter how unique or difficult the problem, there are successful solutions. Identifying the resources available is often the first step in overcoming the problem.

Elected representatives in the Senate and House of Representatives can often be helpful. For example, a young man from Iran with refractory partial seizures who lives with his father and brother in the United States was scheduled to undergo epilepsy surgery. His mother was unable to obtain a visa to enter the United States from Iran. With the support of doctors at the epilepsy center, the local congressional representative was able to secure the visa through the US Department of State.

OTHER NATIONAL RESOURCES

A variety of national organizations serve certain groups of individuals. In many cases, information, services, and advocacy by these organizations are relevant to people with epilepsy who have special needs. When a person has more than one disability, the challenges are often greater. In such cases, tapping into the resources of related organizations can be beneficial. For example, blind people who have uncontrolled epilepsy have special challenges, some of which can be met through organizations that serve the blind.

COMMUNITY RESOURCES

People, organizations, agencies, and other resources available at state or local levels can provide information, advocacy, and services to people with epilepsy and their family members. In many cases, the greatest challenge is identifying these resources. The resources range from financial assistance for food, shelter, and medical care to respite-care programs for parents with severely disabled children. Some of the most important local resources are listed below. Others can be found by calling the EFA national office or the local EFA affiliate, the local or state government, or a comprehensive epilepsy center.

State Department of Education

The state department of education is responsible for providing education to all children in the state. It can provide information about special education programs and services. This office can also be helpful in determining if a child is receiving the needed services to which he or she is entitled.

Board of Education

Each school district has a board of education that sets local policies. The person who coordinates special education or other programs of the local school district can be found there.

Office of Vocational Education for Handicapped Students

Information about existing and new programs for children with disabilities can be obtained from the office of vocational education. This office helps coordinate the distribution of federal funds provided to each state for vocational education for students with special needs.

Protection and Advocacy Offices for Individuals with Disabilities

The protection and advocacy office (the exact title varies from state to state) can provide information on the state's services for people with disabilities. Depending on the state, services may include education, recreational activities, respite programs, residential housing, and legal representation.

Developmental Disabilities Agency

The state developmental disabilities agency allocates federal funds to nonprofit private and public organizations to assist people with developmental disabilities. Some of the services include medical care (evaluation, diagnosis, and treatment), information, social services, protection, social activities, group homes, and advocacy.

State Vocational Rehabilitation Agency

The state vocational rehabilitation agency has numerous local offices that coordinate medical, physical, and occupational therapy; program planning; education; and vocational programs to assist people in obtaining employment.

COMPREHENSIVE EPILEPSY CENTERS

The growth of our understanding about epilepsy has led to the realization that, for some patients, the treatment of epilepsy involves the coordination of several disciplines and may require expertise beyond the capacity of general medical or neurological care. Comprehensive epilepsy centers provide expert care for patients with epilepsy.

The principal doctors at comprehensive epilepsy centers are epileptologists. They are neurologists who, after they complete their training in general neurology, complete additional training in caring for people with epilepsy. This training includes exposure to a multidisciplinary approach to epilepsy-related problems (that is, one that incorporates input from various health care workers). Most programs include extensive training in the interpretation of electroencephalograms (EEGs) and video-EEG recordings. These epilepsy fellowship programs also include training in the use of investigational drugs and epilepsy surgery.

The majority of patients with epilepsy do not require care at comprehensive epilepsy centers. A patient may be referred to an epilepsy center because the nature of the attack is uncertain (Is it epilepsy, or something else?), the type of epilepsy is difficult to classify (Are the seizures partial or primary generalized?), or the seizures or medication adverse effects persist despite optimal treatment. Referral can also be made because employment problems or social disabilities resulting from the epilepsy need expert attention, or an investigational drug or epilepsy surgery is recommended. In most cases, patients are referred to a comprehensive epilepsy center by their neurologist or other doctor.

For some persons, a single consultation at a comprehensive epilepsy center may be worthwhile. For example, a woman with epilepsy who is thinking about starting a family may benefit from speaking with an expert in epilepsy and pregnancy. Although the information provided by the woman's neurologist or epileptologist may be quite similar, it can be comforting simply to hear the answers from another source. In other cases, the expert at the epilepsy center may be aware of more specific or new information before it is known by doctors in the community.

The most common referral to a comprehensive epilepsy center is for people with poorly controlled seizures or troublesome adverse effects of medications. Epilepsy centers can be helpful in recommending optimal use of antiepileptic drugs or changes in lifestyle, such as more sleep, to control seizures or avoid medication adverse effects. All of these recommendations can be made by other doctors, but it may be helpful to have a fresh and new assessment in patients who have difficult-to-control seizures.

For patients with seizures that do not respond to the standard antiepileptic drugs, investigational drugs or surgery may be considered. Investigational drugs are those that have not been approved for general use by the Food and Drug Administration. All new drugs must go through extensive testing of their effectiveness and safety. The process includes clinical trials or testing of the drugs in patients. The clinical trials are supervised by both the drug company and the doctor who actually studies the patients. Before a study is begun, it must be approved by the center's Institutional Review Board, which consists of doctors and other health care professionals, a member of the clergy, a bioethicist, and others. In addition, comprehensive epilepsy centers are the only facilities with the teams and expertise to perform epilepsy surgery (see Chapter 11).

There are differences among epilepsy centers. Some centers care predominantly for children or adults, whereas others care for patients of all ages. Some centers offer only consultation with an epilepsy specialist and certain diagnostic studies such as video-EEG monitoring. Other centers conduct investigational drug trials or specialize in epilepsy surgery. The types of epilepsy surgery performed, the age of patients considered for surgery, and the costs of the surgery may vary considerably at different epilepsy centers. In some cases, one epilepsy center may offer advantages over the other centers.

The EFA's information service provides a list of comprehensive epilepsy centers and their services in various parts of the country. For information, call the EFA (see Appendix 3).

CHAPTER 33

Toward a Cure for Epilepsy

The past decade has witnessed a much greater awareness of epilepsy and an expansion of our nation's health care resources for caring for people with epilepsy. New antiepileptic drugs are helping people with difficult-to-control seizures and providing alternatives for those with troublesome adverse effects of existing medications. Diagnostic and surgical techniques have been improved and are more effective than ever. New therapies for epilepsy are under investigation. The mechanisms leading to seizures and epilepsy are the focus of intensive study.

DECADE OF THE BRAIN

The US Congress declared the 1990s to be the "decade of the brain." Research in epilepsy continues to grow, funded largely by federal grants for medical research. Epilepsy research is active in a wide spectrum of areas, including:

- Investigating neurochemical and cellular changes associated with seizures and the tendency toward having seizures
- Mapping genes linked to epilepsy
- Studying changes in cellular metabolism during and after seizures
- Developing more effective antiepileptic drugs
- Developing and refining advanced techniques for mapping areas of the brain responsible for seizures, so as to improve the results of epilepsy surgery
- Developing and refining new epilepsy surgery procedures
- Understanding the social impact of seizures on children and
- Examining quality-of-life issues in epilepsy

311

SUPPORTING EPILEPSY RESEARCH

Although the largest support is derived from government grants, individuals and small groups can make a significant impact on research in epilepsy. By writing to government representatives and strongly encouraging their support of epilepsy research, individuals can make an important contribution. The Epilepsy Foundation of America (EFA) supports a wide range of programs and services for persons with epilepsy and also provides grants to researchers studying epilepsy. Contributions to the EFA and its local affiliates are important for advancing epilepsy research and support services for people with epilepsy.

Regional comprehensive epilepsy centers not only provide patient care but also often conduct research studies on epilepsy. Support of these centers can be directed toward specific programs such as treatment of children with epilepsy or basic science research studies on epilepsy.

FUTURE ADVANCES IN UNDERSTANDING EPILEPSY

Despite the enormous efforts of the medical and scientific communities to shed light on the causes, diagnosis, and treatment of epilepsy, a cure is not on the horizon, and it is unlikely that dramatic advances in treatment will occur during the remaining years of this century. However, we are likely to see advances in our understanding of the causes of epilepsy, which will lay the foundation for breakthroughs in treatment.

Appendices

Glossary of Terms

Absence Seizure: A primary generalized epileptic seizure, usually lasting less than 20 seconds, characterized by a stare sometimes associated with blinking or brief automatic movements of the mouth or hands; formerly called *petit mal* seizure. Absence seizures usually begin in childhood, are usually easily controlled with medication, and are outgrown by approximately 75% of children. *See* Atypical absence seizure.

ADA: *See* Americans with Diabilities Act.

ADD: *See* Attention deficit disorder.

Adjunct: Something added to another thing in a subordinate position or use; for example, an adjunct drug is one used in addition to another drug, not alone (*add-on therapy*).

Adverse Effects: The undesirable or unfavorable effects of something; for example, the adverse effects of an antiepileptic drug cause troublesome and, occasionally, even serious problems for patients.

AIDS: Acquired immune deficiency syndrome; caused by the human immunodeficiency virus (HIV).

Ambulatory EEG Monitoring: A system for recording the electroencephalogram for a prolonged period (typically 18–24 hours) in an outpatient; the electrodes are connected to a small cassette tape recorder.

Americans with Disabilities Act: A law that makes discrimination against people with disabilities illegal; the act applies to employment, access to public places, and places of accommodation.

Antiepileptic Drug: A medication used to control both convulsive and nonconvulsive seizures; sometimes called an *anticonvulsant*.

Atonic Seizure: An epileptic seizure characterized by sudden loss of muscle tone; may cause the head to drop suddenly, objects to fall from the hands, or loss of leg strength, with falling and potential injury; usually not associated with loss of consciousness.

Attention Deficit Disorder (ADD): An impairment in the ability to focus or maintain attention.

Atypical Absence Seizure: A staring spell characterized by partial impairment of consciousness; often occurs in children with the Lennox-Gastaut syndrome; the EEG shows slow (less than 3 per second) spike-and-wave discharges.

Aura: A warning before a seizure; a simple partial seizure occurring within seconds or minutes before a complex partial or secondarily generalized tonic-clonic seizure, or it may occur alone; also a warning before a migraine headache or a primary generalized seizure.

Autoinduction (of Metabolism): A process in which continued administration of a drug leads to an increase in the rate at which the drug is metabolized.

Automatism: Automatic, involuntary movement during a seizure; may involve mouth, hand, leg, or body movements; consciousness is usually impaired; occurs during complex partial and absence seizures and after tonic-clonic seizures.

Autonomic: Pertaining to the autonomic nervous system, which controls bodily functions that are not under conscious control (for example, heartbeat, breathing, sweating); some partial seizures may cause only autonomic symptoms; changes in autonomic functions are common during many seizures.

Autosomal Dominant: A mode of inheritance in which a gene is passed on by either parent; in most cases, the child has a 50% chance of inheriting the gene; the *expression* of the gene (that is, the development of the physical trait or the disorder) can vary considerably among different individuals with the same gene.

Autosomal Recessive: A mode of inheritance in which an individual has two copies of a gene that requires both copies for *expression*, or development, of the trait. Both parents must be carriers (that is, they have only one copy of the gene and, therefore, do not have the physical trait that the gene confers) or have the trait (that is, have two copies of the same gene).

Axon: The part of the nerve cell (neuron) that communicates with other cells, similar to a telephone wire; the axon is often covered with myelin, an insulating fatty layer, which functions similarly to plastic around a copper wire.

Benign: Favorable for recovery.

Benign Rolandic Epilepsy: An epilepsy syndrome of childhood characterized by partial seizures occurring at night and often involving the face and tongue; the seizures may progress to tonic-clonic seizures, have a characteristic EEG pattern, are easily controlled with medications but may not require treatment, and are outgrown by age 16 years.

Blood Drug Level: The concentration, or amount, of circulating drug in the bloodstream, measured in micrograms (μg) or nanograms (ng) per milliliter (mL). The concentration may be measured as the free or total level, because some of the drug is bound to the protein in the blood and some is not; the *free level* is the amount of drug that is "free" (unbound); the *total level* is the amount of drug that is both bound and unbound to the blood protein; the drug that is free (unbound) is the portion that reaches the brain and exerts an effect on the disorder.

Brand-Name Drug: Medication manufactured by a major pharmaceutical company; the drugs are often expensive but tend to be uniform in the amount of drug and the method of preparation.

Breath-Holding Spells: Episodes in children in which intense crying or an emotional upset is followed by interruption of breathing and sometimes loss of consciousness; the episodes are not harmful, but when prolonged, slight jerking movements may occur.

Catamenial: Referring to the menses or to menstruation; with regard to women with epilepsy, a tendency for seizures to occur around the time of the menses.

Cerebral Palsy: A condition with various combinations of impaired muscle tone and strength, coordination, and intelligence.

Cognitive: Pertaining to the mental processes of perceiving, thinking, and remembering; used loosely to refer to intellectual functions as opposed to physical functions.

Clonic Seizure: An epileptic seizure characterized by jerking movements and involving muscles on both sides of the body.

Complex Partial Seizure: An epileptic seizure that involves only part of the brain and impairs consciousness; often preceded by a simple partial seizure (aura or warning).

Computed Tomography (CT): A scanning technique that uses x-rays and computers to create pictures of the inside of the body; shows the structure of the brain; not as sensitive as MRI.

Consciousness: State of awareness; if consciousness is preserved during a seizure, the person can respond (either in words or actions, such as raising a hand on command) and recall what occurred during the spell.

Convulsion: An older term for a tonic-clonic seizure.

Convulsive Syncope: A fainting episode in which the brain does not receive enough blood, causing a seizure; the episode is not an epileptic seizure but a result of the faint.

CT Scan: *See* Computed tomography.

Daily Dose: The average amount of medication taken over the course of the day to achieve a therapeutic blood level of the drug, usually measured in milligrams (mg) per kilogram (kg) of the patient's body weight (1 kg = 2.2 pounds).

Deficit: A lack or deficiency of an essential quality or element; for example, a neurological deficit is a defect in the structure or function of the brain.

Déjà vu: Feeling as if one has lived through or experienced this moment before; may occur in people without any medical problems or immediately before a seizure (i.e., as a simple partial seizure).

Development: The process of physical growth and the attainment of intelligence and problem-solving ability that begins in infancy; any interruption of this process by a disease or disorder is called *developmental delay.*

Dose-Related Effects: Adverse effects that are more likely to occur at times of peak blood levels of a drug.

EEOC: Equal Employment Opportunity Commission.

EFA: Epilepsy Foundation of America.

Electroencephalogram (EEG): A diagnostic test of brain electrical activity; helpful in diagnosing epilepsy.

Encephalitis: An inflammation of the brain; usually caused by a virus.

Epilepsia Partialis Continua: A continuous or prolonged partial seizure that causes contraction of the muscles; usually restricted to the muscles of the face, arm, or leg; usually not associated with impairment of consciousness.

Epilepsy: A disorder characterized by transient but recurrent disturbances of brain function that may or may not be associated with impairment or loss of consciousness and abnormal movements or behavior.

Epilepsy Syndrome: A disorder defined by seizure type, age of onset, clinical and EEG findings, family history, response to therapy, and prognosis.

Epileptiform: Resembling epilepsy or its manifestations; may refer to a pattern on the EEG associated with an increased risk of seizures.

Epileptogenic: Causing epilepsy.

Epileptologist: A neurologist with specialty training in epilepsy.

Equilibrium Period: *See* Steady state.

Febrile Seizure: A seizure associated with high fever in children aged 3 months to 5 years, usually a tonic-clonic seizure; usually benign.

Fit: An older term for a seizure, usually a tonic-clonic seizure; still used in some places.

Focal Seizure: An older term for a partial seizure.

Focus: The center or region of the brain from which seizures begin; used in reference to partial seizures.

Generalized Seizure: A seizure that involves both sides of the brain and causes tonic and clonic movements (primary or secondary generalized) or another type of primary generalized epilepsy (e.g., absence of atonic seizure).

Generic Drug: A drug that is not sold under a brand name; for example, carbamazepine can be obtained as a generic drug or as Tegretol, its brand name.

Grand mal: An older term for a tonic-clonic seizure.

Half-life: The time required for the amount of a drug in the blood to decline to half of its original value, measured in hours; a drug with a longer half-life lasts longer in the body and, therefore, generally needs to be taken less often than a drug with a shorter half-life.

Hemispherectomy: A surgical procedure to remove a cerebral hemisphere (one side of the brain); the operation is now often modified to remove a portion of the hemisphere and to disconnect the remaining portions.

Heriditary: Passed from one generation to the next through the genes.

HIV: Human immunodeficiency virus; cause of acquired immune deficiency syndrome (AIDS).

Hydrocephalus: A condition associated with obstruction of the cerebrospinal fluid pathways in the brain and accumulation of excess cerebrospinal fluid within the skull.

Hyperventilation: Increased rate and depth of breathing; may be done during the EEG to increase the chances of finding epileptiform or other abnormal activity.

Hypsarrhythmia: An abnormal EEG pattern of excessive slow activity and multiple areas of epileptiform activity; associated with infantile spasms.

Ictal: Referring to the period during a sudden attack, such as a seizure or stroke.

Idiopathic: Referring to a disorder of unknown cause.

Idiosyncratic: Pertaining to an abnormal susceptibility to some drug or other agent, peculiar to the individual.

Incidence: The number of new cases of a disorder occurring in a population during a specified period.

Infantile Spasm: A sudden jerk followed by stiffening; spasms usually begin between age 3 and 12 months and usually stop by age 2 to 4 years, although other seizure types often develop. In some spells, the arms are flung out as the body bends forward ("jackknife seizures"), but in others the movements are more subtle.

Intensive Monitoring: *See* Video-EEG monitoring.

Interictal: Referring to the period between seizures.

Intractable: Difficult to alleviate, remedy, or cure; for example, intractable seizures are difficult to control with the usual antiepileptic drug therapy.

JME: *See* Juvenile myoclonic epilepsy.

Juvenile Myoclonic Epilepsy (JME): A primary generalized epilepsy syndrome, usually beginning at age 5 to 17 years, characterized by myoclonic (muscle-jerk) seizures and possibly also absence and tonic-clonic seizures; responds well to valproate.

Ketogenic Diet: A high-fat, low-carbohydrate diet used to control seizures.

Kindling: An animal model of epilepsy in which small electrical shocks are delivered to the brain at certain intervals (for example, once a day) to cause a progressive tendency toward seizures; eventually, seizures may occur without the electrical shocks.

Lennox-Gastaut Syndrome: A disorder beginning in childhood, characterized by developmental delay or mental retardation, multiple seizure types that do not respond well to therapy, and slow spike-and-wave discharges on the EEG.

Magnetic Resonance Imaging (MRI): A scanning technique that creates pictures of the inside of the body and the brain; uses a strong magnet (does not use x-rays); more sensitive than CT.

Mainstream: Regular (public, private, or parochial) school or classes.

Medical History: The account of a patient's disorder.

Meningitis: A bacterial infection of the membranes surrounding the brain; often diagnosed by a spinal tap (lumbar puncture).

Metabolism: The physical and chemical processes by which substances are produced or transformed (broken down) into energy or products for the uses of the body.

Metabolite: Chemical product derived from breakdown (metabolism) of another chemical; may be biologically *active* or *inactive*. An active metabolite of an antiepileptic drug can be effective in controlling seizures or can cause or contribute to the drug's adverse effects.

Migraine: A headache characterized by throbbing head pain, often greater on one side; may be preceded by a warning (aura) and accompanied by nausea, vomiting, and sensitivity to light and sound. In rare cases weakness, language problems, or other neurological disorders are associated with migraine.

Minor (Motor) Seizure: An older term for seizures that cause contraction of muscles but do not become tonic-clonic seizures; mostly used in certain laws and acts.

Monotherapy: Treatment with a single medication.

Motor: Of, pertaining to, or designating nerves carrying impulses from the nerve centers to the muscles; of or relating to movements of the muscles.

MRI: *See* Magnetic resonance imaging.

Muscle Tone: The level of muscle contraction present during the resting state; with *increased tone* there is stiffness and rigidity; with *decreased tone* there is looseness or floppiness of the limbs and trunk.

Myoclonic Jerk: Brief muscle jerk; may involve muscles on one or both sides of the body; may be normal (for example, as one falls asleep) or caused by a seizure or other disorders.

Myoclonic Seizure: A brief muscle jerk resulting from an abnormal discharge of brain electrical activity; usually involves muscles on both sides of the body, most often the shoulders or upper arms.

Narcolepsy: A condition characterized by sudden and uncontrollable attacks of sleep.

Neuron: A nerve cell.

Neurotransmitter: A chemical substance produced by nerve cells, transported in the axon, and released at the synapse; causes chemical and electrical changes in adjacent cells.

Paroxysmal: Pertaining to a sudden outburst, such as the sudden recurrence or intensification of symptoms or epileptiform activity on the EEG.

Partial Complex Seizure: An alternative term for complex partial seizure.

Partial Seizure: A seizure that involves or arises from part of the brain.

Peak Blood Level: The highest concentration of a drug in the bloodstream.

PET: *See* Positron emission tomography.

Petit mal: An older term for absence seizure; sometimes used incorrectly by the general public to refer to any kind of seizure that is not a convulsion.

Pharmacology: The study of drugs, including their effectiveness, adverse effects, metabolism, interaction with other drugs, and other actions.

Photic Stimulation: Shining, flashing (strobe) lights in the eyes (which may be closed) of a person; used during the EEG to detect photosensitive epilepsy.

Photosensitive Epilepsy: A form of reflex epilepsy in which certain lights, especially flashing lights, can provoke seizures.

Positron Emission Tomography (PET): A diagnostic test that uses a very low and safe dose of a radioactive compound to measure metabolic activity in the brain; can identify areas of decreased metabolism corresponding to the area from which seizures arise; helpful in planning epilepsy surgery.

Postictal: Referring to the period immediately after a seizure; the person may be tired and confused or may immediately return to an awake, attentive state after the seizure.

Predisposition: Tendency or inclination.

Premonitory: Serving as a warning.

Prevalence: The number of cases of a disorder present in a population at a specified time.

Primary Drug: A drug that has stood the test of time in terms of its efficacy and safety in treating a particular disorder; for example, phenytoin and carbamazepine are primary drugs for partial seizures because they have been demonstrated to have very good safety and effectiveness in well-designed and well-controlled studies.

Prognosis: The outlook for a medical condition; the chances the condition will improve, remain unchanged, or worsen.

Progressive: Increasing in scope or severity over time.

Progressive Myoclonic Epilepsy: A rare group of epilepsies, often with a hereditary component, characterized by myoclonic and other types of seizures and progressive neurological impairment; medications help control the seizures, but there is no cure.

Psychic: Pertaining to intellectual or emotional (affective) functions.

Psychogenic (Pseudo) Seizure: A behavioral episode that resembles an epileptic seizure but does not result from abnormal brain electrical activity; psychological in origin, but not resulting from conscious actions; video-EEG monitoring is often used to make the diagnosis.

Psychomotor Seizure: An older term for a complex partial seizure with automatism.

Rasmussen's Syndrome: A disorder with frequent or continuous partial seizures and a progressive abnormality in the brain, possibly the result of a virus.

Reflex Epilepsies: Seizures precipitated by certain conditions or stimuli, such as flashing lights or jazz music.

Refractory: A condition that does not respond easily to treatment.

Secondary Drug: A drug whose efficacy and safety are not as clearly defined as those of a primary drug, usually because it has not been used for as long or as extensively as the *primary*, or first-line, drug or because it was found to be less effective or less safe in controlled studies; some secondary drugs are used in *adjunct*, or *add-on*, therapy.

Seizure: A sudden, excessive discharge of nervous-system electrical activity that usually causes a change in behavior.

Seizure Threshold: Minimal conditions necessary to produce a seizure.

Sensory: Pertaining to the senses (touch, vision, hearing, taste, smell).

Sharp Wave: An EEG pattern indicating the potential for epilepsy; "benign" sharp waves are not associated with seizures.

Sibling: A brother or sister.

Simple Partial Seizure: An epileptic seizure that involves only part of the brain and does not impair consciousness.

Single-Photon Emission Computed Tomography (SPECT): A diagnostic test that uses a very low and safe dose of a radioactive compound to measure blood flow in the brain; not as sensitive as PET.

Slowing: A term used to describe a group of brain waves on the EEG that have a lower frequency than expected for the subject's age and level of alertness and the area of the brain recorded. Slow waves can result from drowsiness or sleep, drugs, or brain injuries and occur during or after seizures.

Social Security Disability Income (SSDI): A federal assistance program for disabled people who have paid Social Security taxes or are dependents of people who have paid.

SPECT: *See* Single-photon emission computed tomography.

Spell: A period, bout, or episode of illness or indisposition; refers to seizures or other disorders that produce brief episodes of behavioral change.

Spike: An EEG pattern strongly correlated with seizures; "benign" spikes are not associated with seizures.

Status Epilepticus: A prolonged seizure (usually defined as lasting longer than 30 minutes) or a series of repeated seizures; a continuous state of seizure activity; may occur in almost any seizure type.

Steady State: A state in which equilibrium has been achieved. In reference to antiepileptic drugs, steady state is achieved when a constant daily dose of a drug produces consistent blood levels of the drug (takes at least five times the half-life of the drug in question).

Sturge-Weber Syndrome: A disorder of blood vessels affecting the skin of the face, eyes, and brain; brain involvement is associated with seizures.

Supplemental Security Income (SSI): A federal assistance program.

Symptomatic: Referring to a disorder with an identifiable cause; for example, severe head trauma can cause symptomatic epilepsy.

Synapse: The junction between one nerve cell and another nerve cell; the axon of one nerve cell releases a neurotransmitter, which diffuses across the synapse and causes changes in the membrane of the adjacent cell.

Syncope: Fainting.

Syndrome: A group of signs and symptoms that collectively define or characterize a disease or disorder; signs are objective findings such as weakness, and symptoms are subjective findings such as a feeling of fear or tingling in a finger.

Temporal Lobe Epilepsy: An older term for partial epilepsy arising from the temporal lobe.

Temporal Lobe Seizure: A simple or complex partial seizure arising from the temporal lobe.

Therapeutic Blood Level: The amount of drug circulating in the bloodstream that brings about seizure control without troublesome adverse effects. "Subtherapeutic" levels are effective in some patients, and "supratherapeutic" or "toxic" levels are tolerated by other patients.

Threshold: The level at which an event or change occurs (*see* Seizure threshold).

Tic: Repeated involuntary contractions of muscles, such as rapid head jerks or eye blinks, as in Tourette's syndrome; may be under partial voluntary control (for example, can be temporarily suppressed); nonepileptic.

Time to Peak Blood Level: The interval between the time a drug is taken and the time it reaches the highest concentration in the blood.

Todd's Paralysis: Weakness after a seizure; originally used to describe muscle weakness on the side of the body opposite the side in which the seizure began (in the brain), but now used to describe a variety of temporary problems after seizures such as blindness, loss of sensation, or loss of speech.

Tone: *See* Muscle tone.

Tonic Seizure: An epileptic seizure that causes stiffening; consciousness is usually preserved. The seizure involves muscles on both sides of the body, and electrical discharge involves all or most of the brain.

Tonic-Clonic Seizure: A convulsion; newer term for grand mal or major motor seizure; characterized by loss of consciousness, falling, stiffening, and jerking; electrical discharge involves all or most of the brain.

Tuberous Sclerosis: A disease in which benign tumors affect the brain, eyes, skin, and internal organs; associated with mental retardation and seizures; inherited as an autosomal dominant trait.

Video-EEG Monitoring: A technique for recording the behavior and the EEG of a patient simultaneously; changes in behavior can be correlated with changes in the EEG; useful for making the diagnosis of epilepsy and localizing the seizure focus.

West's Syndrome: An epileptic syndrome characterized by infantile spasms, mental retardation, and an abnormal EEG pattern (hypsarrhythmia); begins before 1 year of age.

Glossary of Antiepileptic Drugs

Generic Name	Brand Name	Indications
Acetazolamide (a-set-a-**zole**-a-mide)	Diamox	Myoclonic seizures ?Catamenial seizures
Adrenocorticotropic hormone (ACTH)	Cortrosyn	Infantile spasms
Carbamazepine (kar-ba-**maz**-e-peen)	Tegretol (**teg**-ret-ol)	Partial seizures, tonic-clonic seizures
Clonazepam (kloe-**na**-ze-pam)	Klonopin (**klah**-ni-pin)	Myoclonic seizures, absence seizures
Clorazepate (klor-**az**-e-pate)	Tranxene (**tran**-zeen)	Absence seizures, partial seizures
Ethosuximide (eth-oh-**sux**-i-mide)	Zarontin (zar-**on**-tin)	Absence seizures, myoclonic seizures
Felbamate	Felbatol (**fel**-ba-tol)	Partial seizures, tonic-clonic seizures, atonic seizures, tonic seizures
Gabapentin	Neurontin (nur-**an**-tin)	Partial seizures, tonic-clonic seizures
Lamotrigine	Lamictal (lah-**mic**-tal)	Partial seizures, tonic-clonic seizures
Lorazepam (lor-**az**-e-pam)	Ativan	Status epilepticus, seizure clusters
Mephobarbital	Mebaral	Partial seizures, tonic-clonic seizures, myoclonic seizures
Phenobarbital (fee-noe-**bar**-bi-tal)	Luminal (and others)	Partial seizures, tonic-clonic seizures
Phenytoin (**fen**-i-toyn)	Dilantin (die-**lan**-tin)	Partial seizures, tonic-clonic seizures
Prednisone (**pred**-ni-sone)	—	Infantile spasms

Primidone (**pri**-mi-dohn)	Mysoline (**my**-soh-leen)	Partial seizures, tonic-clonic seizures
Trimethadione	Tridione (try-**die**-ohn)	Absence seizures
Valproate (valproic acid; divalproex sodium)	Depakene (de-pa-**keen**) Depakote (**de**-pa-koht)	Absence seizures, tonic-clonic seizures, myoclonic seizures, partial seizures

Resources for People with Epilepsy

Association for the Care of Children's Health
3615 Wisconsin Avenue
Washington, DC 20016
202-244-1801

Association for Children and Adults with Learning Disabilities
4156 Library Road
Pittsburgh, PA 15234
412-341-1515

Association for Retarded Citizens
2501 Avenue J
Arlington, TX 76011
871-640-0204

Children's Defense Fund
25 E Street, NW
Washington, DC 20001
202-628-8787

Council for Exceptional Children
1920 Association Drive
Reston, VA 22091-1589
703-620-3660

The Epilepsy Foundation of America
4351 Garden City Drive
Landover, MD 20785
800-EFA-1000

Epilepsy Information Service
Medical Center Boulevard
Winston-Salem, NC 27157-1078
800-642-0500

Joseph P. Kennedy Foundation
1350 New York Avenue, NW
Suite 500
Washington, DC 20005
202-393-1250

Kids on the Block
9385 C. Gerwig Lane
Columbia, MD 21046
301-368-KIDS

National Epilepsy Library
The Epilepsy Foundation of America
4351 Garden City Drive
Landover, MD 20785
800-EFA-4050

National Information Center for
  Handicapped Children and Youth
7926 Jones Branch Drive
McLean, VA 22102
800-999-5599 or 703-893-6061

Resources for Children with Special
  Skills
200 Park Avenue South
Suite 816
New York, NY 10003
212-677-4650

Sibling Information Center
Department of Educational Psychology
Box U-64
The University of Connecticut
Storrs, CT 06268
203-486-4031

Siblings for Significant Change
823 United Nations Plaza
Room 808
New York, NY 10017
212-420-0776

References and Suggested Readings

Chapter 4

Dostoyevsky, F: The Idiot. Translated by Eva M. Martin. No. 682 in Everyman's Library. Dent, London, 1970, pp 52, 213–214, 222.

Chapter 5

Hauser, WA and Hesdorffer, DC: Epilepsy: Frequency, Causes, and Consequences. Demos Publications, New York, 1990.

Chapter 6

Ferber, R: Solve Your Child's Sleep Problems. Fireside/Simon & Schuster, New York, 1985.

Chapter 12

Sieveking, EH: On Epilepsy and Epileptiform Seizures: Their Causes, Pathology, and Treatment. J Churchill, London, 1858, p 226.

Chapter 17

Bridwell, N: Clifford's Manners. Scholastic, New York, 1987.
Gardener, R: MBD: The Family Book about Minimal Brain Dysfunction. J Aronson, New York, 1973.
Greenspan, S: First Feelings. Viking Penguin, New York, 1985.
Greenspan, S: The Essential Partnership, Viking Penguin, New York, 1990.
Smith, SL: No Easy Answers: The Learning Disabled Child at Home and at School. Phantom Books, Endwell, NY, 1981.
Blank, M, McKirdy, LS, and Payne, PC: Links to Language. Presented at the American Speech-Language, Hearing Association meeting, Atlanta, GA, November 1991.

Chapter 18

Moss, DM: Lee, the Rabbit with Epilepsy. Woodbine House, Kensington, MD, 1989.

Chapters 26, 29, and 30

The Legal Rights of Persons with Epilepsy: An Overview of Legal Issues and Laws, 6th ed. Epilepsy Foundation of America, Landover, MD, 1992.

Index

An "f" following a page number indicates a figure; a "t" indicates a table.

Psychic, defined, 321
Psychogenic (nonepileptic) seizures
Psychogenic seizures — *Continued*
  conditions confused with, 79–80
  defined, 321
Psychosis, 272–273
Puberty. *See also* Adolescent(s)
  epilepsy during, 165–167
  hormonal changes during, 165–166
  metabolic changes during, 166
  psychosocial development changes
    during, 166–167
Public accommodations, for
people with epilepsy, 282
Public Law 94–142, 211, 214–215
Public Law 101–336, 256–260
Public services, for people with epilepsy,
  281–282

Quadriparesis, spastic, 222
Quality of life, 236–237
  epilepsy effects on, 6

Rasmussen's syndrome, 40–41
  defined, 321
Reading, impairment in, causes, 192
Reasonable accommodation, defined,
  258–259
Refractory, defined, 321
Rehabilitation Act of 1973, 265–267
Rehabilitation Act, Section 504, 215–216
Rejection
  of children with epilepsy, 205
  epilepsy and, 170
Relatives, telling them about epilepsy, 197
Relaxation therapy, for epilepsy control,
  146
"Relay station," described, 13
Research, support for, 303, 312
Resources, 295–310
  board of education, 308
  community, 307–309
  comprehensive epilepsy centers,
    309–310
  developmental disabilities agency, 308
  Epilepsy Foundation of America,
    297–306. *See also* Epilepsy
    Foundation of America
  list of, 326–327
  national, 307
  office of vocational education for
    handicapped students, 308
  protection and advocacy offices for
    individuals with disabilities, 308

state department of education, 308
state vocational rehabilitation agency,
  209
Respite care, Epilepsy Foundation of
  America, 306
Responsibility, encouragement of, in
  children with epilepsy, 186
Restraint, following seizures, 264, 283
Reynolds, R., 3
Right hemisphere, 10f
Rigidity, in cerebral palsy, described, 221
Ritalin, for attention deficit disorder, 194
Romantic relationships, epilepsy and,
  243–246
Rugby, epilepsy and, 209

Sadness, depression versus, 270
School Alert program, 305
School nurses, telling them about epilepsy,
  197
Second-injury funds, 268
Second opinions, 69–70
Seizure(s). *See also* Epilepsy
  absence, 20–21, 20t
    atypical, 20t, 21–22
      defined, 315
      zonisamide for, 122
    behavior related to, 190
    defined, 315
    lamotrigine for, 120
  alcohol use and, 54–55
  amphetamines and, 55–56
  antiepileptic drug discontinuation and,
    176–177
  antiepileptic drugs causing, 109t
  arachnoid cysts and, 125
  atonic, 20t, 23
    defined, 315
    lamotrigine for, 120
  autonomic, 20t, 25–26
  behavior problems related to, 190–191
  caffeine and, 56
  causes, 18
  in children, 156–163. *See also* Children,
    seizures in
  classification of, 19–28, 20t
  clonic, 20t, 23
    defined, 317
  complex partial
    behavior related to, 190
    defined, 317
    false arrest following, 283–284
    first aid for, 97–98
    gabapentin for, 119
    lamotrigine for, 120